FRAGRANCE TECHNOLOGY
SYNTHETIC AND NATURAL PERFUMES

FRAGRANCE TECHNOLOGY
Synthetic and Natural Perfumes

Ronald W. James

NOYES DATA CORPORATION

Park Ridge, New Jersey   London, England

1975

Published in the United States of America by
Noyes Data Corporation
Noyes Building, Park Ridge, New Jersey 07656

FOREWORD

The detailed, descriptive information in this book is based on U.S. patents since 1964 relating to the manufacture of synthetic and natural perfumes.

This book serves a double purpose in that it supplies detailed technical information and can be used as a guide to the U.S. patent literature in this field. By indicating all the information that is significant, and eliminating legal jargon and juristic phraseology, this book presents an advanced, technically oriented review of commercial fragrances.

The U.S. patent literature is the largest and most comprehensive collection of technical information in the world. There is more practical, commercial, timely process information assembled here than is available from any other source. The technical information obtained from a patent is extremely reliable and comprehensive; sufficient information must be included to avoid rejection for "insufficient disclosure." These patents include practically all of those issued on the subject in the United States during the period under review; there has been no bias in the selection of patents for inclusion.

The patent literature covers a substantial amount of information not available in the journal literature. The patent literature is a prime source of basic commercially useful information. This information is overlooked by those who rely primarily on the periodical journal literature. It is realized that there is a lag between a patent application on a new process development and the granting of a patent, but it is felt that this may roughly parallel or even anticipate the lag in putting that development into commercial practice.

Many of these patents are being utilized commercially. Whether used or not, they offer opportunities for technological transfer. Also, a major purpose of this book is to describe the number of technical possibilities available, which may open up profitable areas to research and development. The information contained in this book will allow you to establish a sound background before launching into research in this field.

Advanced composition and production methods developed by Noyes Data are employed to bring our new durably bound books to you in a minimum of time. Special techniques are used to close the gap between "manuscript" and "completed book." Industrial technology is progressing so rapidly that time-honored, conventional typesetting, binding and shipping methods are no longer suitable. We have bypassed the delays in the conventional book publishing cycle and provide the user with an effective and convenient means of reviewing up-to-date information in depth.

The Table of Contents is organized in such a way as to serve as a subject index. Other indexes by company, inventor and patent number help in providing easy access to the information contained in this book.

15 Reasons Why the U.S. Patent Office Literature Is Important to You —

1. The U.S. patent literature is the largest and most comprehensive collection of technical information in the world. There is more practical commercial process information assembled here than is available from any other source.

2. The technical information obtained from the patent literature is extremely comprehensive; sufficient information must be included to avoid rejection for "insufficient disclosure."

3. The patent literature is a prime source of basic commercially utilizable information. This information is overlooked by those who rely primarily on the periodical journal literature.

4. An important feature of the patent literature is that it can serve to avoid duplication of research and development.

5. Patents, unlike periodical literature, are bound by definition to contain new information, data and ideas.

6. It can serve as a source of new ideas in a different but related field, and may be outside the patent protection offered the original invention.

7. Since claims are narrowly defined, much valuable information is included that may be outside the legal protection afforded by the claims.

8. Patents discuss the difficulties associated with previous research, development or production techniques, and offer a specific method of overcoming problems. This gives clues to current process information that has not been published in periodicals or books.

9. Can aid in process design by providing a selection of alternate techniques. A powerful research and engineering tool.

10. Obtain licenses — many U.S. chemical patents have not been developed commercially.

11. Patents provide an excellent starting point for the next investigator.

12. Frequently, innovations derived from research are first disclosed in the patent literature, prior to coverage in the periodical literature.

13. Patents offer a most valuable method of keeping abreast of latest technologies, serving an individual's own "current awareness" program.

14. Copies of U.S. patents are easily obtained from the U.S. Patent Office at 50¢ a copy.

15. It is a creative source of ideas for those with imagination.

CONTENTS AND SUBJECT INDEX

INTRODUCTION

The history of perfumes (aromas) dates back at least to the ancient Egyptians; the Bible clearly shows an interrelation between the events of the times and valuable aromas; and Babylon, Nineveh and Carthage were great trading centers for perfumes. Eventually, perfumes, largely through the expansion of the the Roman Empire, were brought to France. Later, the great explorers like Marco Polo, Magellan and Christopher Columbus brought about a tremendous evolution of perfumery through their worldwide efforts to find gold and spices.

It was only some fifty years ago that perfumes were restricted to the realm of the rich and sophisticated men and women of the world. Today, through great progress on the part of the chemical research community and sometimes massive and strongly persuasive and suggestive advertising by the perfumery industry, the names of Chanel, Coty, Nina Ricci, Dior, Matchabelli, Patou, Avon, Fabergé, Rochas, Revlon, Estée Lauder are common household words in many parts of the world.

In the past few decades, the great advances in analytical instrumentation, particularly in the field of separations techniques based on chromatography (paper, thin layer, gas-liquid), coupled with infrared and mass spectrometry and NMR have led to the precise identification of the components of many natural fragrances. Thus the oldest aspirations and dreams of perfumers have been realized in identification and duplication of natural fragrances of flowers and other odiferous substances as they occur in their natural living state.

Today, the supply of fragrances is almost limitless, with less than 5% coming directly from natural sources. Indeed, with over 5,000 raw materials available today, the perfumer can develop fragrances far in the excess of those which occur in nature, limited only by his own imagination. Synthetic perfumes are characterized by uniformity of composition and ready availability. They are relatively inexpensive, and are thus highly desirable and commercially important.

Perfumery materials are not only used directly for perfumes, but are essential for the manufacture of flavors, cosmetics, soaps, toilet preparations and to mask the odors of household cleaners, paints, glues, plastics, insecticides and detergents.

This book describes over 240 processes relating to all phases of the preparation, isolation and refinement of odiferous materials as described in the patent literature. Many of these processes provide new compositions of matter for specific, desirable fragrances, while many other processes result in compounds which enhance a particular note or blend.

1

In most cases, research effort in the fragrance industry has been directed to the duplication or enhancement of a particular perfume or fragrance to materialize a special olfactive impression, for example the smell of the prairie, the green grass, an oriental spice market, the sensuous appeal of a woman, or the aroma of tobacco. The processes described in this book are organized to reflect the major types of perfumes.

The woody odors are typically characteristic of the group of vetiver, sandalwood, cedarwood and guaiac wood. All of these woody odors have a floral and fresh top note. The most popular floral odors include jasmine, rose, lily-of-the valley and violet. Additionally, specific sections are devoted to the other important classes of perfumes which include musk, fruity, camphorous, tobacco, and many other specific fragrances.

WOODY FRAGRANCES

SANDALWOOD

Photochemical Reactions of trans-α-Santalate

R.G. Lewis and W.F. Erman; U.S. Patent 3,626,015; December 7, 1971; assigned to The Procter & Gamble Company describe a photochemical process for obtaining compounds having valuable sandalwood odors from ethyl trans-α-santalate.

East Inidan sandalwood oil has previously been available only from East Indian sandalwood trees. The oil and various individual components of the oil are highly valued perfume bases and used in large quantities throughout the world. The oil, however, is expensive and sometimes is in sporadic supply. For this reason, a continuous effort has been made to synthesize various components of the oil or similar synthetic materials in order to obtain the desirable powerful woody fragrance of sandalwood oil.

cis-α-Santalol, a useful and highly desirable component of sandalwood oil having a desirable sandalwood odor, was synthesized by Lewis and Erman (U.S. Patent 3,478,114). By the process described therein, tricycloekasantalal is reacted with a phosphorane to form alkyl α-santalates. In all cases, the resulting alkyl α-santalate is a mixture of cis and trans isomers with a predominant portion of the mixture of isomers consisting of the trans isomer. This mixture is then reduced to obtain a mixture of cis- and trans-α-santalol.

The synthesis of cis-α-santalol is extremely valuable because it provides a constant source of supply of this highly prized perfume component in consistently acceptable quality. One problem, however, still exists with this synthesis. In nearly all cases, more than 70% of the final mixture of isomers consists of trans-α-santalol, a compound possessing a bland cedar note. This cedar note masks the desirable sandalwood odor to some degree and renders the final product of the synthesis less valuable as a perfume ingredient. Although the isomers can be separated to obtain the desired cis isomer, the separation process, e.g., by gas chromatography or extraction, is expensive. The cost of this separation poses formidable obstacles to commercial utilization of the desirable, synthetically produced cis-α-santalol.

This process is an improvement over the synthesis set forth above. For example, the expensive process of separating the α-santalol isomers is eliminated when the irradiation technique of this process is utilized. For this process, a mixture of trans and cis isomers of ethyl α-santalate rich in the trans isomer of the trans isomer per se, intermediates in the process described in U.S. Patent 3,478,114 referred to above, is utilized as the starting

3

material. By irradiation with ultraviolet light, the mixture of trans and cis isomers or the trans isomer per se of ethyl α-santalate is readily transformed to a mixture of the trans and cis isomers which is enriched in the cis isomer, i.e., a portion of the trans isomer is converted to the cis isomer. The ethyl α-santalate isomers are then reduced to the corresponding trans and cis isomers of α-santalol. With the increase in the amount of cis isomer in the mixture, the powerful sandalwood odor (designated as mild, sweet, woody odor) of cis-α-santalol dominates the bland cedar note of trans-α-santalol. Therefore, no further separation of the isomers is required.

As an added benefit, it has been found that the trans and cis isomers of ethyl α-santalate can be converted by prolonged irradiation of the trans and cis isomers of ethyl $\Delta^{11.12}$-α-santalate. The trans and cis isomers of ethyl $\Delta^{11.12}$-α-santalate are easily reduced to the trans and cis isomers of $\Delta^{11.12}$-α-santalol, both of which have a distinct, powerful, sandalwood odor (designated as mild, creamy, woody odor). The following examples illustrate the process. All percentages and ratios are by weight unless otherwise indicated; temperatures are expressed in degrees centigrade.

Example 1: General Procedure — Data listed in all of the examples were obtained by means of the following techniques unless otherwise indicated. Melting points were determined on a Kofler micro hot stage and are corrected. Boiling points were observed on standard thermometers and are uncorrected. Infrared spectra were recorded on a Perkin-Elmer Infracord spectrophotometer. Nuclear magnetic resonance (nmr) spectra were determined in deuterated chloroform solution or carbon disulfide solution with a Varian model Ha-100 or a Varian Model A-6 spectrometer, using tetramethylsilane as an internal reference. The nmr data are noted by multiplicity (s = singlet, d = doublet, t = triplet, q = quartet and m = unresolved multiplet), integration, coupling constant (in cps), and assignment.

Gas-liquid chromatograms were obtained on an Aerograph model 200 or 202B instrument using two columns: (1) a 5 foot by 0.25 inch column packed with 20% FFAP (commercial polyester packing obtained from Varian Aerograph) on 60 to 80 mesh acid washed chromosorb P.D.M.S.C. (a commercial support from Varian Aerograph) and (2) a 10 foot by 0.25 inch column packed with 20% Reoplex-400 (commercial polyester packing obtained from Varian Aerograph) on 60 to 80 mesh chromosorb W.D.M.C.S. (a commercial siliconized support from Varian Aerograph). The helium flow rate in these columns was maintained at 100 ml/min unless otherwise noted.

All irradiations, unless otherwise indicated, were performed in a conventional photochemical reaction flask equipped with a nitrogen flush and either a quartz or Vycor immersion well. Nitrogen was bubbled through the reaction mixtures and the temperature was maintained in the range of 20° to 35°C by means of a water jacket. The light sources used in the following examples were commercially available mercury lamps. More specific data on the lamps used are tabulated as follows.

	Radiation source	
	Hanovia L–679A[1] (high pressure)	Rayonet RPR–2537A[2] (low pressure)
Total power capacity (watts)	450	[3] 35
Ultraviolet spectral characteristics (watts):		
200 mμ–250 mμ	14.0	[3] 35
250 mμ–300 mμ	21.3	[3] 35
300 mμ–400 mμ	48.4	[3] 35
Total radiated energy	175.8	[3] 35

[1] Obtained from Hanovia Lamp Division, Englehard Industries. For further details, see specification sheet EH–223, 5–1–59, Englehard Industries.
[2] A circular array of 16 lamps as obtained from Southern New England Untraviolet Company. For further details see catalog No. RPR–100, Southern New England Ultraviolet Company.
[3] Watts with principal emission at 253.7 mμ.

Example 2: Irradiation of Ethyl α-Santalates Using a Pyrex Filter — A solution of 860 milligrams (3.27×10^{-3} mols) of a mixture comprised of 5 parts by weight of ethyl trans-α-santalate and 1 part by weight of ethyl cis-α-santalate in 130 milliliters of toluene was degassed with a steady stream of nitrogen for a period of 1 hour in a Vycor vessel fitted with a Pyrex filter. The ethyl α-santalates were prepared by the method described in the patent of Lewis and Erman.

This solution was subjected to ultraviolet light which was generated from a 450 watt Hanovia mercury arc lamp and passed through the Pyrex filter. After 41 hours of continuous irradiation, the ratio of trans to cis isomers of ethyl α-santalate was 6:5 according to gas-liquid chromatographic analysis. Removal of the toluene under reduced pressure left an oily residue which on short path distillation afforded 837 milligrams of a clear oil, boiling point 128° to 135°C (0.6 mm). The distillate was comprised of a mixture of ethyl trans-α-santalate, ethyl cis-α-santalate and ethyl $\Delta^{11.12}$-α-santalate in a weight ratio of 58:39:3 as determined by gas-liquid chromatographic analysis.

The analyses were performed using the instruments and columns described in the general procedure and employing a column temperature of 208°C and a helium flow rate of 60 milliliters per minute. Separation and collection of the trans and cis isomers of ethyl α-santalate by gas-liquid chromatography afforded clear oils whose spectral properties were identical to those described in Example 2 in the patent of Lewis and Erman. This description of spectral properties of the trans and cis isomers of ethyl α-santalate is specifically incorporated by reference.

Example 3: Irradiation of Ethyl α-Santalates Using a Vycor Filter and Cyclohexane Solvent — A solution of 200 milligrams (7.6×10^{-4} mols) of a mixture of 97 parts by weight of ethyl trans-α-santalate and 3 parts by weight of ethyl cis-α-santalate in 150 milliliters of spectroscopically pure cyclohexane was degassed for a period of 1 hour and irradiated with ultraviolet light which was generated from a 450 watt Hanovia mercury arc lamp. Aliquots were removed at specified intervals and analyzed by gas-liquid chromatography. The quantity of aliquot removed, the irradiation period, and the weight percent of each compound in the mixture of compounds in each aliquot is listed in the following table.

		Weight percent of compounds in mixture		
Period of irradiation, minutes	Volume of aliquot, ml.	Ethyl trans-α-santalate	Ethyl cis-α-santalate	Ethyl $\Delta^{11.12}$-α-santalate
2.5	3.0	55	42	3
5	3.0	44	43	13
10	3.0	29	40	37
20	4.0	15	19	66
30	5.0	5	8	87

The gas-liquid chromatography retention time and spectral parameters of ethyl trans-α-santalate and ethyl cis-α-santalate were identical to the retention time and spectral parameters described for these compounds in Example 2 above, and the gas chromatography retention time and spectral parameters of ethyl $\Delta^{11.12}$-α-santalate were identical to the retention time and spectral parameters described for this compound in Example 5 below.

Example 4: Irradiation of Ethyl α-Santalates Using a Vycor Filter and Ethanol Solvent — A solution of 100 milligrams (3.9×10^{-3} mols) of a mixture comprised of 97 parts by weight of ethyl trans-α-santalate and 3 parts by weight of ethyl cis-α-santalate in 150 milliliters of absolute alcohol was degassed for a period of 1 hour and irradiated with ultraviolet light which was generated from a 450 watt Hanovia mercury arc lamp. Aliquots were removed at specified intervals and analyzed by gas-liquid chromatography. The quantity of aliquot removed, the irradiation period, and the weight percent of each compound in the mixture of compounds in each aliquots are listed in the table on the following page.

The gas chromatography retention time and spectral parameters of ethyl trans-α-santalate and ethyl cis-α-santalate were identical to the retention time and spectral parameters described for these compounds in Example 2 above, and the gas chromatography retention

time and spectral parameters of ethyl $\Delta^{11.12}$-α-santalate were identical to the retention
time and spectral parameters described for this compound in example 5 below.

Period of irradiation, minutes	Volume of aliquot, ml.	Weight percent of compounds in mixture		
		Ethyl trans-α- santalate	Ethyl cis-α- santalate	Ethyl $\Delta^{11.12}$-α- santalate
5	5.0	48	36	16
10	5.0	25	36	39

Example 5: Preparation of Ethyl $\Delta^{11.12}$-α-Santalates by Irradiation of Ethyl α-Santalates Using a Vycor Filter and Toluene as Solvent — A solution of 1.65 grams (6.3×10^{-3} mols) of a mixture comprised of 85 parts by weight of ethyl trans-α-santalate and 15 parts by weight of ethyl cis-α-santalate in 130 milliliters of toluene was degassed and irradiated for a period of 6 hours with ultraviolet light which was generated from a 450 watt Hanovia mercury arc lamp. Evaporation of solvent under reduced pressure and distillation of the residual oil afforded 1.02 grams (62% yield) of oil, boiling point 120°C/1.5 millimeters, comprised of ethyl trans-α-santalate (3%), ethyl cis-α-santalate (4%), and the ethyl $\Delta^{11.12}$-α-santalates (93%). Collection of the $\Delta^{11.12}$-α-santalate peak by preparative gas chromatography on the 5 feet by 0.25 inch FFAP column afforded a mixture of ethyl cis- and ethyl trans-$\Delta^{11.12}$-α-santalates, as an oil. Analysis calculated for $C_{17}H_{26}O_2$: C, 77.8; H, 10.0. Found: C, 77.92; H, 10.03.

Example 6: Preparation of $\Delta^{11.12}$-α-Santalols from $\Delta^{11.12}$-α-Santalates — A solution of 417 milligrams (1.6×10^{-3} mols) of ethyl $\Delta^{11.12}$-α-santalates in 10 milliliters of dry ether was added dropwise to a rapidly stirred suspension of 171 milligrams of lithium aluminum hydride in 5 milliliters of dry ether maintained at 0° to 5°C. This suspension was stirred under a nitrogen atmosphere at ice bath temperature (0° to 5°C) for 15 minutes followed by stirring at room temperature for 1 hour. The excess lithium aluminum hydride was destroyed with sodium sulfate decahydrate and the ether was decanted through anhydrous sodium sulfate.

Removal of the ether under reduced pressure and short path distillation of the residual oil afforded 353 milligrams (100% yield) of a clear oil, boiling point 107°C (0.25 mm). Gas-liquid chromatographic analysis of the distillate showed the presence of one major peak, $\Delta^{11.12}$-α-santalol, (75%) and a number of unidentified components (25%). Collection of the major component by preparative gas chromatography (218°C, R_t 420 sec) gave $\Delta^{11.12}$-α-santalol. Analysis calculated for $C_{15}H_{24}O$: C, 81.8; H, 11.1. Found: C, 81.8; H, 11.1. The mixture of trans and cis isomers of $\Delta^{11.12}$-α-santalol had an odor characterized as a mild, creamy, woody odor.

α-Santalol from Tricycloekasantalal

R.G. Lewis and W.F. Erman; U.S. Patent 3,478,114; November 11, 1969; assigned to The Proctor & Gamble Company describe a process for the preparation of α-santalol and certain α-santalate esters in which tricycloekasantalal is used as the starting material.

α-Santalol is a highly valued perfume base and is used in large quantities throughout the world. Previously, the only practical method for obtaining α-santalol was to isolate it from naturally occurring sources, e.g., from East Indian sandalwood oil, a primary source of α-santalol. See, for example, Bradfield et al, *Journal of the Chemical Society* (British), 79, page 390 (1935). However, the supply of East Indian sandalwood oil and other sources of α-santalol is limited and a possible shortage in the foreseeable future is predicted.

It has been generally accepted in the prior art that α-santalol, isolated from naturally occurring sources, exists exclusively in the form of trans-α-santalol. See for example, G. Brieger, *Tetrahedron Letters*, 2123 (1963). Compared with the products of this process on the basis of advanced analytical techniques, α-santalol isolated from naturally occurring sources appears to be cis-α-santalol. By means of this process, however, trans-α-santalol, cis-α-santalol, or a mixture of these two isomers, can be selectively synthesized as desired. The process for preparing α-santalol comprises reacting tricycloekasantalal with a phosphorane to form alkyl α-santalate and reacting the alkyl α-santalate with a reducing agent to form α-santalol. The term alkyl α-santalate refers to alkyl trans-α-santalate, alkyl cis-α-santalate, and mixtures where alkyl is selected from the group consisting of methyl, ethyl, propyl, butyl, and pentyl. This process for the preparation of α-santalol is illustrated below for a preferred example, i.e., where alkyl is ethyl.

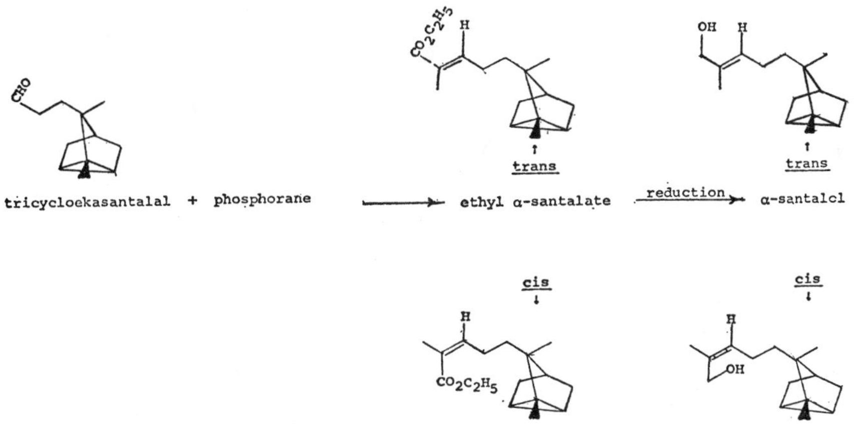

tricycloekasantalal + phosphorane ⟶ ethyl α-santalate $\xrightarrow{\text{reduction}}$ α-santalol

The following examples illustrate the process. All percentages and ratios are by weight unless otherwise specified. Data listed in all of the examples were obtained by means of the following instruments and techniques. Melting points were determined on a Kofler micro hot stage. Boiling points were observed on standard thermometers. Infrared spectra were recorded on a Perkin-Elmer Infracord spectrophotometer. Microanalyses were performed. The nmr spectra were obtained with a Varian Associates A-60 or a Varian Associates HA-100 instrument in deuterated chloroform or carbon disulfide using tetramethylsilane as an internal reference.

Gas-liquid chromatograms (glc) were obtained on an Aerograph Model 200 analytical instrument using one of two columns. Column A: 20% General Electric SF-96 silicone on 60-80 mesh chromosorb with H.M.D.S. (a conventional silicone coating), 10' by 0.25" outside diameter; Column B: 20% Reoplex-400 (a conventional polyester packing) on 60-80 mesh chromosorb with H.M.D.S., 10' by 0.25" outside diameter. The flow rate in either column was 60 milliliters per minute.

Example 1: Preparation of trans-α-Santalol — To a solution of 1.53 grams of (carbethoxyethylidene)triphenylphosphorane in 5 milliliters of methylene chloride was added a solution of 340 milligrams of tricycloekasantalal in 5 milliliters of dry methylene chloride and the resulting solution was stirred for 66 hours at room temperature under a nitrogen atmosphere. The methylene chloride was removed under reduced pressure (20 to 25 millimeters), and the remaining residue was extracted with six 30 milliliter portions of boiling n-hexane. The n-hexane extracts were combined and the total volume was reduced to 50 milliliters.

This material was then passed through 10 grams of activity IV alumina with 500 milliliters of n-hexane. The n-hexane was removed under reduced pressure (20 to 25 millimeters) leaving 577 milligrams of a light yellow oil. Analysis of this oil on column A at 200°C indicated the presence of four major components, i.e., a saturated ester by infrared (R_t 200 sec), an alcohol by infrared (R_t 310 sec), ethyl cis-α-santalate (R_t 935 sec), and ethyl trans-α-santalate (R_t 1275 sec). Further purification and separation by glc gave 23 milligrams of ethyl cis-α-santalate as a light yellow oil and 225.0 milligrams of ethyl trans-α-santalate as a clear oil. Ethyl trans-α-santalate: $[\alpha]_D^{25}$ + 32.75°. Analysis calculated for $C_{17}H_{26}O_2$: C, 77.8; H, 10.0. Found: C, 77.8; H, 9.7. Ethyl cis-α-santalate: $[\alpha]_D{}^{25}$ +8.17°. Analysis calculated for $C_{17}H_{26}O_2$: C, 77.8; H, 10.0. Found: C, 77.9; H, 10.0.

A solution of 140 milligrams of the ethyl trans-α-santalate in 3 milliliters of dry diethyl ether was added dropwise to 2 milliliters of diethyl ether containing 54 milligrams of lithium aluminum hydride. The resulting mixture was stirred under a nitrogen atmosphere for 1 hour while maintaining the temperature at 25°C. The ether solution was filtered, dried over anhydrous sodium sulfate, again filtered and the ether removed under reduced pressure (20 to 25 millimeters) to produce 117.5 milligrams of a clear viscous oil. Analysis of this oil on column B at 203°C indicated the presence of trans-α-santalol (92%, R_t 790 seconds). Further purification and separation by glc gave 66.1 milligrams of pure trans-α-santalol as a clear oil: $[\alpha]_D{}^{25}$ + 18.09°. Analysis calculated for $C_{15}H_{24}O$: C, 81.8; H, 11.0. Found: C, 81.8; H, 11.2.

Example 2: Preparation of cis-α-Santalol — A solution of 1.01 grams of tricycloekasantalal and 6.0 grams of (carbethoxyethylidene)triphenylphosphorane in 25 milliliters of dry methanol was stirred for 16 hours at 26°C under a nitrogen atmosphere. The methanol was removed under reduced pressure (20 to 25 millimeters). Further purification and separation by glc gave 223 milligrams of ethyl cis-α-santalate and 1.07 grams of ethyl trans-α-santalate. The analytical data for these compounds were equivalent to that obtained for the same compounds in Example 1.

A solution of 99.1 milligrams of the ethyl cis-α-santalate in 3 milliliters of dry diethyl ether was added dropwise to a solution of 30 milligrams of lithium aluminum hydride in 3 milliliters of diethyl ether. The resulting solution was stirred for 1 hour under a nitrogen atmosphere while the temperature was maintained at about 25°C. The solution was filtered and dried over sodium sulfate. The ether was removed under reduced pressure (20 to 25 millimeters) to afford 84.3 milligrams of a clear viscous oil. Analysis of this oil on column B at 203°C showed the presence of cis-α-santalol (85%, R_t 640 sec). Further separation, purification and collection by glc yielded 46.2 milligrams of pure cis-α-santalol as a clear viscous oil: $[\alpha]_D{}^{25}$ + 18.33°. Analysis calculated for $C_{15}H_{24}O$: C, 81.8; H, 11.0. Found: C, 81.5; H, 11.1.

A commercially available sample of naturally occurring α-santalol, which had been separated from East Indian sandalwood oil, was obtained from Givaudan-Delawana, Inc. The infrared spectrum, nmr spectrum, and glc retention time of this material was identical to the same data for the cis-α-santalol prepared in Example 2.

Additionally, seven commercially available samples of α-santalol from East Indian sandalwood oil and one commercially available sample of α-santalol from Australian sandalwood oil were shown by glc to be identical to the cis-α-santalol prepared in Example 2.

Example 3: Preparation of α-Santalol — Ethyl α-santalate prepared in accordance with Example 2 (comprising a mixture of ethyl trans-α-santalate and ethyl cis-α-santalate) was twice distilled, boiling point 136° to 139°C/0.76 millimeters. To a solution of 309 milligrams of lithium aluminum hydride in 20 milliliters of diethyl ether was added dropwise with stirring 1.774 grams of the distilled ethyl α-santalate in 30 milliliters of diethyl ether. The resulting mixture was stirred for 1.3 hours at 26°C under a nitrogen atmosphere.

Excess sodium sulfate decahydrate was added to the solution which was then filtered. The ether was removed under reduced pressure (20 to 25 millimeters) to afford a clear oil. This oil was distilled to yield 1.35 grams of distillate, boiling point 113° to 119°C/0.5 millimeters. The distillate was analyzed on a EgSSX (10' by 0.25") chromatographic column at 180°C and was shown to contain cis-α-santalol (13%, R_t 11 min, 55 sec) and trans-α-santalol (71%, R_t 13 min, 30 sec).

3-Normethyl-β-Santalol

H.C. Kretschmar and W.F. Erman; U.S. Patent 3,673,261; June 27, 1972; assigned to

The Procter & Gamble Company describe synthetic perfume compounds which are valuable synthetic perfume components and have a desirable sandalwood odor. These compounds are bicyclo[2.2.1]heptane compounds, two of which have olefinic unsaturation in the side chain giving rise to cis and trans isomers, e.g., 2-methylene-3-exo(trans-4'-methyl-5'-hydroxypent-3'-enyl)bicyclo[2.2.1]heptane, 2-methylene-3-exo(cis-4'-methyl-5'-hydroxypent-3'-enyl)-bicyclo[2.2.1]heptane, and a third compound which contains no unsaturation in the side chain, e.g., 2-methylene-3-exo(4'-methyl-5'-hydroxypentyl)bicyclo[2.2.1]heptane. The first of these compounds, 2-methylene-3-exo(trans-4'-methyl-5'-hydroxypent-3'-enyl)bicyclo[2.2.1]heptane has the structural formula shown below. This compound may be referred to either using its bicyclic nomenclature or the term, trans-3-normethyl-β-santalol.

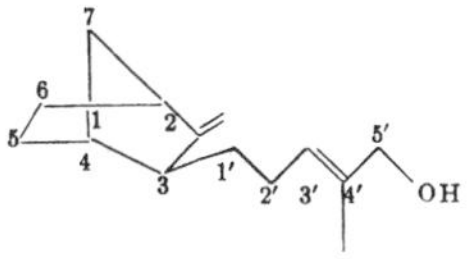

The second of these bicyclic compounds, 2-methylene-3-exo(cis-4'-methyl-5'-hydroxypent-3'-enyl)bicyclo[2.2.1]heptane, has the following structural formula. This compound may be referred to using either its bicyclic nomenclature or cis-3-normethyl-β-santalol.

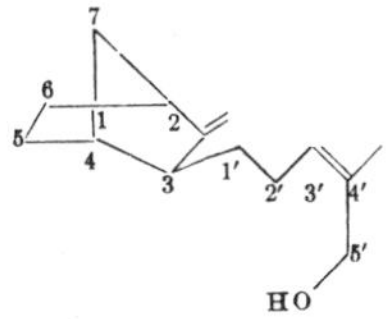

The third compound, 2-methylene-3-exo(4'-methyl-5'-hydroxypentyl)bicyclo[2.2.1]heptane, has the structural formula shown below. This compound may be referred to using either the bicyclic nomenclature given above or the term, 3-normethyldihydro-β-santalol.

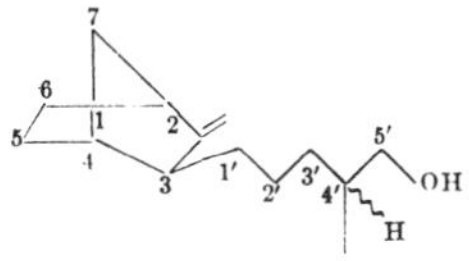

All of the above normethyl-β-santalol derivatives are valuable as perfume components useful in the preparation of perfumes having an odor described as sandalwood. The processes comprise three routes. In each of these processes the first step is the same and involves the reaction of 2-methylbicyclo[2.2.1]hept-2-ene with acrolein. The three routes all describe synthetic reactions using the reaction products obtained from the reaction of 2-methylbicyclo[2.2.1]hept-2-ene and acrolein. For example, Route 1 describes a process for preparing cis- and trans-3-normethyl-β-santalol. Route 2 describes a process for preparing 3-normethyl-β-santalol. Route 3 describes a process for preparing a similar compound, 3-normethyldihydro-β-santalol. Complete synthesis procedures and analytical results are described in the patent.

β-Santalol from 3-Methylnorcamphor

H.C. Kretschmar and W.F. Erman; U.S. Patent 3,662,008; May 9, 1972; assigned to The

Procter & Gamble Company describe a process for preparing β-santalol, a component of sandalwood oil, having a valuable sandalwood odor and useful in perfume compositions. The process involves an 8-step synthesis from 3-methylnorcamphor. β-Santalol is prepared by alkylating 3-methylbicyclo[2.2.1] heptan-2-one having the structural formula:

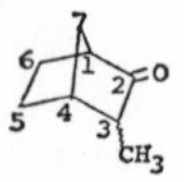

in strong base selected from the group consisting of a sodium, lithium or potassium amide, or hydride, or trityl sodium, potassium, or lithium with allyl chloride, bromide, or iodide to obtain endo-3-methyl-exo-3(1'-prop-2'-enyl)bicyclo[2.2.1] heptan-2-one.

This compound is reacted with a methylmetallic compound selected from the group consisting of methyllithium and methylmagnesium bromide, followed by a hydrolysis to obtain exo-2-methyl-endo-3-methyl-endo-2-hydroxy-exo-3(1'-prop-2'-enyl)bicyclo[2.2.1] heptane, which is then brominated with bromine to obtain exo-2-methyl-endo-3-methyl-endo-2-hydroxy-exo-3(2',3'-dibromopropyl)bicyclo[2.2.1] heptane.

This compound is dehydrobrominated with a strong base (sodium, potassium, lithium amide) to obtain exo-2-methyl-endo-3-methyl-endo-2-hydroxy-exo-3(1'-prop-2'-ynyl)bicyclo[2.2.1] heptane which is then dehydrated with a dehydrating agent selected from the group consisting of thionyl chloride, phosphorus oxychloride, boron trifluoride, aluminum oxide, sulfuric acid and p-toluenesulfonic acid to obtain endo-3-methyl-exo-3(1'-prop-2'-ynyl)-2-methylene-bicyclo[2.2.1] heptane.

This product is then reacted with a compound selected from the group consisting of di(sec-iso-amyl)borate, di(menthyl-1-en-9-yl)borane, di(cyclohexyl)borane, and di(iso-butyl)-aluminum hydride followed by an alkaline peroxide oxidation to obtain endo-3-methyl-exo-3-(3'-oxopropyl)-2-methylene-bicyclo[2.2.1] heptane, which is next reacted with (carbethoxy-ethylidene)triphenylphosphorane to obtain endo-3-methyl-exo-3(cis-4'-carbethoxypent-3'-enyl)-2-methylene-bicyclo[2.2.1] heptane and endo-3-methyl-exo-3(trans-4'-carbethoxypent-3'-enyl)-2-methylene-bicyclo[2.2.1] heptane.

These two compounds are then reduced with a reducing agent selected from the group consisting of lithium alumium hydride or sodium, potassium, or lithium in an alcohol sovent to obtain endo-3-methyl-exo-3(cis-5'-hydroxy-4'-methylpent-3'-enyl)-2-methylene-bicyclo-[2.2.1] heptane and endo-3-methyl-exo-3(trans-5'-hydroxy-4'-methylpent-3'-enyl)-2-methylene-bicyclo[2.2.1] heptane.

The product of the process described above is a mixture of endo-3-methyl-exo-3(cis-5'-hydroxy-4'-methylpent-3'-enyl)-2-methylene-bicyclo[2.2.1] heptane (cis-β-santalol) and endo-3-methyl-exo-3(trans-5'-hydroxy-4'-methylpent-3'-enyl)-2-methylene-bicyclo[2.2.1] - heptane (trans-β-santalol). As used here, the term β-santalol without the designation cis or trans is intended to refer to the mixture of the two geometric isomers. β-Santalol, the product of the above process, possesses a desirable, woody sandalwood fragrance and, thus, has utility as a perfume per se and is useful as a component in perfume compositions. The cis isomer and the trans isomer can be separated and are individually useful as odorants per se and as components in perfume compositions. In addition, the intermediates produced in the above process are useful as odorants per se having a distinctive fragrance in addition to their utility as intermediates in the process.

Example: Perfume compositions containing mixtures of the cis- and trans-isomers of β-santalol and containing cis-β-santalol and trans-β-santalol are prepared by intermixing the components shown on the following page. The compositions exhibit highly desirable and useful odors.

Composition A
Sandal

Mixture of cis- and trans-β-santalol*	40.0
Geranium bourbon	15.0
Vetivert	3.0
Patchouli	1.0
Olibanum	1.0
Coumarin	2.5
Citronellol	15.0
Phenyl ethyl alcohol	7.5
Musk xylol	0.6
Musk ambrette	0.4
Peru balsam	4.0
Ambre synthetic	3.5
Cassia	1.0
Cinnamic alcohol	0.5
Jasmine synthetic	1.5
α-Ionone	3.5

*A mixture of the cis- and trans-isomers of β-santalol in a ratio of 1:4.8

Composition B
Rose de chine

Geranium bourbon	20
Geraniol	30
Rose Otto synthetic	4
Cis-β-santalol	3
Patchouli	8
Cedarwood	8
Musk xylol	6
Terpineol	15
Phenyl ethyl alcohol	6

In related work, *H.C. Kretschmar and W.F. Erman; U.S. Patent 3,679,756; July 25, 1972; assigned to The Procter & Gamble Company* describe another process for preparing β-santalol from 3-methylnorcamphor comprising the steps of: (1) alkylating 3-methylnorcamphor with β-bromopropionaldehyde ethylene glycol acetal; (2) reacting the reaction product of Step (1) with a methylmetallic compound such as methyllithium, followed by acid hydrolysis; (3) reacting the reaction product of Step (2) with (carbethoxyethylidene)triphenylphosphorane; (4) dehydrating the reaction product of Step (3) with a dehydrating agent, such as thionyl chloride; and (5) reducing the reaction product of Step (4) with a reducing agent, such as lithium aluminum hydride to obtain β-santalol.

Dihydro-β-Santalol

W.I. Fanta and W.F. Erman; U.S. Patent 3,673,263; June 27, 1972; assigned to The Procter & Gamble Company describe a process for obtaining dihydro-β-santalol, which has a valuable sandalwood odor, from 3-endo-methyl-3-exo(4'-methyl-5'-hydroxypentyl)norcamphor.

The process comprises the steps of: (1) reacting 3-endo-methyl-3-exo(4'-methyl-5'-hydroxypentyl)norcamphor having the general formula:

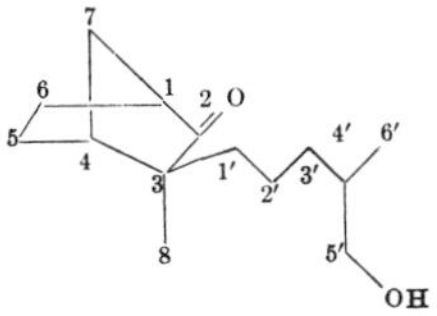

with an organometallic compound selected from the group consisting of methyl Grignards and methylmetallic compounds to obtain an organometallic salt of 2-exo-3-endo-dimethyl-3-exo(4'-methyl-5'-hydroxypentyl)norborneol having the general formula:

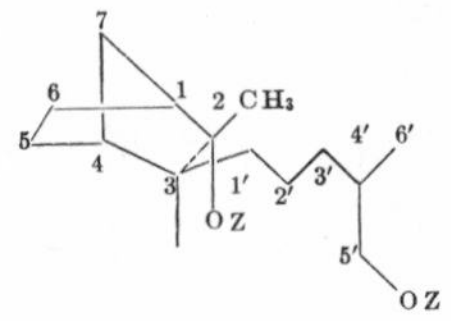

where Z is selected from the group of cations consisting of sodium, potassium, lithium, magnesium bromide, magnesium iodide, and magnesium chloride; (2) hydrolyzing the reaction product of Step (1) to obtain 2-exo-3-endo-dimethyl-3-exo(4'-methyl-5'-hydroxy-pentyl)norborneol having the general formula:

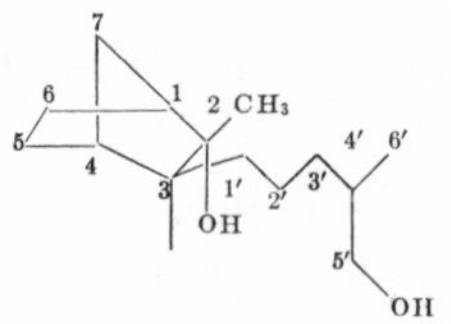

and (3) dehydrating 2-exo-3-endo-dimethyl-3-exo(4'-methyl-5'-hydroxypentyl)norborneol with a compound selected from the group consisting of Lewis acids, oxalic acid, p-toluene-sulfonic acid, sulfuric acid, hydrochloric acid, and hydrobromic acid to obtain dihydro-β-santalol having the general formula:

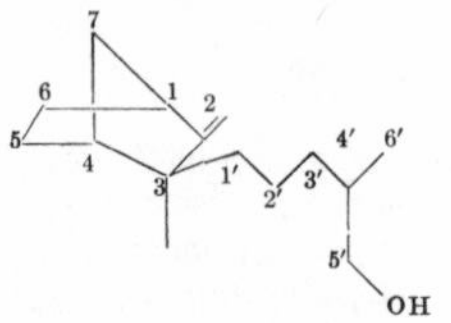

Example: Preparation of Dihydro-β-Santalol from 3-Endo-Methyl-3-Exo(4'-Methyl-5'-Hydroxypentyl)Norcamphor — (a) The starting compound, 3-endo-methyl-3-exo(4'-methyl-5'-hydroxypentyl)norcamphor, is prepared according to the process set forth in Example 1 of U.S. Patent 3,579,479. In this process, 2-methyl-4-pentenol is borated with boric acid to form tris(2-methyl-4-pentenyl) borate. The borate is hydrobrominated by a free radical addition and then hydrolyzed to obtain 2-methyl-5-bromopentanol. The bromo-pentanol is borated with boric acid and, subsequently, this product is reacted with the enolate of 3-methylnorcamphor and then hydrolyzed to form 3-endo-methyl-3-exo(4'-methyl-5'-hydroxypentyl)norcamphor.

(b) A 250 milliliter flask fitted with a mechanical stirrer and an addition funnel was charged with 33 milliliters of 3 M ethereal methyl magnesium bromide solution (0.10 mol) and 100 milliliters (71.5 grams) of diethyl ether. A nitrogen atmosphere was introduced and a solution of 5.6 grams (0.025 mol) of 3-endo-methyl-3-exo(4'-methyl-5'-hydroxypentyl)-norcamphor in 50 milliliters (35.8 grams) of diethyl ether was added over 15 minutes. The resulting mixture was stirred rapidly at reflux for 5 hours. The reaction product was hydrolyzed by the cautious dropwise addition of 20 milliliters of an aqueous saturated sodium sulfate solution. The ethereal layer was drawn off and the remaining semisolid, inorganic material was washed well with several portions of ether. The combined organic layers were washed once with an aqueous sodium sulfate solution, dried over magnesium sulfate, and the solvent was removed by distillation to afford 7.7 grams of viscous oil. Distillation gave 5.58 grams (93%) of 2-exo-methyl-3-endo-methyl-3-exo(4'-methyl-5'-hydroxypentyl)norborneol, boiling point 132°C (0.18 mm).

(c) A dry 50 milliliter flask fitted with condenser and septum was charged with a solution containing 5.58 grams (0.023 mol) of 2-exo-methyl-3-endo-methyl-3-exo(4'-methyl-5'-hydroxypentyl)norborneol in 23 milliliters of anhydrous diethyl ether. A nitrogen atmosphere was introduced and 2.3 milliliters of a 47% boron trifluoride etherate (0.019 mol) solution was added as rapidly as possible. The resulting dark solution was refluxed for 2 hours and cautiously added to an excess of saturated aqueous sodium bicarbonate solution. The ether layer was removed and the aqueous solution was extracted with ether.

The ether extracts were combined with the original ether layer and washed with 2 portions of brine. The ether solution was dried with magnesium sulfate. Subsequent solvent removal afforded 6.27 grams of light yellow oil which on distillation gave 4.55 grams (87%) of colorless dihydro-β-santalol which showed 98% purity by gas-liquid partition chromatography and which had a desirable, strong sandalwood odor. Dihydro-β-santalol could be further purified by column chromatography (Florisil-elution with 2 to 5% ether in hexane) or redistillation, boiling point 106° to 107°C (0.1 mm), on larger scale.

In related work, *W.I. Fanta and W.F. Erman; U.S. Patent 3,580,954; May 25, 1971; assigned to The Procter & Gamble Company* describe a process for preparing 3-endo-methyl-3-exo(4'-methyl-5'-hydroxypentyl)norcamphor from 2-methyl-4-pentenol.

The process comprises the steps of: (1) borating 2-methyl-4-pentenol having the general formula:

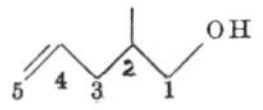

with a compound selected from the group consisting of boric acid, boric anhydride and mixtures thereof to obtain tris(2-methyl-4-pentenyl) borate having the general formula:

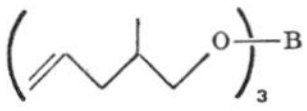

(2) hydrobrominating tris(2-methyl-5-bromopentyl) borate with hydrogen bromide in the presence of a free radical catalyst to form tris(2-methyl-5-bromopentyl) borate which is then hydrolyzed to obtain 2-methyl-5-bromopentanol having the general formula:

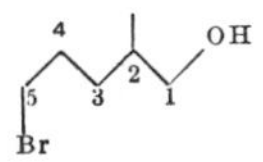

(3) etherifying 2-methyl-5-bromopentanol with dihydropyran to obtain the 2-methyl-5-bromopentyl tetrahydropyranyl ether having the general formula:

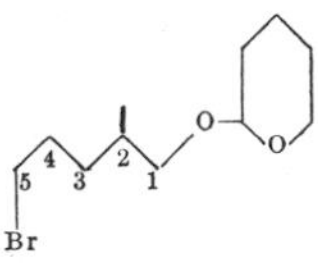

(4) reacting 2-methyl-5-bromopentyl tetrahydropyranyl ether with a mixture prepared from 3-methylnorcamphor having the general formula shown on the following page:

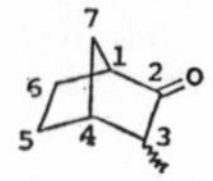

and a strong base to obtain tetrahydropyranyl ether of 3-endo-methyl-3-exo(4'-methyl-5'-hydroxypentyl)norcamphor having the general formula:

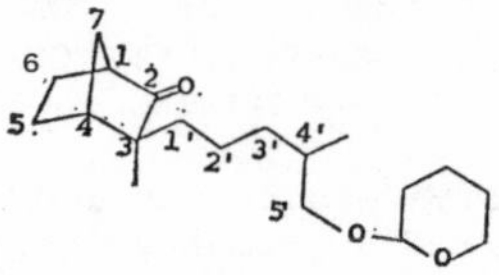

and (5) treating tetrahydropyranyl ether of 3-endo-methyl-3-exo(4'-methyl-5'-hydroxypentyl)-norcamphor with a catalytic amount of an acid selected from the group consisting of p-toluenesulfonic acid and hydrochloric acid to obtain 3-endo-methyl-3-exo(4'-methyl-5'-hydroxypentyl)norcamphor having the general formula:

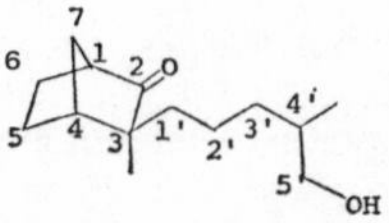

3-Endo-methyl-3-exo(4'-methyl-5'-hydroxypentyl)norcamphor has utility as a perfume component and as an intermediate in the synthesis of dihydro-β-santalol, a very valuable sandalwood substitute.

Example 1: Preparation of 3-Endo-Methyl-3-Exo(4'-Methyl-5'-Hydroxypentyl)Norcamphor from 2-Methyl-4-Pentenol — (Step 1) The preparation of tri(2-methyl-4-pentenyl)borate from 2-methyl-4-pentenol is as follows. A 500 milliliter flask fitted with a Dean-Stark trap and condenser was charged with a solution of 25 grams (0.25 mol) of 2-methyl-4-pentenol in 250 milliliters of benzene and 5.25 grams (0.083 mol) of boric acid. The reaction was refluxed under nitrogen until the theoretical amount of H_2O (4.5 ml) had collected. The solution was cooled slightly and the solvent was removed at reduced pressure to afford 27.2 grams (100%) of colorless oil. This material, tri(2-methyl-4-pentenyl)borate, was used directly without further purification.

Results substantially similar to this are obtained when 0.042 mol of boric anhydride are substituted for the 0.083 mol of boric acid in that the hydroxyl groups of the 2-methyl-4-pentenol are protected in the subsequent step. Substantially similar results are also obtained when toluene and xylene are substituted for benzene on an equal weight basis.

(Step 2) The preparation of 2-methyl-5-bromopentanol from tri(2-methyl-4-pentenyl)borate is as follows. A dry 500 milliliter flask fitted with a subsurface gas inlet and reflux condenser was charged with a solution of about 0.25 mol of crude tri(2-methyl-4-pentenyl)borate in 250 milliliters of hexane and 500 milligrams of benzoyl peroxide. The mixture was cooled to 0°C and excess anhydrous hydrogen bromide, about 2.5 mols, was passed in rapidly over a period of 50 minutes. The reaction mixture was stirred for an additional hour; the excess gas was removed by a nitrogen sweep. The reaction product was hydrolyzed and the benzoyl peroxide and hydrogen bromide were removed with a saturated aqueous solution of sodium bicarbonate followed by a brine wash.

The solution was dried with magnesium sulfate and the hexane was removed by distillation to afford 41.52 grams of 2-methyl-5-bromopentanol. This material can be used directly in the next step of this process. However, it was further purified by distillation to afford 36.8 grams (86%) of clear 2-methyl-5-bromopentanol, boiling point 70°C (0.1 mm).

(Step 3) The preparation of 2-methyl-5-bromopentyl tetrahydropyranyl ether from 2-methyl-5-bromopentanol is as follows. A dry 50 milliliter flask was charged with a mixture of 10.5 grams (0.059 mol) of 2-methyl-5-bromopentanol and 6.2 grams (0.074 mol) of dihydropyran (distilled). The flask was fitted with a drying tube, cooled to 0°C, and the solution was treated with 25 drops of phosphorus oxychloride. The resulting reaction mixture was stirred at room temperature for 3 hours and then added to 100 milliliters of 2% aqueous sodium hydroxide.

The reaction product was isolated with diethyl ether. The ether isolated was washed with brine, dried over magnesium sulfate and the solvent removed to give 15.44 grams of crude 2-methyl-5-bromopentyl tetrahydropyranyl ether. Distillation afforded 14.95 grams (96%) of colorless 2-methyl-5-bromopentyl tetrahydropyranyl ether, boiling point 83° to 85°C (0.02 millimeter). The 2-methyl-5-bromopentyl tetrahydropyranyl ether isolated had an odor characterized as a mild, sweet woody odor. This odor characteristic is useful in a wide variety of perfume compositions.

(Step 4) The preparation of tetrahydropyranyl ether of 3-endo-methyl-3-exo(4'-methyl-5'-hydroxypentyl)norcamphor from 2-methyl-5-bromopentyl tetrahydropyranyl ether is as follows. A 500 milliliter flask fitted with a condenser and addition funnel was charged with 4.9 grams (0.125 mol) of a 61% mineral oil dispersion of sodium hydride. A nitrogen atmosphere was introduced followed by 60 milliliters of benzene (distilled). A solution of 12.4 grams (0.1 mol) of 3-methylnorcamphor in 60 milliliters of redistilled benzene was added and enolate formation took place over 2 hours at reflux (80° to 100°C). To this refluxing reaction mixture was added a solution of 26.5 grams (0.1mol) of 2-methyl-5-bromopentyl tetrahydropyranyl ether in 60 milliliters of redistilled benzene.

Reflux was continued for an additional 61 hours after which time the cooled mixture was added to brine and the product isolated with diethyl ether. The combined ether extracts were washed with brine and dried over magnesium sulfate. Removal of solvent afforded 33.52 grams of yellow oil. The crude oil contained several grams of unreacted starting materials which were smoothly removed by distillation, boiling point 30° to 100°C (0.02 mm).

The residual oil, 20.78 grams (67%), was composed mainly of tetrahydropyranyl ether of 3-endo-methyl-3-exo(4'-methyl-5'-hydroxypentyl)norcamphor and was treated as described in the following step. The residual oil can be distilled to afford pure tetrahydropyranyl ether of 3-endo-methyl-3-exo(4'-methyl-5'-hydroxypentyl)norcamphor, 135° to 140°C (0.02 millimeter). The tetrahydropyranyl ether of 3-endo-methyl-3-exo(4'-methyl-5'-hydroxypentyl)norcamphor isolated above has an odor characterized as a mild, herbaceous, woody odor. This odor characteristic is useful in a wide variety of perfume compositions.

(Step 5) The preparation of 3-endo-methyl-3-exo(4'-methyl-5'-hydroxypentyl)norcamphor is as follows. A solution of 20.78 grams (0.067 mol) of crude tetrahydropyranyl ether of 3-endo-methyl-3-exo(4'-methyl-5'-hydroxypentyl)norcamphor and 1.5 grams (0.008 mol) of p-toluenesulfonic acid monohydrate in 250 milliliters of ethanol was refluxed under nitrogen for 2 hours. The cooled reaction product was added to brine and the product was isolated with ether.

Removal of magnesium sulfate dried solvent afforded 19.12 grams of crude 3-endo-methyl-3-exo(4'-methyl-5'-hydroxypentyl)norcamphor which on subsequent distillation gave 14.0 grams (96%) of product. Further purification by distillation, boiling point 127° to 130°C (0.07 mm), and gas-liquid partition chromatography gave 3-endo-methyl-3-exo(4'-methyl-5'-hydroxypentyl)norcamphor. 3-Endo-methyl-3-exo(4'-methyl-5'-hydroxypentyl)norcamphor isolated above had an odor characterized as sweet, fruity (strawberry, pineapple, melon, berry, apple) floral note.

Example 2: Perfume Compositions —Perfume compositions containing 3-endo-methyl-3-exo(4'-methyl-5'-hydroxypentyl)norcamphor are prepared by intermixing the components shown below. The compositions exhibit highly desirable and useful odors.

Composition A, Strawberry Base

Components:	Percent by Weight
3-Endo-methyl-3-exo(4'-methyl-5'-hydroxypentyl)norcamphor	10
Ethyl acetate	30
Ethyl benzoate	3
Ethyl butyrate	20
Ethyl nitrate	10
Ethyl pelargonate	5
Ethyl formate	10
Amyl acetate	4
Benzyl acetone	3
Methyl naphthyl ketone	1
Methyl salicylate	2
Cinnamon oil	1
Coumarin	1

Composition B, Pineapple Base

Components:	Percent by Weight
Amyl butyrate	50
Ethyl butyrate	20
Ethyl acetate	5
Acetaldehyde	6
Chloroform	5
Lemon oil	2
3-Endo-methyl-3-exo(4'-methyl-5'-hydroxypentyl)norcamphor	1
Propyl valerate	10
Vanillin	1

In related work, *W.I. Fanta and W.F. Erman; U.S. Patent 3,579,479; May 18, 1971; assigned to The Procter & Gamble Company* describe a process for preparing 2-methyl-5-bromopentanol and 3-endo-methyl-3-exo(4'-methyl-5'-hydroxypentyl)norcamphor from 2-methyl-4-pentenol. The process comprises the steps of (1) borating 2-methyl-4-pentenol with boric acid and/or boric anhydride to obtain tri(2-methyl-4-pentenyl)borate; (2) hydrobrominating the tri(2-methyl-4-pentenyl)borate in the presence of a free radical catalyst and subsequently hydrolyzing the reaction product to obtain 2-methyl-5-bromopentanol; (3) borating the 2-methyl-5-bromopentanol with boric acid and/or boric anhydride to obtain tri(2-methyl-5-brompentyl)borate; (4) alkylating 3-methylnorcamphor with the tri(2-methyl-5-bromopentyl)borate and subsequently hydrolyzing the reaction product to obtain 3-endo-methyl-3-exo(4'-methyl-5'-hydroxypentyl)norcamphor.

W.I. Fanta and W.F. Erman; U.S. Patent 3,580,953; May 25, 1971; assigned to The Procter & Gamble Company also describe another process for preparing 3-endo-methyl-3-exo(4'-methyl-5'-hydroxypentyl)norcamphor from 2-methyl-4-pentenol. The process comprises the steps of: (1) esterifying 2-methyl-4-pentenol; (2) hydrobrominating the ester in the presence of a free radical catalyst; (3) reducing the hydrobrominated ester to 2-methyl-5-bromopentanol; (4) borating the 2-methyl-5-bromopentanol with boric acid and/or boric anhydride to obtain tri(2-methyl-5-bromopentyl)borate; and (5) alkylating 3-methylnorcamphor with the tri(2-methyl-5-bromopentyl)borate and subsequently hydrolyzing the reaction product to obtain 3-endo-methyl-3-exo(4'-methyl-5'-hydroxypentyl)norcamphor.

Pyranyl Ether of 3-Endo-Methyl-3-Exo(4'-Methyl-5'-Hydroxypentyl)Norcamphor

A process described by *W.I. Fanta and W.F. Erman; U.S. Patent 3,624,106; November 30, 1971; assigned to The Procter & Gamble Company* relates to the compound, tetrahydropyranyl ether of 3-endo-methyl-3-exo(4'-methyl-5'-hydroxypentyl)norcamphor.

The process for preparing the above noted compound and converting it to 3-endo-methyl-3-exo(4'-methyl-5'-hydroxypentyl)norcamphor comprises the steps of: (1) esterifying 2-methyl-4-pentenol having the general formula:

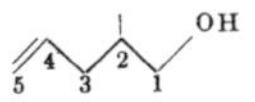

to obtain the ester of 2-methyl-4-pentenol having the general formula:

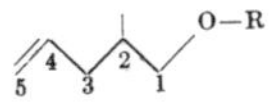

where R is an acyl group containing from 2 to about 5 carbon atoms; (2) hydrobrominating the ester of Step (1) with hydrogen bromide in the presence of a free radical catalyst to obtain a 2-methyl-5-bromopentyl ester having the general formula:

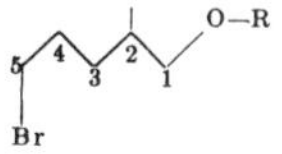

(3) reducing the hydrobrominated ester of Step (2) with a reducing agent to obtain 2-methyl-5-bromopentanol having the general formula:

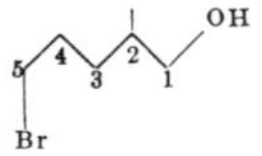

(4) etherifying 2-methyl-5-bromopentanol with dihydropyran to obtain the 2-methyl-5-bromopentyl tetrahydropyranyl ether having the general formula:

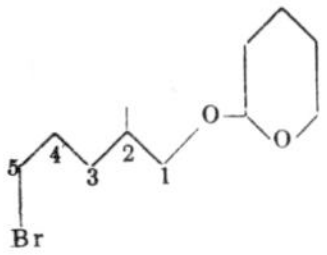

(5) reacting 2-methyl-5-bromopentyl tetrahydropyranyl ether with a mixture prepared from 3-methylnorcamphor having the general formula:

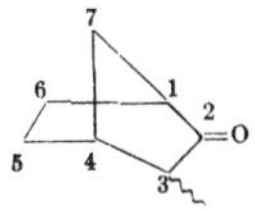

and a strong base to obtain the compound, tetrahydropyranyl ether of 3-endo-methyl-3-exo(4'-methyl-5'-hydroxypentyl)norcamphor having the general formula shown on the following page:

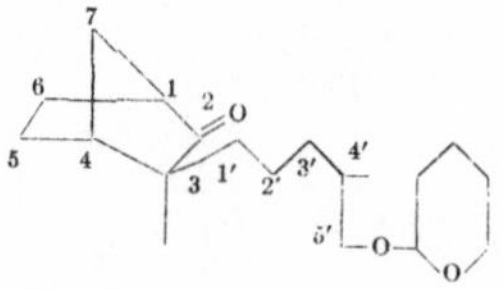

and (6) treating tetrahydropyranyl ether of 3-endo-methyl-3-exo(4'-methyl-5'-hydroxy-pentyl)norcamphor with a catalytic amount of an acid selected from the group consisting of p-toluenesulfonic acid and hydrochloric acid to obtain 3-endo-methyl-3-exo(4'-methyl-5'-hydroxypentyl)norcamphor having the general formula:

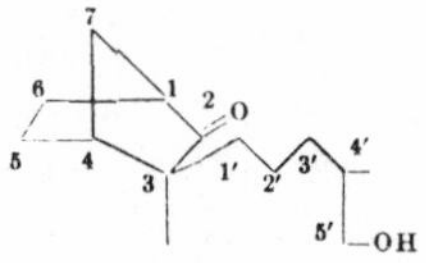

Bicyclo[2.2.1] Heptyl Carbinols by Grignard Reaction

W.J. Houlihan; U.S. Patent 3,250,815; May 10, 1966; assigned to Universal Oil Products Company has found that woody, earthy type odors are possessed by bicyclo[2.2.1]heptyl carbinols and their esters having the general formula:

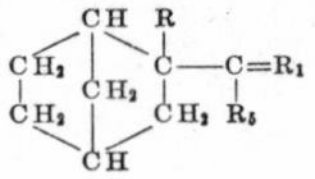

where R is hydrogen or a lower alkyl group containing from 1 to 3 carbon atoms, R_1 is an oxygen atom forming a keto group or:

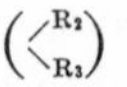

$$\left(\begin{smallmatrix} R_2 \\ R_3 \end{smallmatrix}\right)$$

where R_2 is hydrogen or lower alkyl group containing from 1 to 3 carbon atoms and R_3 is a hydroxy group or:

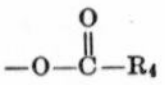

$$-O-\overset{\overset{\textstyle O}{\|}}{C}-R_4$$

where R_4 is a lower alkyl group containing from 1 to 3 carbon atoms and R_5 is a saturated or unsaturated isoamyl group.

The compounds of the process are prepared by reacting a 2-acyl-2-R-bicyclo[2.2.1]heptane (Compound I) with a Grignard reagent of the formula R"MgX to produce the corresponding bicyclo[2.2.1]heptyl carbinol (Compound II). This latter compound can be hydrogenated to produce the corresponding diene (Compound III) or to produce the corresponding ene (Compound IV).

These latter compounds can be oxidized to produce the corresponding ketones (Compounds V and VI) when R' is hydrogen and acylated to produce the corresponding esters (Compounds VII and VIII). These steps can be chemically represented as shown on the following page:

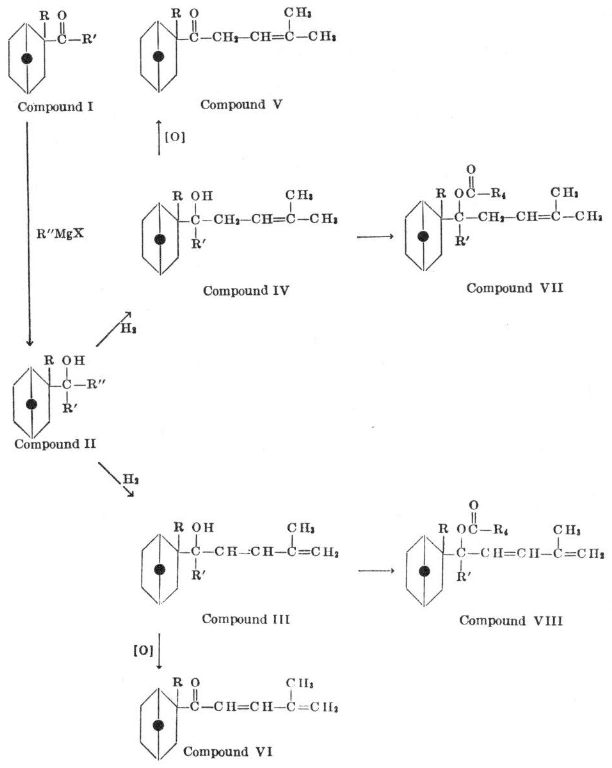

R O
‖
⬡—C—R'

Compound I

R O   CH₃
‖ |
⬡—C—CH₂—CH=C—CH₃

Compound V

↑ [O]

R'' MgX

R OH   CH₃
| |
⬡—C—CH₂—CH=C—CH₃
|
R'

Compound IV

→

O
‖
R OC—R₄   CH₃
| |
⬡—C—CH₂—CH=C—CH₃
|
R'

Compound VII

R OH
|
⬡—C—R''
|
R'

Compound II

H₂

H₂

R OH   CH₃
| |
⬡—C—CH=CH—C=CH₂
|
R'

Compound III

→

O
‖
R OC—R₄   CH₃
| |
⬡—C—CH=CH—C=CH₂
|
R'

Compound VIII

[O]

R O   CH₃
‖ |
⬡—C—CH=CH—C=CH₂

Compound VI

where R' is a hydrogen or a lower alkyl group, R" is saturated or unsaturated isoamyl group, X is a halo group and R is as indicated above.

Example 1: A Grignard reagent is prepared from ethyl bromide (55 grams, 0.5 mol) and magnesium (12.2 grams, 0.5 mol) in diethyl ether (500 grams). With good stirring a solution of 2-methylbut-1-ene-3-yne (33 grams, 0.5 mol) in diethyl ether (100 grams) is added dropwise in 0.75 hour. Gassing (ethane) is observed at the start of addition and continues for about 4.5 hours. A solution of 2-methyl-2-formylbicyclo[2.2.1]heptane (56 grams, 0.4 mol) in diethyl ether (100 milliliters) is added rapidly. The mixture is refluxed for 1.5 hours and then allowed to stand overnight at room temperature.

The complex is hydrolyzed with saturated ammonium chloride, filtered and dried. Distillation through a claisen head gives 55.5 grams (67.3%) of 2-methyl-2-(4'-methylpent-2'-yne-4'-ene-1'-ol)bicyclo[2.2.1]heptane, boiling point 118° to 122°C at 3 mm. The compound has an earthy green, sweet, slight anise note.

Example 2: A solution of 2-methyl-2-(4'-methyl-pent-2'-yne-4'-ene-1'-ol)bicyclo[2.2.1]heptane (15.2 grams, 0.075 mol), Ionol (1 crystal) and isopropanol (20 milliliters) is hydrogenated in the presence of a lindlar catalyst (0.050 gram) at 25.5°C and an initial pressure of 26.2 psi. After 1.0 molar equivalent of hydrogen is absorbed (1.5 hours) the reaction is filtered and distilled. There is obtained 12.8 grams (81%) of 2-ethyl-2-(4'-methylpenta-2',4'-diene-1'-ol)bicyclo[2.2.1]heptane, boiling point 107° to 108°C at 2.0 mm. The compound has an earthy green, sweet, slight anise odor.

Example 3: A solution of 2-methyl-2-(4'-methylpent-2'-yne-4'-ene-1'-ol)bicyclo[2.2.1] heptane (15.2 grams, 0.075 mol), Ionol (1 crystal) and isopropanol (35 milliliters) is hydrogenated in the presence of 5% palladium-carbon catalyst (1.0 gram) at 24°C and initial pressure of 27.0 psi. The temperature is not allowed to exceed 30°C during hydrogen-uptake. After 2.0 molar equivalents of hydrogen is absorbed (0.5 hour) the reaction is cooled, filtered and distilled. There is obtained 11.1 grams (72%) of 2-methyl-2-(4'-methylpent-3'-ene-1'-ol)bicyclo[2.2.1] heptane, boiling point 104° to 110°C at 2.0 mm. The compound has an earthy green, sweet, slight anise note.

The compounds have a green earthy odor which is refreshingly wood-like. They can find wide application in a variety of products, particularly in perfume and cologne of the oriental type. A typical formula for a perfume is as follows:

	Parts
Amylbicyclo[2.2.1] heptyl carbinol	20.00
Methyl eugenol	10.00
50% Oakmoss absolute	7.50
Diphenyl oxide	5.00
50% Galbanum resinoid	2.50
Octyl isobutyrate	2.50
Gamma-heptanolide	2.50
5% Dibutyl sulfide	0.75
Geranium Moraccan	0.51
Octyl acetate	1.25

Dihydro-β-Santalal

A process described by *K.M. Pieper and T.W. Gibson; U.S. Patent 3,673,256; June 27, 1972; assigned to The Procter & Gamble Company* relates to dihydro-β-santalal, 3-endo-methyl-3-exo(4'-methylpentanalyl)-2-methylenebicyclo[2.2.1] heptane, which is a valuable synthetic perfume component having a desirable sandalwood odor. Dihydro-β-santalal has the structural formula shown below.

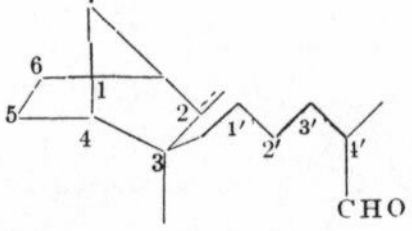

The process for preparing dihydro-β-santalal comprises the step of oxidizing dihydro-β-santalol, 3-endo-methyl-3-exo(4'-methyl-5'-hydroxypentyl)-2-methylenebicyclo[2.2.1] heptane, with an oxidizing agent selected from the group consisting of chromic acid and chromium trioxide-pyridinium complex. The process can be summarized according to the equation shown below.

dihydro-β-santalol   dihydro-β-santalal

11-Hydroxy-2,13,13-Trimethyltricyclo[6.4.0.1^{2,5}] Tridecane

J. Dorsky and W.M. Easter, Jr.; U.S. Patent 3,499,937; March 10, 1970; assigned to The

Givaudan Corporation describe a polycyclic alcohol which has been prepared in pure form by careful fractionation. It is a viscous, colorless oil with a strong sandalwood odor. The formula, 11-hydroxy-2,13,13-trimethyltricyclo[6.4.0.1^{2,5}] tridecane, may be represented as follows.

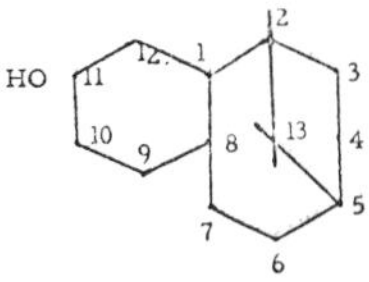

The alcohol is a mixture which contains at least 4 isomers as indicated by the number of peaks appearing on its gas-liquid chromatogram. In general, therefore, the product comprises at least 55% by weight of the polycyclic alcohol, $C_{16}H_{28}O$, the balance, if any, being a material having the formula:

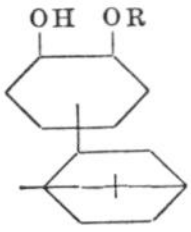

where R is a lower aliphatic hydrocarbon radical having up to 5 carbon atoms or cycloaliphatic hydrocarbon radical having up to 2 carbon atoms in the side chain. The side chain may be joined to the cycloaliphatic nucleus at any of the available positions and mixtures of the resulting position isomers may be used. The process comprises hydrogenating a material having the formula:

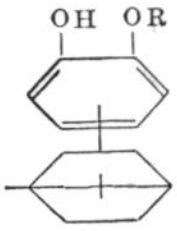

To obtain a composition having about 55% by weight of the polycyclic alcohol, $C_{16}H_{28}O$, it usually takes about 5 repetitions of the hydrogen absorption and venting cycles. Products formed by hydrogenolysis include water, alcohols, such as methanol, and hydrocarbons such as methane. Their removal by venting is essential for the completion of the reaction. The following examples illustrate the process. Unless otherwise stated, the parts are by weight, and the temperature is in degrees centigrade.

Example 1: Preparation of Bornylguaiacol — Camphene (815 grams) is added from a heated dropping funnel over 1 hour or more at 100° to 150°C to guaiacol (745 grams) and Filtrol (48 grams), an acid clay alkylation catalyst. The mixture is stirred for 1 hour after the camphene has been added and is washed to a pH of 7. On distillation, bornylguaiacol (1,000 grams) is obtained, boiling point 167° to 173°C/2 to 3 mm.

Example 2: Preparation of 11-Hydroxy-2,13,13-Trimethyltricyclo[6.4.0.1^{2,5}] Tridecane — Bornylguaiacol (1,000 grams) and Raney nickel catalyst (25 grams) are charged to a high pressure, steel hydrogenator and hydrogenation is conducted at 600 psi and 175°C. Absorption is rapid until about 1.5 mols hydrogen per mol bornylguaiacol is consumed. Thereafter, absorption is slow and it is not possible to complete the hydrogenation even by raising the pressure to 2,000 psi. The pressure is then reduced to atmospheric by venting and vacuum (200 mm Hg) is applied to distill off volatile by-products which stop the hydrogenation. Hydrogen pressure is built up to 600 psi and very rapid absorption occurs for about 30 minutes. This procedure is repeated about 10 times until the refractive index of the product is 1.508 to 1.505 and the methoxyl content is less than 2%.

Water, methanol and methane are formed by hydrogenolysis. Their removal by venting is essential for completion of the reaction. One mol of water and one-tenth mol of methanol per mol of bornylguaiacol hydrogenated can be collected by cooling the vented gas. A total of about 4.5 mols hydrogen is consumed per mol of bornylguaiacol. Of this, 3.0 mols is required to saturate the benzene ring and the remainder for hydrogenolysis of the methoxyl and hydroxyl groups. The crude hydrogenated product weighs 925 grams. Distillation at 2 mm yielded the following fractions.

No.	B.P.	n_D^{20}	Grams
1.	111–113	1.493–1.494	55
2.	140–160	1.506–1.508	810
3.	>160	1.52	45
4.	Residue		15

No. 1 is a practically odorless hydrocarbon, $C_{16}H_{28}$ formed by complete hydrogenolysis. Found (percent): C, 87.12; H, 12.80. Calculated (percent): C, 87.20; H, 12.80. No. 2 is a polycyclic alcohol, $C_{16}H_{28}O$. Found (percent): C, 81.13; H, 11.54; CH_3O, 0.0; hydroxyl value by acetylation, 240. Calculated (percent): C, 81.32; H, 11.92; CH_3O, 0.0; hydroxyl value, 237. It is a viscous, colorless oil with a strong sandalwood odor. No. 3 is a mixture containing No. 2 and unreacted bornylguaiacol.

Example 3: Preparation of Composition Containing About 55% of Polycyclic Alcohol of Example 2 and About 45% of Bornylhexahydroguaiacol — Bornylguaiacol is hydrogenated as in Example 2 except that the venting procedure is repeated only until the methoxyl content has been reduced to about 5.0%. About 5 ventings are required. The refractive index of the product is about 1.510. Distillation yields about 820 grams of product, boiling point 140° to 160°C, 2 mm, containing about 5.3% methoxyl. It has been found that compositions which contain 50% by weight of this polycyclic alcohol exhibit little effectiveness as perfume materials. Compositions which contain 60% or more of the polycyclic alcohol, which are produced by this process, possess unexpected high perfume value.

CEDARWOOD

2-Isopropoxycamphane and 2-(β-Hydroxyethoxy)Camphane

B.J. Kane; U.S. Patent 3,354,225; November 21, 1967; assigned to The Glidden Company describes a class of camphane derivatives having advantageous odor characteristics. Cedar oil (sometimes termed cedarwood oil or cedar leaf oil, depending upon the source from which it is obtained) is well known in commerce as a valuable essential oil which is used to impart a cedar-like odor to a variety of compositions such as, for example, furniture polishes, paint, soaps, insect repellents, disinfectants, shoe dressings, floor waxes, auto waxes, aerosol compositions employed to mask airborne odors, and the like.

Cedar oil is composed primarily of a liquid portion consisting of cedrene, a compound having the empirical formula $C_{15}H_{24}$ and a solid crystalline portion consisting of cedrol, a compound having the empirical formula $C_{15}H_{26}O$. Cedar oil is obtained commercially from the leaves or wood of cyprus and cedar trees (*Juniperus virginiana*) or from wood of the West Indies and South America tree (*Cedrela odorata*) by expensive time consuming extraction and distillation procedures such as those procedures conventionally employed in the production and manufacture of essential oils which are obtained from natural sources.

This process provides a class of compounds distinctly different from cedrene, cedrol or mixtures. The compounds can be economically synthesized and these compounds have odor and other properties which will enable them to replace the difficultly obtainable cedar oil in areas of commerce and in compositions where cedar oils are presently employed. The compounds are camphane derivatives and are analogs, homologs, or isomers of known compounds. The compounds are of the formula shown on the following page:

```
            CH₃
             |
             C
         ___/|\___
       /    |     \
  H₂C       |      C—O—R
       |    |     /| H
   CH₃—C—CH₃    /
       |    |  CH₂
  H₂C       |  /
       \___ | /
            C
            |
            H
```

where R is selected from the group consisting of:

```
         H
         |
     H—C—H                H   H
         |                |   |
        —C—H    and     —C—C—OH
         |                |   |
     H—C—H              . H   H
         |
         H
```

One of the compounds falling within the scope of the above formula is 2-isopropoxycamphane, a compound characterized in having a boiling point of 138°C at 100 mm pressure and 84°C at 10 mm pressure, a specific gravity of 0.882 and an index of refraction (n_{15}) of 1.4538.

Another compound falling within the scope of the above formula is 2-(β-hydroxyethoxy)-camphane. This compound is characterized in having a boiling point of 121°C at 10 mm of pressure and a boiling point of 86°C at 1 mm of pressure, a specific gravity (25/25) of 0.990 and an index of refraction (n_{15}) of 1.4800.

The above compounds, which distinctly differ in structure, chemical and physical properties from the compounds associated with cedar oil, surprisingly have the odor and insect repellency commonly associated with that material.

The compounds may be prepared by reacting camphene with an appropriate alcohol, (e.g., isopropyl alcohol or ethylene glycol), in the presence of a suitable catalyst. Suitable catalysts include mineral acids such as, for example, phosphoric and sulfuric acids and water-insoluble, strong cation exchange resins. These cation exchange resins are porous electrolytes having an enormous nondiffusible anion and a single diffusible cation. Such cation exchange resins include, for example, those cation exchange resins described in U.S. Patents 2,340,111, 2,366,007 and 2,366,008. It is preferred that the cation be a sulfonic acid group which includes nuclear sulfonic acid groups as well as alkylene sulfonic acid groups. The following examples illustrate the process; all parts and percentages are by weight unless otherwise specified.

Example 1: Preparation of 2-Isopropoxy-Camphane — To a reaction zone there was added 100 grams of camphene, 130 grams of isopropanol and 20 grams of Amberlyst 15, an acidic nuclear sulfonic cation exchange resin based on a styrene-divinyl benzene copolymer and in the hydrogen form and having a highly porous (macro reticulated) structure. The contents of the reaction zone were stirred with a mechanical stirrer and heated to and maintained at a temperature of 84° ± 2°C.

The stirring was continued at the above temperature for 24 hours after which the liquid reaction product was decanted from the ion exchange resin and fractionally distilled at reduced pressure to yield the following distillate fractions: Forty-nine and two-tenths grams of substantially pure 2-isopropoxy-camphane were obtained along with 50 grams of isopropanol, 25.6 grams camphene and 30.4 grams of a mixture of camphene and 2-isopropoxy-camphane. The boiling point of the pure 2-isopropoxy-camphane was determined at 100 mm pressure and found to be 138°C and the specific gravity was determined at 0.882. The index of the refraction of the compounds was also determined at 1.4538 (n_{15}). The pure material had a pronounced cedar-like odor in contrast to the n-propoxycamphane which had a camphor/banana-like odor.

Example 2: Preparation of 2-(β-Hydroxyethoxy)Camphane — To a reaction vessel there was added 100 grams of camphene, 91 grams of ethylene glycol, 88 grams of acetone and 30 grams of Amberlyst 15, the acidic anion exchange resin employed in Example 1. The contents of the reaction vessel were stirred with a mechanical stirrer and heated to and maintained at 74° ± 2°C.

The stirring was continued at the above temperature for 60 hours after which the liquid reaction product was separated from the ion exchange resin by filtration and was fractionally distilled between temperatures of 45° to 120°C and between pressures of 100 to 0.2 millimeter to yield the following distillate fractions: 69 grams of substantially pure 2-(β-hydroxyethoxy)camphane, 55 grams of acetone, 23 grams of ethylene glycol, 17 grams of camphene and 17 grams of a mixture consisting substantially of camphene and 2-(β-hydroxyethoxy)camphane. The boiling point of the pure 2-(β-hydroxyethoxy)camphane was determined at 10 mm pressure and found to be 121°C. The specific gravity of the product was determined to be 0.990 at 25°C and the index of refraction was determined and found to be 1.480 at 15°C.

The pure material had a pronounced cedar-like odor in contrast to the 2-ethoxy-camphane which had a camphoraceous odor. Although the compounds of this process may be prepared by reacting camphene and alcohol in the presence of mineral acids, the procedures set forth in the foregoing examples are preferred methods of preparation.

Example 3: The following five liquid compositions were prepared by dispersing 2-isopropoxy-camphane in the quantities indicated in the below listed liquid diluents.

	Composition Number				
Ingredients	1	2	3	4	5
	Percent				
2-isopropoxy-camphane	20	25	30	20	10
2-(β-hydroxyethoxy)-camphane					10
Ligroin	80				40
Ethyl Alcohol		75			
Mineral Oil			70		40
Isopropyl Alcohol				80	

The foregoing compositions were useful in imparting a cedar odor to products such as furniture polishes, paint, soaps, insect repellents, dog repellents, disinfectants, shoe dressings, floor and auto waxes and as sprays to mask cooking odors.

Cedrol Ethers

J.H. Blumenthal; U.S. Patent 3,373,208; March 12, 1968; assigned to International Flavors & Fragrances Inc. describes cedrol ethers which are various lower aliphatic ethers of cedrol such as the methyl, ethyl, propyl, allyl, butyl and methallyl ethers of cedrol. These materials may be illustrated by the structural formula:

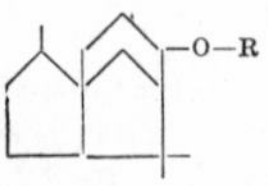

where R is methyl, ethyl, propyl, butyl, allyl or methallyl. The production of cedrol ethers involves reacting an alkali metal derivative of cedrol with an alkyl or alkenyl halide or with a neutral sulfuric acid ester such as dimethyl or diethyl sulfate, or with an alkyl ester of an aryl sulfonic acid.

Example 1: To a refluxing mixture of 575 grams of xylene and 164 grams of sodium hydride (54% suspension in mineral oil) was added a solution of 575 grams of cedrol (recrystallized) in 2,875 milliliters of dry xylene. The mixture was refluxed until gas evolution ceased. To the refluxing mixture was added 253 grams of dimethyl sulfate over a period of 30 minutes. The mixture was refluxed for another 7 hours.

After cooling, the reaction mass was poured into a solution of 285 grams of water and 100 grams of 50% aqueous sodium hydroxide. The oil layer was separated and washed neutral with water. The solvent was stripped off to yield 640 grams of crude cedryl methyl ether. GLC indicated one peak with the absence of the starting alcohol. Fractionation yielded 577 grams of cedryl methyl ether, representing a yield of 94%. Analysis for $-OCH_3$ found: 13.02%; theory: 13.12. This material is useful as a perfume and has an amber-woody odor.

Example 2: To a mixture of 200 grams of dry xylene and 57 grams of sodium hydride (54% suspension) at reflux was added a solution of 222 grams of recrystallized cedrol in 1,000 grams of dry xylene. The reaction mixture was refluxed for 2 hours and 169 grams of allyl bromide was dropped in at reflux over 30 minutes. The reaction mixture was refluxed for another 3 hours, cooled and poured into water. The oil layer was separated and washed with water and the solvent distilled off under vacuum.

The residue was rushed-over. The distillate weighed 200 grams and GLC indicated one major (80%) and one minor peak (20%). The minor peak had the same retention time as cedrol (85% yield based on cedrol which reacted). Fractionation yielded cedryl allyl ether. This material is useful as a perfume and has a woody-amber odor with a fruity nuance.

Example 3: The following is an example of a perfume formula embodying cedryl methyl ether and producing a perfume having a woody-amber fragrance.

	Parts
Bergamot oil CP	100
Orange oil fla. CP	100
Bitter orange oil WI	50
Lemon oil cal. CP	20
Mandarin oil	20
Lime oil exp. WI	10
Ocimene	10
2-Tert-butylcyclohexyl acetate	10
Cedryl methyl ether	50

Octahydro-1,3a,6-Trimethyl-1H-1,6a-Ethanopentaleno[1,2-c] Furan

J.H. Blumenthal, G. Stork and E.T. Theimer; U.S. Patent 3,281,432; October 25, 1966; assigned to International Flavors & Fragrances Inc. describe a tetracyclic oxide which has a woody, amber odor useful in perfumery. This compound is octahydro-1,3a,6-trimethyl-1H-1,6a-ethanopentaleno[1,2-c]furan, and has the formula:

In carrying out the process, one prepares a cedryl hypohalite by reacting cedrol with a hypohalous acid. The hypohalites thus prepared are next converted to halohydrins, preferably by exposing them to the action of actinic light. The halohydrins may then be treated with a base such as sodium hydroxide to produce the desired product.

Example 1: Preparation of Octahydro-1,3a,6-Trimethyl-1H-1,6a-Ethanopentaleno[1,2-c]-Furan — In a 12-liter, 3-necked flask equipped with stirrer, thermometer and addition funnel and wrapped in metal foil to exclude light there are placed 9,000 grams of aqueous sodium hypochlorite solution (4.6% available chlorine). A solution of 1,040 grams (4.7 mols) of recrystallized cedrol, 24,000 cc of carbon tetrachloride and 700 grams of glacial acetic acid is added at 0°C over a period of 15 minutes. The reaction mixture is stirred at 0°C for 2 hours. The carbon tetrachloride solution is separated, washed twice with cold sodium bicarbonate solution and dried over magnesium sulfate. The hypochlorite solution should be kept cold and protected from light as it is very labile and may decompose violently if allowed to stand in sunlight.

The carbon tetrachloride solution of cedryl hypochlorite prepared as described above is placed in a 5-liter, 3-necked flask previously purged with nitrogen. A slow stream of nitrogen is continually passed through the flask during the reaction. With good stirring, the solution is cooled to about 5°C, using a Dry Ice bath, and the light source, a 150 watt incandescent bulb placed about 1 inch from the flask, turned on. The temperature of the reaction mixture is maintained between 10° and 19°C by external cooling.

After 45 minutes, the test for active chlorine is negative. The carbon tetrachloride is removed by distillation and the residue refluxed with methanolic sodium hydroxide for 3 hours. Water is added and the methanol distilled off. The residual oil layer is separated and washed neutral with salt solution. The crude oil weighs 974 grams and contains 40% of the desired product. The pure oxide as entitled above is obtained by fractionation, boiling point 122°C at 4.5 mm. The main feature of the IR spectrum is a strong absorption at 9.55 microns, typical of the tetrahydrofuran structure. Salient features of the nmr spectrum of this compound are tabulated below. The spectrum is measured on the Varian-A spectrometer. Chemical shift values are reported in ppm; tetramethyl silane (internal standard) taken as O.

Proton	Chemical Shift
$\overset{-O}{H-\underset{\|}{C}-H}$	3.40 p.p.m.
$CH_3-\underset{\|}{C}-O-$	1.09 (s)
$CH_3-\underset{\|}{C}-$	0.98 (s)
$CH_3-\underset{\|}{\overset{\|}{C}}-\\ \quad H$	0.82 (d)

Example 2: Preparation of Octahydro-1,3a,6-Trimethyl-1H-1,6a-Ethanopentaleno[1,2-c]-Furan — A solution containing cedryl hypochlorite in carbon tetrachloride is prepared as in Example 1. The solution is flash distilled by dropwise addition to a still pot maintained at 110°C. During distillation, the hypochlorite is converted to the crude chlorohydrin. This mixture is heated at 110°C for 2½ hours to produce the desired product above entitled. The product is isolated by fractional distillation as described in Example 1.

Aliphatic Cyclododecanol Ethers

T. Leidig; U.S. Patent 3,281,474; October 25, 1966; assigned to Haarmann & Reimer GmbH, Germany has found that cyclododecanol ethers which contain up to 4 carbon atoms in the ether radical are suitable as odoriferous compounds. The aliphatic ether radical may be either saturated or unsaturated. The following are examples of ether radicals: methyl, ethyl, n-propyl, n-butyl, allyl, methylallyl and crotyl radicals. Examples of suitable compounds according to the process and their properties are set forth in the table on the following page.

Ether group	B.P.	D_4^{20}	n_D^{20}	Odour
Methyl ether	95–98° C./2 mm	0.911	1.4742	Cedar and ambret.
Ethyl ether	117–119° C./3 mm	0.905	1.4740	Cedarwood.
n-Propyl ether	124–127° C./3 mm	0.896	1.4694	Cedarwood, tobacco.
Isopropyl ether	114–118° C./3 mm	0.907	1.4759	Cedar with musk.
n-Butyl ether	127–129° C./3 mm	0.892	1.4696	Cedarwood.
Isobutyl ether	133–138° C./4 mm	0.903	1.4728	Cedar-like, precious wood with note of ambret.
Allyl ether	129–131° C./3 mm	0.912	1.4839	Tobacco, cigar chest.
Crotyl ether	134–140° C./3 mm	0.910	1.4838	Cedar with musk note.
Methallyl ether	130–135° C./3 mm	0.912	1.4814	Vetiver, cellar odour.

The odiferous compounds have a typical smell of cedar with a characteristic note of musk. The compounds may be obtained, for example, by reacting the alkali compounds of cyclododecanol with alkyl or alkenyl halides or neutral sulfuric acid esters.

Example: Precious Wood Complex —

250 parts by weight of cyclododecanol methyl ether
200 parts by weight of cyclododecanol ethyl ether
 50 parts by weight of cyclododecanol methallyl ether
 20 parts by weight of γ-iraldein
 80 parts by weight of delta iraldein
 50 parts by weight of oryclone
 50 parts by weight of vetiveryl acetate
170 parts by weight of liquid cedryl acetate
 30 parts by weight of guaiyl acetate
100 parts by weight of cedar ketone

VETIVER

Isolongifolene Ketone

J.B. Hall; U.S. Patent 3,718,698; February 27, 1973; assigned to International Flavors & Fragrances Inc. describes a process for producing isolongifolene ketone and its epimer which comprises treating isolongifolene with a peroxygen compound under acidic conditions to obtain a substantially fully saturated ketone, as well as the saturated epimer. The ultimate starting material in the process is longifolene, a cyclic terpene having the structural formula:

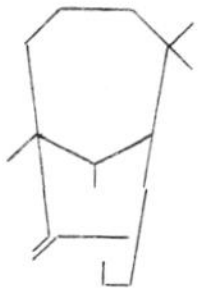

Longifolene is widely distributed in nature, notably among species of the genus Pinus. One of these sources of longifolene is so-called Indian turpentine oil obtained from *Pinus longifolia* Roxb. It occurs in such Indian turpentine oil in amounts of about 30% and is preferably purified before use herein to higher purities of 80% or more. The specific starting material for use in the process is isolongifolene having the formula shown on the following page.

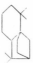

The isomer of longifolene is readily obtained according to methods known in the art.
For example, it can be obtained by treating longifolene with boron trifluoride. Since
the purity of the ultimate product can more readily be obtained with relatively pure
isolongifolene, it is desirable that the isolongifolene used have a purity of 80% or more.

The process is carried out by treating isolongifolene with a peroxygen source such as
hydrogen peroxide in the presence of an acidic material which is desirably an organic
anhydride or acid. The peroxygen source preferably has a substantial content of active
oxygen, and hydrogen peroxide of at least 30% H_2O_2 content is desirable. Lower per-
alkanoic acids are preferred peracids in the practice of this process. Such peracids desirably have strengths of 30% or more. An especially preferred peroxygen source for use
in this process is 50% or stronger hydrogen peroxide.

Example 1: Preparation of Isolongifolene — A clean, dry 50-gallon stainless steel reactor
is charged with 250 pounds of longifolene, agitated, and swept with nitrogen. The nitrogen
pressure is maintained at 5 psig, and 2.8 pounds of boron trifluoride etherate is charged
to the reactor during 1 hour. During this time, the reactor temperature is maintained at
25° to 30°C by a water jacket. After all of the etherate is added, the reaction is maintained at 30°C for 1 hour.

The reaction mixture is then neutralized with 200 pounds of 5% aqueous sodium hydroxide
solution and washed at room temperature (20° to 30°C) for one-half hour. The aqueous
and organic layers so formed are separated, and the lower aqueous layer is discarded.
The organic layer is then washed with 40 pounds of 10% aqueous sodium chloride at
room temperature for one-half hour. The lower aqueous layer is separated to provide a
washed organic phase containing isolongifolene.

Preparation of Saturated Isolongifolene Ketone — A 12-liter reaction flask fitted with a
stirrer, thermometer and condenser is charged with 3,264 grams (16 mols) of isolongifolene
and 3,600 grams (70 mols) of formic acid (90%). The mixture is agitated while 1,088
grams (16 mols) of 50% hydrogen peroxide is added at 44° to 49°C during 1 hour. The
mixture is then stirred for another 3 hours at 44° to 49°C.

The reaction mass is then washed with 2.5 liters of 10% aqueous sodium chloride and then
with 1 liter of 5% aqueous sodium hydroxide. The organic layer is separated from the
aqueous layer to obtain saturated isolongifolene ketone substantially free of unsaturated
ketone. This ketone can be separated, if desired, from a smaller amount of lactone and
the unreacted starting material by distillation at 3 mm Hg and about 112°C to obtain a
colorless liquid having a rich, woody odor.

The purified saturated isolongifolene ketone is subjected to infrared (IR) spectroscopy
and shows a carbonyl absorption at 1,695 cm^{-1}, gem-dimethyl absorption at 1,368 and
1,387 cm^{-1}, and an absorption attributable to a methylene group adjacent to a carbonyl
group at 1,410 cm^{-1}. Nuclear magnetic resonance (nmr) data show a singlet attributable
to 3 methyl protons at 0.89 ppm, a singlet attributable to 3 methyl protons at 0.93 ppm,
a singlet attributable to 3 methyl protons at 0.98 ppm, a singlet at 1.16 ppm attributable
to 3 methyl protons, broad band attributable to methylene and methine protons at 1.23
to 2.04 ppm, and protons in a position alpha to a carbonyl group at 2.10 to 2.30 ppm.
The foregoing parts refer to the frequency shift measured in a carbon tetrachloride solution
on a Varian Model HA-100 spectrometer.

Preparation of Stable Saturated Isolongifolene Ketone-Epimer — The crude saturated iso-longifolene ketone obtained above is charged to the 12-liter reaction flask, together with 4 liters of methanol and 168 grams of 50% aqueous sodium hydroxide. The reaction mixture is stirred at reflux for 2½ hours.

After addition of 1,800 milliliters of water, the methanol is recovered under atmospheric pressure at 85°C. The water layer is extracted once with a liter of toluene, and the toluene extract is combined with the organic layer, which combination is then washed with 1 liter of 10% aqueous sodium chloride until it is neutral. The toluene is stripped, and 100 grams of Primol refined mineral oil is added. The mixture is then flash distilled at 2 mm Hg with a pot temperature of 135° to 208°C and a head temperature of 115° to 154°C. This yields 3,916 grams of distillate. The distillate is fractionated at 3 mm Hg and a 9:1 reflux ratio after 50 grams of Primol and 8 grams of Ionox antioxidant are added. The material boils at 121°C under 2.8 mm Hg.

The isomer product so obtained is a colorless liquid having a full bodied, rich, precious wood fragrance note. It can be employed with tobacco fragrances, pine aromas, and sweet grass type aromas. IR spectroscopy of material shows a carbonyl absorption at 1,715 cm^{-1}, gem dimethyl absorptions at 1,370 and 1,392 cm^{-1}, and a methyl group adjacent to a carbonyl group at 1,420 cm^{-1}.

NMR shows a singlet attributable to 3 methyl protons at 0.97 ppm, a singlet attributable to 3 methyl protons at 1.05 ppm, a singlet attributable to 6 methyl protons at 1.20 ppm, a multiplet at 1.25 to 2.00 attributable to methylene and methine protons, and a multiplet attributable to 3 protons alpha to a carbonyl group at 2.00 to 2.25 ppm. The nmr figures are obtained under the same conditions as set forth above.

Example 2: The epimer produced in Example 1 is used to prepare a chypre perfume according to the following formula.

Ingredient	Amount (parts)
Santalol	60
Coumarin	90
Musk ketone	30
Musk ambrette	20
Ambreine absolute	25
Tarragon oil	25
Angelica root oil	5
Clary sage	30
Epimer from Example 1	60
Linalool oil	30
Patchouli oil	20
Isoeugenol	35
Methylionone	50
Oakmoss absolute	60
Bergamot oil	225
Jasmine absolute	20
Rose absolute	15
Methyl salicylate	2
Lavender oil	3
Vanillin	15
Heliotropin	35
Ylang oil, Manila	70
Cinnamyl acetate	25
Benzoin resinoid	50

The presence of the epimer in the foregoing perfume composition provides a full bodied, rich, precious wood note and maintains a good formula balance, even in the absence of the vetivert oil customarily used in such formulations.

Isolongifolene Acetate

A.J. Curtis, B.G. Jaggers and J.F. Janes; U.S. Patent 3,647,847; March 7, 1972; assigned to Bush Boake Allen Limited, England describe isolongifolene esters of the formula:

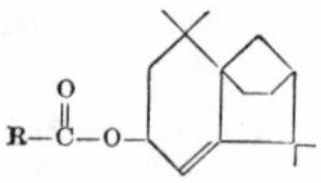

where R is a C_1 to C_5 alkyl group prepared by allylic substitution, e.g., oxidation, of iso-longifolene followed by replacement of the substituent by an RCO_2- group. The esters have valuable perfumery properties particularly as replacements for vetiverol derivatives.

Example 1: Isolongifolene (102 grams), acetic acid (100 milliliters) and cuprous chloride (0.2 gram) were introduced into a 500 milliliter flask fitted with a stirrer. The flask was heated to 80°C and 49 grams tert-butyl perbenzoate were added over 2 hours. The mixture was heated at 80°C or a further 8 hours and then diluted with petroleum ether and washed consecutively with water, sodium carbonate solution (10%) and water. The extract was allowed to stand over anhydrous sodium sulfate overnight and the petroleum ether was removed by evaporation over a steam bath.

Distillation of the oil yielded a mixture of isolongifolenyl acetates, refractive index at 25°C was 1.5000, density at 25°C was 1.0108 g/cc, boiling point at 2 mm mercury pressure was about 131°C. Saponification of 5 grams of the acetate mixture produced as above, using a solution of sodium hydroxide in aqueous ethanol, yielded 3 grams of a mixture of alcohols having a refractive index of 1.5099 at 25°C.

Example 2: Isolongifolene (204 grams) and anhydrous sodium carbonate (80 grams) were placed in a 500 milliliter flask fitted with a stirrer and cooling jacket. Chlorine was slowly passed into the mixture at such a rate that the temperature was maintained below 30°C. When the chlorination was finished, the isolongifolenyl chlorides produced were filtered free from the inorganic salts.

The chlorides were then placed in a 2 liter flask fitted with a stirrer and were heated with acetic acid (1.000 milliliter) and sodium acetate (100 grams) for 48 hours at 80°C. The mixture was diluted with water and extracted with petroleum ether. The combined extracts were washed with water, sodium bicarbonate solution (10%) and again with water. The resulting petroleum ether extract was then dried over anhydrous sodium sulfate and the solvent removed by evaporation over a steam bath. Distillation of the oil yielded a mixture of acetates as in Example 1.

Example 3: A woody base suitable for incorporation into a wide variety of perfumery compositions in concentrations ranging from 0.1 to 20% of the compounded composition was prepared from the following ingredients.

	Parts
Cedarwood oil (American)	500
Isolongifolenyl acetate	200
Olibanum resin	50
Methylionone	50
Vetivert oil (Bourbon)	20
Coumarin	20
Bois de Rose oil	10
Patchouli oil (Penang)	10
Sandalwood oil (East Indian)	10

Hydroxymethyl Longifolene and Acyloxymethyl Longifolene

A.J. Curtis, J.F. Janes and B.G. Jaggers; U.S. Patent 3,745,131; July 10, 1973; assigned to Bush Boake Allen Limited, England have found that ω-hydroxymethyl longifolene and the lower ω-acyloxymethyl longifolene derivatives such as ω-acetoxymethyl longifolene are valuable ingredients of compounded perfumery concentrates.

Firstly this is because in such concentrates and perfumed materials these compounds have the most surprising effect that this incorporation in some way makes the basic note of the perfume last longer, that is, the compounds appear to have some fixative effect on the other more volatile perfumery ingredients of the composition and such other ingredients appear to be lost less rapidly from the composition. Secondly, these longifolene derivatives have the effect of blending together the individual odors of the other perfumery ingredients of the composition resulting in the composition as a whole having a more harmonious perfume note and therefore a more immediate impact on the connoisseur without the need to allow the composition to mature.

Example 1: Perfume with Woody Base —

Constituents of Perfumery Composition	Parts by Weight
Cedarwood oil (American)	400
Methylionone	100
Patchouli oil (Seychelles)	400
Vetiver oil (Bourbon)	100

Such a composition gives the odor effect of a mixture of the individual ingredients with the note of the cedarwood oil predominating. After application to a substrate, the notes of different constituents predominate at different times. The addition of 50 parts of ω-hydroxymethyl longifolene had the effect of blending together the mixture and at the same time accentuated the warm woody note of the Patchouli oil. This character was maintained throughout an extended dry out period.

On the other hand, when 50 parts of ω-acetoxymethyl longifolene was used instead, it blended the mixture similarly but resulted in the typical root-like character of the Vetiver oil as well as the note of the Patchouli oil being accentuated. Again the total odor characteristics were maintained through an extended dry out period.

Example 2: Perfume of Sophisticated Aldehyde Base —

Constituents of Perfumery Composition	Parts by Weight
Undecylenic aldehyde	20
γ-Nonalactone	10
Methyl nonyl acetaldehyde	10
Hydroxycitronellal	50
Methylionone	100
Patchouli oil (Seychelles)	50
Sandalwood oil (East Indian)	160
Vetiveryl acetate	500

It was found that the addition of 50 parts of either ω-hydroxymethyl longifolene or w-acetoxymethyl longifolene caused a blending together of the various aldehydic notes which was otherwise achieved only after several months of maturation of the composition. This effect was maintained throughout an extended dry out period as also was the overall character of the perfume.

Cyclododecadienecarboxylic Acid Esters

W.F. Erman; U.S. Patent 3,318,945; May 9, 1967; assigned to The Procter & Gamble

Company describes aliphatic esters of 4,8-cyclododecadiene-1-carboxylic acids where the aliphatic substituent contains from 1 to about 4 carbon atoms, e.g., a radical selected from the group consisting of methyl, ethyl, propyl, isopropyl, n-butyl and t-butyl.

It has been found that the cyclododecadienecarboxylic acid esters possess powerful lasting woody odors reminiscent of vetiver oil. Vetiver oil and its derivatives are well known perfume compositions. It has also been found that these compounds are non-toxic, are not sensitizers and, in fact, are quite mild. Some compounds prepared by this process are methyl 4-cis-8-trans-cyclododecadiene-1-carboxylate, methyl 4-trans-8-cis-cyclo-dodecadiene-1-carboxylate, ethyl 4-trans-8-cis-cyclododecadiene-1-carboxylate, ethyl 4,8-trans,trans-cyclododecadiene-1-carboxylate, propyl 4,8-trans,trans-cyclododecadiene-1-carboxylate, isopropyl 4-cis-8-trans-cyclododecadiene-1-carboxylate, isopropyl 4,8-trans,trans-cyclododecadiene-1-carboxylate, n-butyl 4-trans-8-cis-cyclododecadiene-1-carboxylate and t-butyl 4-cis-8-trans-cyclododecadiene-1-carboxylate.

The starting material for the preparation of the compounds is 1,5,9-cyclododecatriene. This compound is known in the prior art, being prepared by the trimerization of butadiene with alkyl metal type catalysts. A suitable method for its preparation is found in *Ange-wante Chemie,* volume 69, No. 11:397 (June 7, 1957). Of the four theoretically possible stereo isomers of 1,5,9-cyclododecatriene, only two have thus far been isolated. These are the cis,trans,trans and the trans,trans,trans isomers as shown below.

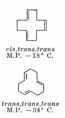

cis,trans,trans
M.P. —18° C.

trans,trans,trans
M.P. —34° C.

Both of these two isomeric forms are suitable starting materials for purposes of this process. In general terms, the synthesis route to the ester compounds proceeds as follows. The 1,5,9-cyclododecatriene is reacted with hydrogen bromide, in the presence of a free radical catalyst, producing monobrominated cyclododecadienes. The three possible bromo compounds, i.e., 1-bromo-4-cis-8-trans-cyclododecadiene, 1-bromo-4-trans-8-cis-cyclododeca-diene, and 1-bromo-4,8-trans,trans-cyclododecadiene, are then converted to the carboxylic acid esters.

The methyl ester derivatives, for instance, methyl 4-cis-8-trans-cyclododecadiene-1-car-boxylate, methyl 4-trans-8-cis-cyclododecadiene-1-carboxylate, and methyl 4,8-trans,trans-cyclododecadiene-1-carboxylate are prepared by treatment of the bromo compounds with magnesium to form a Grignard reagent, subsequent carboxylation with carbon dioxide followed by diazomethane alkylation. The other lower aliphatic esters, i.e., ethyl, propyl, isopropyl, n-butyl and t-butyl, are prepared from the corresponding diene carboxylic acids by treatment of the acid chloride with the appropriate alcohol. These procedures are illustrated in detail in the following examples, where all temperatures are in degrees centigrade.

Example: Ozone (0.2976 grams, 6.2×10^{-3} mols, 1.0 mol percent) was added over a period of 13 minutes and 36 seconds at a rate of 4.5×10^{-4} mols per minute into a solution of 100.0 grams (0.616 mol) of 1,5,9-cis,trans,trans-cyclododecatriene in 100 milliliters of anhydrous methylene chloride cooled to –63°C. After removal of residual oxygen by flushing with helium for 10 minutes, dry hydrogen bromide was bubbled into the olefin at a rate of 2.0 cubic feet per hour for a period of 10 minutes. A temperature rise of 38°C (–63° to –25°C) was noted during this addition.

The bulk of the excess HBr was removed from the system by flushing with helium for 5 minutes, the reaction mixture diluted with 400 milliliters of ether, and poured into 200 milliliters of cold 5% aqueous sodium bicarbonate. The organic layer was partitioned, washed with cold water, dried over magnesium sulfate and the solvent removed under reduced pressure to afford 134.0 grams of light yellow liquid. A 67 gram portion of this liquid was distilled from an 18 inch spinning band column to afford 62.35 grams (83%) of a monobromocyclododecadiene reaction product, boiling point 111°C/1.2 mm. Analysis calculated for $C_{12}H_{19}Br$: C, 59.3; H, 7.9; Br, 32.9. Found: C, 59.2; H, 7.7; Br, 33.1.

To a mixture of 16.96 grams (0.698 mol) of magnesium and 25 milliliters of tetrahydro-furan, freshly distilled over lithium aluminum hydride, was added 20.0 grams of the mono-bromocyclododecadiene reaction product prepared. After a short induction period, the reaction mixture warmed to 60°C. An additional 135.0 grams of monobromo compound (total = 155.0 grams, 0.638 mol) dissolved in 450 milliliters of dry tetrahydrofuran was added dropwise over a 2 hour period as the temperature fluctuated between 30° and 60°C. After the addition was complete, the reaction mixture was heated at reflux for 30 minutes, then cooled to 0°C.

The dropping funnel was replaced with a gas inlet tube that extended below the surface of the reaction mixture and anhydrous carbon dioxide was bubbled in, with vigorous stirring, for 4 hours while the temperature was maintained at 0°C. The product was hydrolyzed by the dropwise addition of 500 milliliters of 5% sulfuric acid to the reaction mixture maintained at 0°C. The product was extracted with three 200 milliliter portions of ether and the ethereal layer washed well with water. The acidic product was extracted with three 200 milliliter portions of 10% sodium hydroxide, the basic extracts washed with ether and acidified with concentrated hydrochloric acid to pH 1.

The product was dissolved in ether, the ethereal solution washed with water, dried over magnesium sulfate and the ether removed under reduced pressure to yield 53.0 grams (40%) of the mixture of carboxylic acids. The carboxylic acid mixture was dissolved in 200 milliliters of ether and cooled to 0°C. To this mixture was added a solution of 14.0 grams (0.33 mol) of diazomethane in 500 milliliters of ether. The mixture was stored for 2 hours at 0° to 5°C, and the excess diazomethane decomposed by thorough washing with 10% hydrochloric acid. The ethereal solution was washed with water, dried over magnesium sulfate and evaporated under reduced pressure to afford 59.0 grams (40%) of the mixture of methyl cyclododecadienecarboxylates.

Analysis by gas chromatography through a 10' by ¼" stainless steel column packed with 30% succinic acid-triethylene glycol polymer on 60/80 mesh acid washed chromasorb at 197°C and helium flow rate of 42 milliliters per minute indicated the presence of two isomeric methyl 4,8-cis,trans-cyclododecadiene-1-carboxylates and the 4,8-trans,trans-cyclododecadiene-1-carboxylate in the ratio 33.4:41.2:26.4. The mixture of methyl 4,8-cis,trans-cyclododecadiene-1-carboxylates was separated from the trans,trans isomer by fractional distillation, boiling point 131°C/4.2 mm. Analysis calculated for $C_{14}H_{22}O_2$: C, 75.6; H, 10.0. Found: C, 75.5; H, 10.0.

As confirmation of structure, 1.5 grams (0.0062 mol) of the above methyl cyclododeca-dienecarboxylate mixture dissolved in 100 milliliters of absolute alcohol was hydrogenated in a Parr hydrogenator at 50 psi initial hydrogen pressure in the presence of 0.500 gram of 10% palladium on charcoal catalyst over a period of 4 hours at 27°C. After filtration of catalyst and removal of solvent, the residual methyl cyclododecanecarboxylate was dissolved in 100 milliliters of 10% alcoholic potassium hydroxide and stored for 16 hours at room temperature.

The alcohol was removed under reduced pressure, the water layer acidified and extracted with ether. The ethereal layer was washed with water, dried over magnesium sulfate, solvent removed under reduced pressure, and the residue recrystallized from petroleum ether to afford 1.40 grams (99%) of cyclododecanecarboxylic acid, as colorless needles, melting point 95° to 97.5°C. The product was recrystallized from petroleum ether for analysis, melting point 97° to 99°C. Analysis calculated for $C_{13}H_{24}O_2$: C, 73.5; H, 11.4. Found: C, 73.2; H, 11.3. The trans,trans isomer was identified by comparison of the gas chromatographic retention time with that of a sample of the trans,trans isomer prepared from 1,5,9-trans,trans,trans-cyclododecatriene.

β,2-Dimethyl-5-Isopropylstyrene

H.J. Toet, J.T.M.F. Maessen and L.M. van der Linde; U.S. Patent 3,461,085; August 12, 1969; assigned to N.V. Chemische Fabriek Naarden, Netherlands describe perfume compositions which have the general formula:

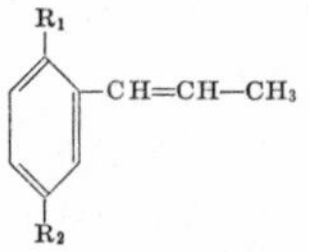

in which R_1 is methyl or ethyl and R_2 is a branched or straight chain alkyl group containing 3 to 5 carbon atoms and which may be propyl, isopropyl, butyl, isobutyl, tert-butyl, pentyl and isopentyl. The preferred group for R_2 is isopropyl. This group of styrene derivatives, especially β,2-dimethyl-5-isopropylstyrene, have high odor value per se and in perfume compositions. The odors are reminiscent of vetivert, galbanum, and angelica oil. Examples of perfume compositions according to the process are as follows.

Example 1:

	Parts by Weight
Hyacinth composition:	
Isoamyl salicylate	340
Phenylethyl alcohol	250
Cinnamic alcohol	150
Citronellol	100
Phenylacetaldehyde dimethylacetal	50
Hydratropic aldehyde	30
β,2-Dimethyl-5-isopropylstyrene	25
Petitgrain oil	25
Citronellyl acetate	25
Galbanum oil	5

Example 2:

	Parts by Weight
Petitgrain composition:	
Menthanyl acetate	250
Linalyl acetate	200
Linalool	200
Geraniol	150
α-Terpineol	65
β-Methyl-2-ethyl-5-isopropylstyrene	50
Geranyl acetate	50
1-Limonene	35

AMBERGRIS-IONONES

4-(9,10-Dehydro-2,2-Dimethyldecahydronaphth-1-yl)-3-Buten-2-one

W.C. Meuly and P.S. Gradeff; U.S. Patent 3,480,677; November 25, 1969; assigned to

Rhodia Inc. have found that substituents higher than the methyl group in the 2-position of the ionone ring give a variety of products with valuable odor properties. Further, it has been found that ionones of outstanding odor properties may be obtained if, in addition to a substituent in the 2-position of the ionone ring, one or two substituents are also introduced into the 3-position. The ionones of this process have the general formula shown below.

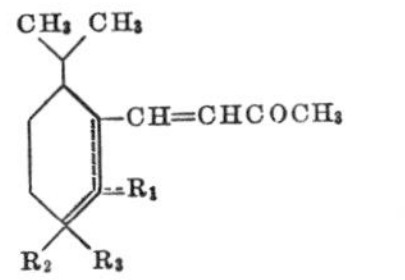

The dotted line in the formula indicates that the double bond is located in the 1-position or in the 2-position of the ring, or that it may be in the exo position, between the carbon atom in the 2-position and the side chain, so that the products may be beta–ionones or alpha–ionones or gamma–ionones.

In the above formula, R_1 is a lower alkyl group containing between 1 and 4 carbon atoms, R_2 is H or a lower alkyl group containing between 1 and 3 carbon atoms, and R_3 is H or CH_3. When R_1 is methyl, R_2 is an alkyl group greater than ethyl and R_3 is hydrogen. When, however, both R_1 and R_2 are methyl, then also R_3 is methyl. The ionones of the process are further characterized by the fact that R_1 and R_2 together may form a trimethylene or tetramethylene bridging group. The ionones described herein are listed in the table below.

Ionone Homologue	R_1	R_2	R_3
4-[(9-10)dehydro-2,2-dimethyl-decalin-1-yl]-3-buten-2-one	$-CH_2CH_2CH_2CH_2-$		H
4-(2-butyl-3,6,6,-trimethyl-cyclohexen-2-yl)-3-buten-2-one	C_4H_9	CH_3	H
4-(2-ethyl-3-propyl-6 6-dimethyl-cyclohexen-2-yl)-3-buten-2-one	C_2H_5	C_3H_7	H
4-(2,6,6-trimethyl-3-isopropyl-cyclohexen-2-yl)-3-buten-2-one	CH_3	$(CH_3)_2CH-$	H
4-(2-isobutyl-6,6-dimethyl-cyclohexen-2-yl)-3-buten-2-one	i-butyl	H	H
4-2,3,3,6,6-pentamethyl cyclohexen-1-yl)-3-buten-2-one	CH_3	CH_3	CH_3
4-(2-isopropyl-6,6-dimethyl-cyclohexen-1-yl)-3-buten-2-one	$(CH_3)_2CH-$	H	H

The compounds exist predominantly in the alpha ionone structure. The gamma isomer structure, present in variable amount, is detected by nuclear magnetic resonance and infrared analysis. When two substituents are present in the 3-position, the alpha structure may not exist, and the beta ionone structure is present.

According to one process for the preparation of the ionones, an unsaturated carbinol is oxidized to the aldehyde, condensed with acetone under alkaline conditions to give a pseudoionone, which is then cyclized to the ionone under the action of a strong acidic reagent, specifically, phosphoric acid or sulfuric acid. The unsaturated carbinols are tertiary carbinols of the type of linalool and exhibit valuable properties as perfuming agents. The aldehydes, oxidation products of the carbinols, also have valuable perfuming properties, in addition to being intermediates for the synthesis of the ionones of this process.

Example: This example illustrates the stepwise preparation of 4-(9,10-dehydro-2,2-dimethyl-decahydronaphth-1-yl)-3-buten-2-one. (a) To 194 grams (1 mol) of 1-vinyl-2-(3-methyl-2-buten-1-yl)-1-cyclohexanol in 250 grams of acetone, there is added, under reflux over a period of 5 hours, 178 grams of $Na_2Cr_2O_7 \cdot 2H_2O$ in 700 grams of 25% sulfuric acid. After refluxing for an additional 35 minutes and cooling, the aqueous layer is discarded, and the organic layer is washed with 5% NaOH, water, dried and evaporated to remove the acetone. The crude product, 182 grams, contains 55.2% of 2-(3-methyl-2-buten-1-yl)cyclohexyliden-acetaldehyde, boiling point 121° to 125°C/0.8 mm.

The substance possesses a rich, earthy and fruity note, which makes it useful for oriental type perfumes. The lasting power is greatly superior to citral, since it still exhibits a powerful odor after 5 days on a blotter, while citral under the same conditions, fades within 24 hours.

(b) To a refluxing solution of 194 grams of 1-vinyl-2-(3-methyl-2-buten-1-yl)cyclohexanol and 250 grams of acetone, there is added, under stirring, a mixture of 178 grams of $Na_2Cr_2O_7 \cdot 2H_2O$ in 706 grams of 25% sulfuric acid, over a period of 5 hours. After refluxing for one additional hour, the lower layer is discarded. To the organic layer, 400 grams of acetone and a solution of 30 grams of 98% NaOH in 350 cc of water are added and the mixture stirred 20 hours at room temperature. The pseudoionone is obtained by neutralization with acetic acid, evaporation of acetone, extraction with cyclohexane and fractionation. The crude product (186 grams) on distillation yields 5-[2-(3-methyl-2-buten-1-yl)-1-cyclohexyliden]-3-penten-2-one (93% pure), boiling point 140° to 145°C/1 mm.

(c) The preparation of 4-(9,10-dehydro-2,2-dimethyldecahydronaphth-1-yl)-3-buten-2-one is as as follows. The general procedure for the cyclization with phosphoric acid consists of slowly adding under stirring the pseudoionone to 5 parts of 85% phosphoric acid at 10°C; the reaction mixture is then poured into ice, the product extracted with benzene and the extract washed, dried and distilled. Application of this procedure, to 61 grams of the pseudoionone obtained in (b) above, gives 25 grams of the ionone, boiling point 129° to 131°C/0.3 mm.

Ultraviolet analysis indicates the absence of carbon to carbon conjugated double bond, that is, the absence of a beta-ionone structure. Nuclear magnetic resonance spectrum indicates that the substance is the alpha-ionone isomer, with minor amount of the gamma isomer.

The substance has a very interesting odor, which is only partly that of other ionones. It has a soft, warm, woody, earthy character, resembling ambergris. Like ambergris, it is extremely tenacious and constitutes an excellent fixative for perfumes. Its odor strength is more that 3 times greater than beta-ionone. While the odor of ionone remains less than 2 days on blotting paper, this product is of almost unchanged intensity after 6 days. Because of its strength and stability, the substance is particularly valuable in soaps.

Dimethylperhydronaphthospirofuran Compounds

S. Chodroff and R.S. Vazirani; U.S. Patent 3,417,107; December 17, 1968; assigned to Norda Essential Oil and Chemical Co., Inc. describe a compound which has a dimethyl perhydronaphthospirofuran structure having a unique woody-ambergris note and valuable fixative properties.

It has been found that a product possessing a uniquely attractive ambergris note as well as a high degree of persistence in the form of an isomeric mixture of dimethylperhydronaphthospirofurans can be obtained in a multiple step procedure. In the first step, mycrene is condensed with itaconic acid or preferably with a derivative thereof such as a lower alkyl (C_1 to C_5) ester, desirably in the presence of hydroquinone or some other conventional antioxidant such as a phenolic compound which minimizes wasteful polymerization of the diolefin. The methylpentenylcyclohexene moiety of the resulting product is cyclized in the presence of a strongly acidic cyclizing catalyst such as boron trifluoride etherate, concentrated phosphoric acid, sulfuric acid, etc. thereby forming a dimethyl octahydronaphthalene structure which has the itaconic residue (in the form of a carboalkoxy radical, —COOR, and of a methanocarboalkoxy radical, —CH_2COOR), attached to one carbon atom of the cyclohexene ring.

This itaconic residue is reduced to the corresponding methanohydroxy and ethanohydroxy radicals, —CH_2OH and —CH_2CH_2OH, preferably in the presence of a selective reducing agent such as a dialkyl aluminum hydride, lithium aluminum hydride or, less desirably, by high pressure hydrogenation in the presence of a catalyst such as copper chromite. The resulting methanohydroxy and ethanohydroxy radicals are dehydrated in the presence of an acid dehydration catalyst such as sulfuric acid, phosphoric acid or, preferably, toluene sulfonic acid to form a spirotetrahydrofuran ring therefrom. The octahydronaphthalene ring is then fully saturated by selective catalytic hydrogenation, e.g., in the presence of a palladium catalyst.

Alkyl-Substituted Ionones

J.J. Beereboom; U.S. Patent 3,679,754; July 25, 1972; assigned to Pfizer Inc. has found it possible to convert α-ionone, β-ionone and mixtures of these to various alkyl-substituted δ-ionone derivatives in high yield by the use of a process which entails alkylating the ionone starting materials in the presence of a basic condensing agent so as to form the corresponding δ-ionone derivative.

Example 1: To a stirred solution of 44.8 grams (0.4 mol) of potassium t-butoxide in 200 milliliters of dry dimethyl sulfoxide, there were added 67.3 grams (0.35 mol) of β-ionone in a dropwise manner during the course of 30 minutes at 25°C. After stirring for an additional 30 minutes, 30.3 grams (0.60 mol) of methyl chloride gas was bubbled into the mixture during the course of 45 minutes. The resulting reaction mixture was then stirred at 25°C for 16 hours and thereafter poured into 1 liter of cold water. After acidification with glacial acetic acid, the resulting aqueous solution was extracted with several 100 milliliter portions of diethyl ether and the product subsequently isolated therefrom by means of evaporation under reduced pressure. Vacuum distillation of the residual liquid then afforded 57.6 grams of isomethyl-δ-ionone, boiling point 80° to 86°C/0.3 mm Hg.

The semicarbazone derivative, prepared in the usual manner by conventional organic procedure from the above ionone, was recrystallized several times from methanol-benzene to give 49 grams of pure isomethyl-δ-ionone semicarbazone, melting point 175° to 177°C. Analysis calculated for $C_{15}H_{25}N_3O$: C, 68.4; H, 9.6; N, 16.0. Found: C, 68.4; H, 9.4; N, 15.8.

The pure ketone was subsequently regenerated from the semicarbazone by mixing the latter with an equal part by weight of phthalic anhydride and thereafter steam distilling. Upon extraction with diethyl ether, the product was recovered and subsequently isolated by means of vacuum distillation to give 36.2 grams (49%) of pure isomethyl-δ-ionone, boiling point 93° to 95°C/1.3 mm Hg. Analysis calculated for $C_{14}H_{22}O$: C, 81.5; H, 10.8. Found: C, 81.6; H, 10.8.

Example 2: To a stirred solution of 112 grams (1.0 mol) of potassium t-butoxide dissolved in 400 milliliters of dry dimethyl sulfoxide, there were added in a dropwise manner 168.2 grams (0.88 mol) of β-ionone during the course of 30 minutes. The solution was then stirred for an additional 30 minutes and subsequently treated, in a dropwise manner, with 137 grams (0.88 mol) of ethyl iodide dissolved in 100 milliliters of dimethyl sulfoxide at 25°C. The reaction mixture was then stirred for 1 hour at 25°C and for an additional hour at 60°C, and thereafter poured into 2 liters of cold water. After acidification with glacial acetic acid, the resulting aqueous solution was extracted with three 500 milliliter portions of diethyl ether.

The combined ethereal extracts were then subsequently washed with successive portions of water and saturated sodium chloride solution, respectively, before drying over anhydrous sodium sulfate. The dried ethereal solution was then filtered and evaporated under reduced pressure to give 194 grams of amber liquid that was subsequently distilled in vacuo to afford 147 grams of crude isoethyl-δ-ionone, boiling point 90° to 94°C/1 mm Hg.

The semicarbazone obtained from 142 grams of the above crude product was prepared in the usual manner and subsequently recrystallized from ethanol to give 74.5 grams of pure isoethyl-δ-ionone semicarbazone, melting point 168° to 170°C. Analysis calculated for $C_{16}H_{27}N_3O$: C, 69.3; H, 9.8; N, 15.2. Found: C, 69.6; H, 9.8; N, 15.0. The pure ketone was then regenerated from the semicarbazone by the standard phthalic anhydride steam distillation procedure and subsequently purified by means of vacuum distillation to give 49 grams of pure isoethyl-δ-ionone, boiling point 100°C /3 mm Hg.

Irones from 1,1-Dimethyl-2-(3-Oxobutyl)Cyclopropane

According to a process described by *A. Eschenmoser, D. Felix and M. Stoll; U.S. Patent 3,413,351; November 26, 1968; assigned to Firmenich et Cie, Switzerland* irones are prepared by treating 1,1-dimethyl-2-(3-methyl-7-oxo-3,5-octadien-1-yl)cyclopropane with an acidic reagent so as to cause the opening of the cyclopropane ring and the cyclization of the product to form irone.

Example 1: Sixty grams of zinc iodide were dissolved in 200 milliliters of absolute ether in a humidity free nitrogen atmosphere in a 3 neck flask. Five hundred milliliters of ethereal diazomethane solution (about 0.8 N) were dropped into the zinc iodide solution in the course of 45 minutes while cooling with ice. The bis(iodomethyl) zinc content of the reaction solution was determined iodometrically. The solution was about 0.19 molar which corresponds to a yield of about 71% based on zinc iodide.

Seven hundred milliliters of the reagent solution were concentrated to about 150 milliliters in a rotary evaporator at a bath temperature of –5° to –10°C with exclusion of humidity; 16.7 grams of 6-methyl-5-hepten-2-one were then added to the concentrated solution in a nitrogen atmosphere, and the whole was agitated. The yellowish solution was then slowly heated to room temperature and then refluxed for 2 hours (bath temperature, 50°C). The reaction mixture was then poured onto ice, taken up in ether, the ethereal extract extracted several times with ice water, then with diluted ammonia and finally with ice water until neutral.

After drying of the extract over sodium sulfate and removal of the ether, the crude product was distilled from a Claisen flask in the vacuum of a water jet pump. 14.82 grams of distillate of boiling point 51.5° to 85°C at 13 torr were obtained. This distillate contained 82% of 1,1-dimethyl-2-(3-oxobutyl)cyclopropane. The cyclopropane derivative purified by repeated distillation and gas chromatography was a colorless volatile oil whose odor was similar to that of methylheptenone and which had the following properties: n_D^{20} = 1.4310, d_4^{20} = 0.858. Analysis calculated for $C_9H_{16}O$: C, 77.09%; H, 11.50%. Found: C, 77.06%; H, 11.57%.

Example 2: 10.5 grams of geranyl acetate were mixed at low temperature in the manner described in Example 1 with 150 milliliters of bis(iodomethyl) zinc solution containing 0.12 mol of $Zn(CH_2I)_2$. The mixture was heated to room temperature and then refluxed for 2 hours. After working up in the manner described in Example 1, there were obtained 11.2 grams of crude product yielding on distillation in a high vacuum 9.1 grams of distillate of boiling point 110° to 120°C/0.1 torr, n_D^{20} = 1.4591. This distillate contained about 81% of 1,1-dimethyl-2-(3-methyl-5-acetoxy-3-penten-1-yl)cyclopropane.

Example 3: 9.1 grams of citral were mixed at 0°C with 150 milliliters of bis(iodomethyl) zinc solution containing 0.12 mol of bis(iodomethyl) zinc. The mixture was heated to room temperature and refluxed for 2 hours. After working up in the manner described in Example 1 and distillation of the crude product in a high vacuum there were obtained 6.2 grams of yellow oil, boiling point 63° to 70°C/0.1 torr, n_D^{20} = 1.4783. This distillate contained 72% of 1,1-dimethyl-2-(3-methyl-5-oxo-3-penten-1-yl)cyclopropane.

In related work, *A. Eschenmoser, D. Felix and M. Stoll; U.S. Patent 3,470,241; Sept. 30, 1969; assigned to Firmenich & Cie, Switzerland* describe additional studies with cyclopropane intermediates for irones. According to the process, the 1,1-dimethyl-2-(3-methyl-7-oxo-3,5-octadien-1-yl)cyclopropane serving as an intermediate in the preparation of irone is obtained by reacting pseudo-ionone in an inert and humidity free atmosphere with bis(iodomethyl) zinc.

The process consists of adding dropwise an ethereal solution of zinc iodide to an ethereal solution of diazomethane. The formation of bis(iodomethyl) zinc is accompanied by the evolution of nitrogen gas. Pseudo-ionone is then added to the ethereal solution of the reagent at about –5° to –10°C. All these operations are carried out in an inert and humidity free atmosphere, e.g., under nitrogen.

Continuous Production of Pseudoionones

W. Hoffmann, H. Pasedach and R. Fischer; U.S. Patent 3,745,189; July 10, 1973; assigned to Badische Anilin- & Soda-Fabrik AG, Germany describe a continuous process for the production of pseudoionones having the general Formulas (Ia), (Ib) and (Ic):

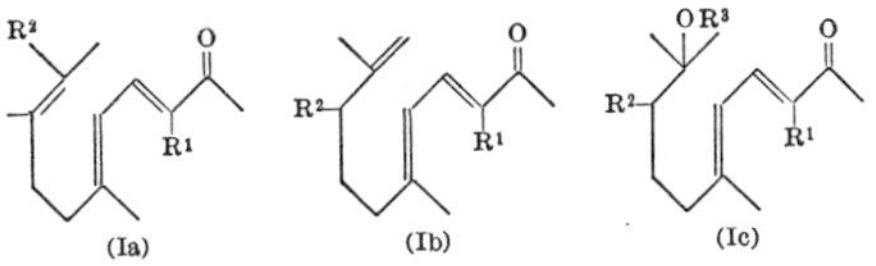

(Ia)   (Ib)   (Ic)

in which R^1 and R^2 denote hydrogen atoms or methyl groups, and R^3 denotes an alkyl group having from 1 to 4 carbon atoms, starting from dehydrolinalools having the general Formulas (IIa), (IIb) and (IIc):

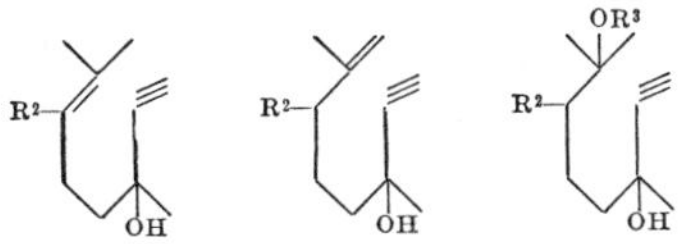

(IIa)   (IIb)   (IIc)

and an acetoacetic ester having the general Formula (III)

(III)

$$CH_3CO-CH-COOR^3$$
$$|$$
$$R^1$$

The continuous reaction of the compounds (IIa), (IIb) and (IIc) with (III) to form the compounds (Ia), (Ib) and (Ic) at temperatures of from 100° to 400°C in the presence or absence of catalytic amounts of a weak acid is generally known. However, contaminants which are difficult to remove form in addition to the desired compounds. Moreover, the space time yields are so low that they do not meet the requirements placed on industrial processes.

It has been found that the production of pseudoionones (Ia), (Ib) and (Ic) by reacting a dehydrolinalool (IIa), (IIb) or (IIc) at from 150° to 300°C with an acetoacetic ester (III) can be carried out in a very economical and advanced continuous manner by effecting the reaction in at least two reactors arranged in series, the temperature in the first reactor being from 160° to 190°C and the temperatures in the subsequent reactors being in each case from 1° to 50°C higher than in the preceding reactor, the residence times of the reaction material in the reactors being equal or substantially equal and between 10 minutes and 5 hours.

The starting compounds (IIa), (IIb) and (IIc) are known and can be obtained, for example, by ethynylation of the appropriate ketones. Alkyl esters of acetoacetic acid having from 1 to 4 carbon atoms in the alkyl radical are suitable as the acetoacetic esters (III), preferably the methyl and ethyl esters. The starting compounds react together stoichiometrically, but it is advisable to use the acetoacetic ester in an excess of up to four times the molar amount in order to achieve more rapid conversion. The following examples illustrate the process.

Example 1: Four glass flasks each provided with a distillation head and having a capacity of 250 ml, the reaction chamber of each flask being limited to 150 ml by an overflow, are arranged in series.

A solution of 116 g of 3,7-dimethyl-7-octen-1-in-3-ol, 177 g of methyl acetoacetate and 2 grams of adipic acid is introduced continuously per hour into this apparatus. The reaction temperature is adjusted to 180°C in the first reactor and to 185°, 190° and 195°C in the subsequent reactors. The residence time is 30 minutes per reactor. The reflux-discharge ratio is so adjusted at the distillation heads that only methanol distils off. The amounts of methanol and carbon dioxide obtained per hour from the four reactors are as follows.

Reactor Number	1	2	3	4
Methanol (gram)	15	7	4	3
Carbon dioxide (liter)	4	5	4	3

About 240 g of reaction mixture is obtained per hour. 6,10-dimethyl-3,5,10-undecatrien-2-one is obtained therefrom by distillation in an 86% yield.

Example 2: 6,10-Dimethyl-10-methoxy-3,5-undecadien-2-one is obtained in an 84% yield from an hourly supply of 133 g of 3,7-dimethyl-7-methoxy-1-octyn-3-ol, 167 g of methyl acetoacetate and 2 g of benzoic acid in the manner described in Example 1.

1-(4-Oxopent-1-enyl)-1,3-Dimethylcyclohex-2-ene

W. Hoffmann, H. Pasedach and H. Pommer; U.S. Patent 3,734,967; May 22, 1973; assigned to Badische Anilin- & Soda-Fabrik AG, Germany describe the compounds 1-(4-oxopent-1-enyl)-1,3-dimethylcyclohex-2-ene (Ia) and 1-(4-oxopent-1-enyl)-1,3-dimethylcyclohex-3-ene (Ib) and their methyl homologs. It has been found that these compounds (Ia) and (Ib), which have the general formulas:

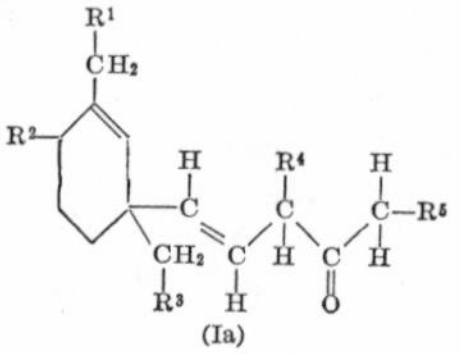

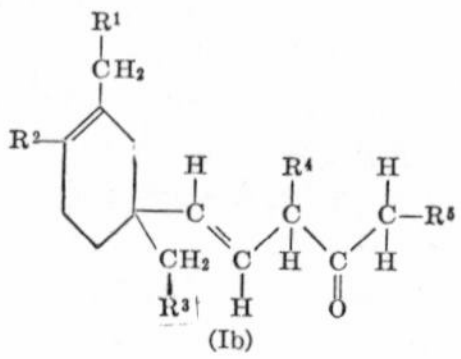

where the radicals R^1, R^2, R^3, R^4 and R^5 may each be a hydrogen atom or a methyl group, are obtained in a reaction by allowing formic acid to act on a 6,10-dimethylundeca-3,5,10-trien-2-one having the general Formula (II)

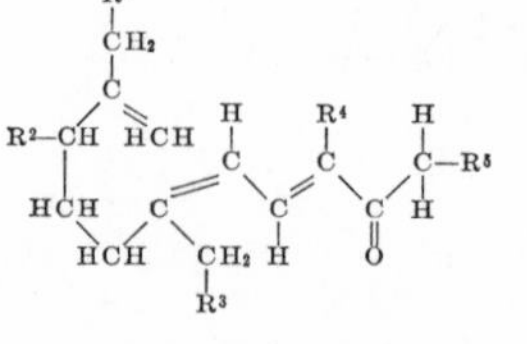

where R^1, R^2, R^3, R^4 and R^5 have the above meanings. Preferred starting materials (II) are α-pseudoionone (R^1 to R^5 all denoting hydrogen atoms) and its monomethyl or dimethyl homologs. The compounds (II) are known or accessible by known methods.

Formic acid effects a catalytic cyclization of the compounds (II), as a rule to form a mixture of about equal parts of (Ia) and (Ib). The reaction concerned is an anomalous reaction because cyclization of α-pseudoionone and β-pseudoionone with sulfuric acid or phosphoric acid is known to give α-ionone and β-ionone and in cyclization of β-pseudoionone with formic acid α-ionone is formed. In the nomenclature of (Ia) and (Ib), α-ionone would be referred to as 1-(3-oxobut-1-enyl)-2,2,6-trimethylcyclohex-5-ene and β-ionone would be referred to as 1-(3-oxobut-1-enyl)-2,2,6-trimethylcyclohex-6-ene.

The products are valuable perfumes which in their fundamental character resemble the structurally related ionones and their homologs, but differ clearly therefrom in their shades, some of which are original, for example, raspberry. The process is illustrated by the following examples.

Example 1: 1-(4-Oxopent-1-enyl)-1,3-Dimethylcyclohex-2-ene and 1-(4-Oxopent-1-enyl)-1,3-Dimethylcyclohex-3-ene — 500 g of 6,10-dimethyl-3,5,10-trien-2-one (pseudoionone) is added in the course of 30 minutes at 50°C to 2,500 g of pure formic acid while stirring and the mixture is kept at this temperature for another 30 minutes. 500 g of ice is then added, the aqueous phase formed is extracted several times with hexane, the extracts are united with the original organic phase, and the combined mixture is washed and neutralized several times with sodium hydrogen carbonate solution and water and then worked up conventionally by distillation. The yield of the abovementioned mixtures of isomers (about equal parts of each) is 75%. The physical characteristics are shown below and both isomers have a pleasant raspberry odor.

	Boiling Point (0.1 mm)	n_D^{25}
For the mixture	65° to 70°C	1.4876
For the 2-ene isomer	65° to 66°C	1.4873
For the 3-ene isomer	69° to 70°C	1.4879

Example 2: 1-(4-Oxopent-1-enyl)-1-Ethyl-3-Methylcyclohex-2-ene and 1-(4-Oxopent-1-enyl)-1-Ethyl-3-Methylcyclohex-3-ene — These compounds are obtained as described in Example 1 from 100 g of 6-ethyl-10-methylundeca-3,5,10-trien-2-one and 250 g of formic acid in a yield of 68%. The physical characteristics are as follows for the mixture: boiling point 105° to 110°C at 2 mm; n_D^{25} is 1.4916. The odor of the mixture is sweet and iris-like.

WOODY—GENERAL

Tetramethyl Octalones

J.H. Blumenthal; U.S. Patent 3,265,739; August 9, 1966; assigned to International Flavors & Fragrances Inc. describe two tetramethyl substituted unsaturated bicyclic ketones (I) and (II) and the ketone obtained by hydrogenation of the double bond thereof, (III).

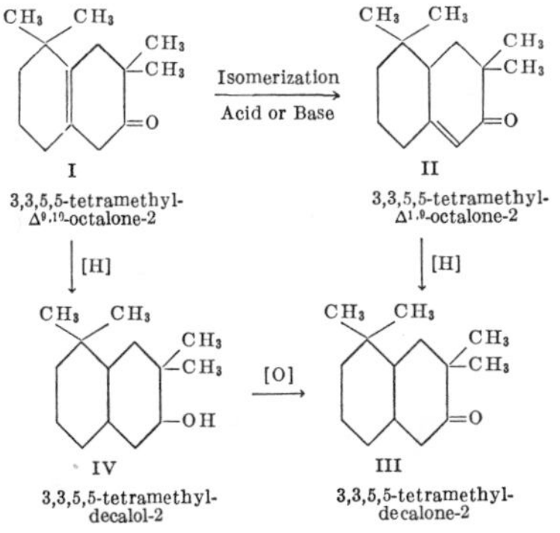

I
3,3,5,5-tetramethyl-
Δ⁹,¹⁰-octalone-2

II
3,3,5,5-tetramethyl-
Δ¹,⁹-octalone-2

IV
3,3,5,5-tetramethyl-
decalol-2

III
3,3,5,5-tetramethyl-
decalone-2

The above compounds, except the intermediate alcohol (IV), possess odors which are useful as perfume materials. The following examples illustrate the process. All temperatures are in degrees centigrade. All pressures herein are in millimeters of mercury unless otherwise indicated.

Example 1: To a mixture of 420 g of concentrated sulfuric acid (96%) and 500 ml of hexane which had been cooled to –10°C was added with good stirring a precooled solution of 168 g (0.82 mol) of geranyl isobutyronitrile prepared as described below, in an equal volume of hexane over a period of 20 minutes, while maintaining the temperature of the reaction at –10°C.

The cooling bath was removed and the mixture stirred until the temperature reached 0°C (about 10 minutes). The reaction mixture was then poured with stirring into a mixture of 800 g of ice and 800 g of water. The mixture was adjusted with sodium hydroxide to pH 5 while maintaining the temperature under 30°C. It contained an oil and an aqueous layer. The oil layer was separated and the aqueous layer, after standing for 30 minutes, was extracted twice with hexane.

The combined organic layers were washed twice with 10% H_2SO_4 and then washed neutral with salt solution, 5% sodium bicarbonate and salt solution. The solvent was removed and the residue distilled at 1 mm without a column (boiling point range 90° to 100°C) to yield 93 g of material testing 95% as ketone (52% yield of crude product).

The vapor phase chromatogram (vpc) showed the presence of one major (90%) and one minor peak (10%). Fractionation at 2 mm through a 12" packed column gave a good separation of the isomeric ketones. The main fraction was ketone (I); boiling point 95°C at 2 mm Hg n_D^{20} 1.4930. NMR absorption data confirmed the structures of the ketone as follows.

	Tau Value
Multiplicity:	
Singlet	9.03
Singlet	8.98
Multiplet	8.63, 8.47
Multiplet	8.17
Singlet	7.85
Singlet	7.35

The infrared curve shows the presence of nonconjugated ketone (I) and a trace of ketone (II). The product has a fine, woody perfume. Geranyl isobutyronitrile may be prepared by the condensation of isobutyronitrile with the allylic chloride obtained by the addition of HCl to myrcene (U.S. Patent 2,882,323) by means of sodamide.

Example 2: To 2,400 g of polyphosphoric acid at 50°C was added with stirring in about 1 hour, 410 g (2 mols) of geranyl isobutyronitrile. The temperature was allowed to rise during the addition to 105°C. The reaction mixture was stirred for 2 hours at 100° to 105°C and then was poured with stirring into 7,200 g of warm water. The mixture was adjusted to a pH of 5 by addition of 30% sodium hydroxide and then stirred at 70° to 80°C for 1 hour.

Two layers formed. The lower layer was separated and the upper layer washed twice with 300 g of aqueous HCl (1:1); then successively with salt solution, 5% sodium carbonate and salt solution. The solvent was distilled off and the residue flash distilled at 3 mm. The distillate was fractionated through a 12 plate column at 3 mm. The main cut which solidified on standing weighed 257 g and tested 97% ketone (60% of theory). Recrystallization from aqueous ethanol yielded ketone (II), a white crystalline solid, melting at 58°C, which showed one peak by vpc. Its UV absorption was that expected of a conjugated ketone of this type with a λ_{max} of 240 mμ, ϵ = 15,900. The product had a woody, tobacco-like perfume. NMR absorption data confirmed the structure of the ketone as follows.

	Tau Value
Multiplicity:	
Doublet	9.23, 9.05
Singlet	9.01
Multiplet	8.55, 8.45, 8.36
Multiplet	8.00, 7.85
Singlet	4.42

Acyl Cyclododecenes

J.H. Blumenthal; U.S. Patent 3,754,036; August 21, 1973; assigned to International Flavors & Fragrances Inc. describes fragrance materials which are prepared by acylation cylation of trimethylcyclododecatriene. The cyclic hydrocarbons treated according to this process are trialkyl-substituted cyclododecenes, preferably such cyclododecenes having from 1 to 3 unsaturated carbon-to-carbon bonds.

The lower alkyl groups having from 1 to 3 carbon atoms are contemplated, and the preferred alkyl substituent is methyl. The substances produced by trimerizing such methyl butadienes as isoprene, piperylene (1,3-pentadiene) or mixtures of isoprene and piperylene to obtain cyclic derivatives are a convenient source of such materials. Thus, cyclododecenes for use in the process include 1,5,9-trimethylcyclododecatriene-1,5,9; 1,5,9-trimethylcyclododecatriene-1,5,10; and other such trimethylcyclododecatrienes.

The acylation can be carried out with an excess of acetic anhydride which performs the function of a vehicle in the reaction mass, although a substantial excess of the anhydride may cause a high degree of polyacylation. In order to minimize such polyacylation, an excess of the trialkyl cyclododecene can be used in the reaction mixture.

The reaction is preferably carried out in the presence of an acidic catalyst. It has been found that Friedel-Crafts acylation agents are especially desirable as catalysts. Thus, boron trifluoride, stannic chloride, ferric chloride, and zinc chloride are preferred catalysts. The following examples illustrate the process.

Example 1: Into a 5 liter reaction flask equipped with a stirrer, thermometer, reflux condenser, addition funnel and drying tube are charged the following materials: 1,250 ml acetic anhydride; 1,550 ml BF_3-etherate; and 500 g 1,5,9-trimethylcyclododecatriene-1,5,9 as described below.

The flask is charged initially with acetic anhydride and BF_3-etherate and then cooled to $0°C$. At $0°C$, the trimethylcyclododecatriene is added. The reaction mass is stirred and made homogeneous, and is then poured onto 4,000 g of ice. Thereafter, sodium hydroxide (5% aqueous) is added to neutralize the mass. The two resulting phases are separated, and the aqueous phase is extracted with benzene.

The benzene extract is bulked with the main organic phase, and the benzene solvent is then stripped off. The weight of the resulting oil is 645 g. The oil is then distilled. The ketonic product thus obtained has a boiling range of $180°$ to $210°C$ at 2 mm Hg and a persistent woody-amber fragrance.

Example 2: Into a 500 ml reaction flask equipped with a stirrer, thermometer, reflux condenser and addition funnel are added the following: 100 g methylene chloride (CH_2Cl_2); 100 g 1,5,9-trimethylcyclododecatriene-1,5,9; 10 g stannic chloride; and 60 g acetic anhydride. The methylene chloride and trimethylcyclododecatriene are initially placed into the flask. Then the stannic chloride is added at temperatures between $25°$ and $30°C$. Immediately subsequent to the stannic chloride addition, acetic anhydride is added at temperatures between $20°$ and $30°C$. The reaction is then allowed to proceed for a period of 2 hours between temperatures of $22°$ and $28°C$.

At the end of the 2 hour period, the reaction mass is worked up. 100 ml benzene is added to the mass, and the mass is then washed with one volume of sodium chloride solution, whereupon two phases are formed. The organic phase is separated and washed with one volume of 5% sodium bicarbonate and then with one volume of 10% sodium chloride solution. The benzene is stripped out of the organic phase. The net weight of the resulting ketonic product prior to distillation is 83.0 g. After distillation, the preferred material has a boiling point of 126° to 134°C at 1 mm Hg and a persistent woody-amber fragrance note.

Acylated Trimethylcyclododecatrienes

S. Lemberg; U.S. Patent 3,718,697; February 27, 1973 describes fragrance-imparting materials which are (C-15 polycyclic alkyl)-lower alkyl ketones produced by acylating with cyclization trimethylcyclododecene and recovering the acylated cyclized products. In addition, hydrogenated products can be obtained by hydrogenating the trimethylcyclododecene or the acylated cyclized trimethylcyclododecene. The products are suitable for incorporation into a wide variety of perfumes and fragrance-modifying compositions. The following examples illustrate the process.

Example 1: Into a 1 liter reaction flask equipped with stirrer, thermometer, reflux condenser, funnel and heating mantle, are placed 160 g of acetic anhydride and 52 g of polyphosphoric acid. The mixture is heated to 75°C and 200 g of 1,5,9-trimethylcyclododecatriene-1,5,9 is added during a 2 hour period while the temperature is maintained at 75° to 80°C.

Subsequent to the addition of the cyclododecatriene, the reaction mass is stirred at 75° to 80°C for a period of 7 hours. The reaction mass is then allowed to come to room temperature and two volumes of ice water are added. The resulting mixture is extracted with two volumes of benzene followed by three washes with aqueous sodium bicarbonate and three with saturated aqueous sodium chloride.

The benzene solution is then dried over magnesium sulfate, and the solvent is evaporated to obtain 173 g of crude product. This product is subsequently stripped in an 8 inch packed column and redistilled at 134° to 186°C at 0.2 mm Hg on a 2 foot column. The distillate is a (C-15 polycyclic alkyl)-methyl ketone. The IR spectrum shows an acetate absorption band at 1,350 cm^{-1},

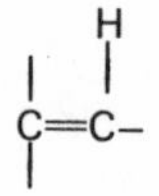

$$\underset{\underset{|}{C}=\underset{|}{C}-}{\overset{\overset{H}{|}}{}}$$

absorption at 830 cm^{-1}, and carbonyl absorption at 1,710 cm^{-1}. The material so obtained has a woody, amber fragrance with an emphatic amber character.

Example 2: The procedure of Example 1 is carried out in a 5 liter flask with 2,700 g acetic anhydride, 390 g of polyphosphoric acid, and 1,500 g of the trimethylcyclododecatriene. This material has substantially the same physical and chemical properties as the distillate produced in Example 1. The NMR spectrum shows the characteristics set forth below.

Assignment	Chemical Shift (ppm)	Number of Protons
C=CH	5.00 (multiplet)	1.8
=C—C(H)—C=O =C—CH₂—C=	3.00–2.50 (multiplet)	1.4
=C—CH₂ CH₃—C=O	2.10, 2.03, 1.98 (singlets)	9.1
=C—CH₃ —CH₂—	1.72–1.33	13.7

Example 3: The procedure of Example 1 is carried out with a mixture of 800 g of acetic anhydride, 260 g polyphosphoric acid, and 1,000 g of 1,5,9-trimethylcyclododecatriene-1,5,9. The gross weight of the product prior to distillation is 1,040 g. The product has substantially the same characteristics chemically and physically as set forth in Examples 1 and 2. The following composition is prepared.

Ingredient	Amount (grams)
Cassia absolute	60
Methyl ionone	60
Jasmine extra	60
Neroli oil, bigarade	60
Patchouli oil	60
Vanillin	60
Violet perfume base	60
Distilled cyclized acylate of Example 1	60
Lemon oil	60
Rose geranium oil	120
Lavender oil, French	120
Sweet orange oil	80
Musk extract, 3%	50
Civet extract, 3%	50

The blend is tested and found to have the same desirable characteristics of richness and persistence provided by the very expensive vetivert oil, and it further possesses a woody, amber-like quality. The material of Example 1 thus permits replacement of, or substitution in, traditional materials such as sandalwood, vetivert, and patchouli.

Monoepoxidized Cyclododecatrienes

G. Ohloff and K.H.S. Elte; U.S. Patent 3,723,478; March 27, 1973; assigned to Firmenich & Cie, Switzerland have found that mixtures of isomeric monoepoxides of trimethylcyclododecatrienes prepared by monoepoxidizing a mixture of 3,4,8- and 4,8,12-trimethyl-1,5,9-cyclododecatrienes or a mixture of 1,5,9- and 2,5,9-trimethyl-1,5,9-cyclododecatrienes possess valuable odoriferous properties and also have a fixative effect in mixtures with other odoriferous substances. Certain ketones and lactones derivable from the monoepoxides also have useful odoriferous characteristics.

Cyclic Diketones

B.P. Corbier and P.J. Teisseire; U.S. Patent 3,578,715; May 11, 1971; assigned to SA des Etablissements Roure-Bertrand Fils & Justin Dupont, France describe diketones of the general formula

(1)

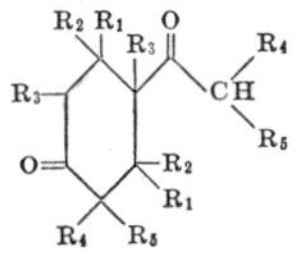

and their lower enolethers, enolesters or ketals. In general Formula (1), R_1 and R_2 represent lower alkyl or cyclo lower alkyl groups or, together a lower alkylene group, preferably containing up to 5 carbon atoms, such as methyl, ethyl, propyl, butyl, cyclopropyl, tetramethylene or pentamethylene, while R_3, R_4 and R_5 represent hydrogen atoms or lower alkyl groups, for example, those containing 1 to 5 carbon atoms, such as methyl, ethyl, propyl, butyl.

The compounds of Formula (1), their enolethers, enolesters and ketals are distinguished by interesting odors, woody odors in particular, and accordingly are suitable for use as odorants, for example, in perfumes, soaps, detergents, cleansing agents and other scented compositions. The process comprises reacting a ketone of the general formula:

(2)

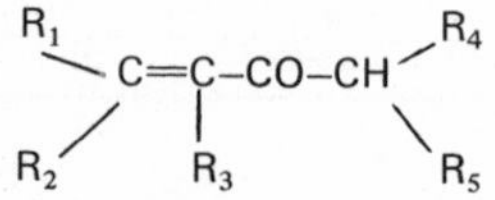

$$R_1 \underset{R_2}{\overset{}{\diagdown}} C = \underset{R_3}{\overset{}{C}} - CO - CH \underset{R_5}{\overset{R_4}{\diagup}}$$

in which R_1 through R_5 are as defined above, with a lower alkyl orthoformate in the presence of an acid catalyst and, if desired, subjecting the reaction product to hydrolysis, ketalization, enol etherification ór enol esterification.

The following compounds, for example, are characterized by their distinctive odors. The monoethylenolether corresponding to the formula:

(3)

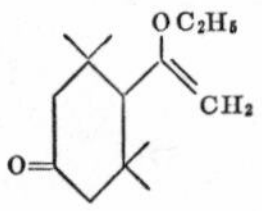

i.e., 4-(1-ethoxyvinyl)-3,3,5,5-tetramethylcyclohexanone, has a woody odor accompanied by an animal flavor. The bisethylenolether corresponding to the formula:

(4)

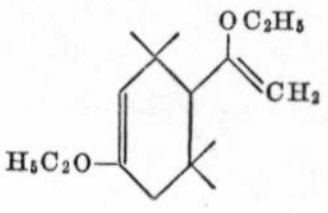

i.e., 1-ethoxy-4-(1-ethoxyvinyl)-3,3,5,5-tetramethylcyclo-1-hexene, has a pleasant woody smell. The monoethylenolether corresponding to the formula:

(5)

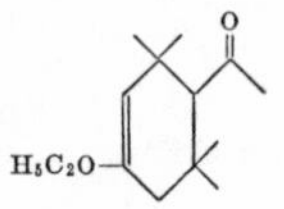

i.e., 1-ethoxy-4-acetyl-3,3,5,5-tetramethylcyclo-1-hexene has a highly refined, woody smell, as has the ethylene ketal corresponding to the formula:

(6)

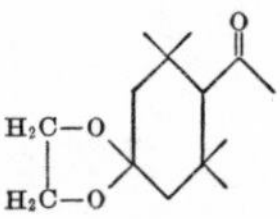

i.e., 4-acetyl-1,1-ethylenedioxy-3,3,5,5-tetramethylcyclohexane. In the following examples, the temperatures are given in degrees centigrade (°C).

Example 1: 1 ml of boron trifluoride etherate is added to 490 g (5 mols) of mesityl oxide. The temperature of the reaction mixture is increased to 50°C, 148 g (1 mol) of ethylorthoformate being added to it over a period of 4 hours. The temperature is kept at 50°C for 4 hours, after which 5 g of powdered sodium carbonate are added and the mixture stirred for 30 minutes.

The resulting product is washed once with 100 ml of a 10% sodium carbonate solution and twice with 100 ml of a 30% brine solution. A mixture of ethyl alcohol, ethyl formate and excess mesityl oxide is obtained by distillation at normal pressure. Rectification yields approximately 70 g of a mixture boiling between 75° to 84°C, from which 4-(1-ethoxyvinyl)-

3,3,5,5-tetramethylcyclohexanone [see also Formula (3)] can be isolated. Boiling point: 80° to 82°C/2 mm Hg.

Example 2: 1 ml of boron trifluoride etherate is added to 117.6 g (1.2 mols) of mesityl oxide. The temperature of the reaction mixture is increased to 50°C, 148 g (1 mol) of ethyl orthoformate being added to it over a period of 2 hours. The temperature is kept at 30°C for 24 hours, after which the reaction mixture is worked up as described in Example 1. The following compounds are obtained as the main products in practically the same quantities: (a) 1-ethoxy-4-(1-ethoxyvinyl)-3,3,5,5-tetramethylcyclo-1-hexene [see also Formula (4)]; boiling point: 74° to 76°C/2 mm Hg; (b) the 4-(1-ethoxyvinyl)-3,3,5,5-tetramethylcyclohexanone of Formula (3) described in Example 1.

Example 3: Some odorant compositions containing a mixture of 4-(1-ethoxyvinyl)-3,3,5,5-tetramethylcyclohexanone (Substance A) and 1-ethoxy-4-(1-ethoxyvinyl)-3,3,5,5-cyclo-1-hexene (Substance B), are described in the following.

	Parts by Weight
Mixture of Substances A and B	100
Benzyl salicylate	200
p-Cresylacetate (10%) in diethyl phthalate	10
C_{16}-aldehyde in diethyl phthalate (10%)	10
Geraniol extra	40
Benzyl acetate	50
α-Ionone	100
Diethylacetophenone	25
Phenyl oxide	10
Linalyl acetate	150
Cinnamic alcohol	30
Coumarin	50
Mixtures of Substances A and B	150
Diisobutyl carbinol acetate	200
Eugenol extra	50
Methylnonyl acetaldehyde (10%) in diethyl phthalate	30
C_{16}-aldehyde (10%) in diethyl phthalate	10
Phenylethyl acetate	30
Amyl cinnamic aldehyde	20
Benzyl acetate	40
α-Ionone	100
Hydroxycitronellal	70
Geranium-Bourbon essence	70
Geraniol extra	30
Citronellol	30
Coumarin	20

Perhydro-1,4,9,9-Tetramethyl-4,7-Methanoazulenones

J.D. Grossman, B.D. Mookherjee, R.S. de Simone and E.T. Theimer; U.S. Patent 3,748,284; July 24, 1973; assigned to International Flavors & Fragrances Inc. describe certain perhydro-1,4,9,9-tetramethyl-4,7-methanoazulenones and processes for their production. These materials are ketones having the formula:

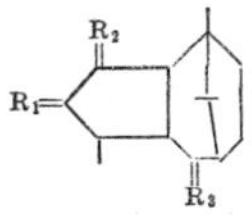

where one of R_1, R_2 and R_3 is oxygen and each of the other two represents two hydrogen atoms. The azulenones of the process provide a superior amber, precious wood, camphoraceous fragrance note and are much more intense than those previously known. The compound can be considered as perhydro derivatives of methanoazulene and are octahydro-1,4,9,9-tetramethyl-4,7-methanoazulen-3(2H)-one, (I); octahydro-1,4,9,9-tetramethyl-4,7-methanoazulen-2(3H)-one, (II); octahydro-1,4,9,9-tetramethyl-4,7-methanoazulen-8(7H)-one, (III); and mixtures thereof.

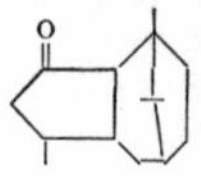

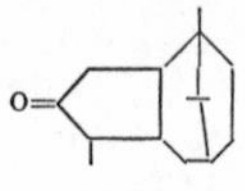

The ketones can be prepared by a process which comprises treating a saturated alcohol having the structure

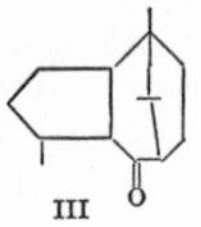

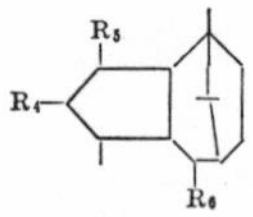

or mixtures of such alcohols where one of R_4, R_5 and R_6 is OH and the other two are H with an agent which will oxidize a secondary hydroxyl to a carbonyl and provide the ketones having the structure

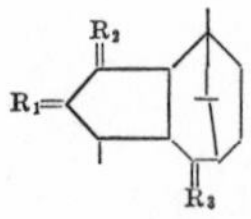

where R_1, R_2 and R_3 are as described above. The following examples illustrate the process.

Example 1: Hydroboration of β-Patchoulene Followed by Oxidative Hydrolysis to Produce Secondary Alcohol Mixture — A 20 liter reaction vessel is charged with 2,500 ml of tetrahydrofuran and 640 g of sodium borohydride, and 2,800 g of boron trifluoride etherate is added dropwise to the mixture. 1,850 g of 1,4,9,9-tetramethyl-$\Delta^{3a,8a}$-octahydro-4,7-methanoazulene (beta-patchoulene) is added to the reaction mass, and the mass is refluxed at atmospheric pressure for 8 hours.

After cooling to 25°C, 300 ml of water is added over a 30 minute period while the mass is maintained at 25°C. 6.3 grams of 3.0M aqueous sodium hydroxide is then added with stirring during 45 minutes. 1,500 ml of a 50% solution of H_2O_2 is added at 25°C over 75 minutes.

After the addition is complete, the organic layer is separated, the aqueous phase is extracted twice with equal volumes of diethyl ether, and the ether extracts and the organic layer are combined, washed twice with equal volumes of 5% sodium chloride solutions, dried over anhydrous magnesium sulfate, filtered and concentrated on a flash evaporator. The yield of crude secondary alcohol mixture, containing secondary alcohols of the structure

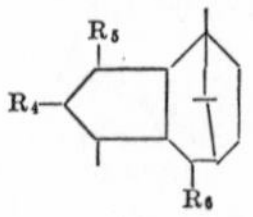

where R_4, R_5 and R_6 are defined as above, is 2,364 g. Gas-liquid phase chromatography (GLC) (8' x ¼' – 20% Carbowax 20M polyethylene glycol coated on Anakron ABS silanized acid washed calcined diatomaceous earth column; flow rate, 100 ml/min; chart speed, 15"/hr) indicates 82.2% of the 2-ol; 12.7% 3-ol; and 5.1% 8-ol.

Example 2: Oxidation of the Secondary Alcohol to the Ketone — A 10 liter reaction vessel is charged with 888 g of chromium trioxide, 3.8 liters of glacial acetic acid and 1,600 milliliters of water. A solution of 2,254 g of the alcohol mixture prepared in Example 1 in 2.2 liters of acetic acid is added dropwise to the mixture, while the temperature is kept at 25° to 30°C. The mixture is stirred until the exotherm ceases.

A solution of 250 g of chromium trioxide in 600 ml of glacial acetic acid and 100 ml of water is then added to the reaction mass. The mass is maintained at 25° to 30°C with stirring for 12 hours. At this point the reaction is 95% complete as indicated by GLC, and the acetic acid is distilled off and the resulting crude oil washed twice with equal volumes of 5% sodium chloride-5% $NaHCO_3$ solution, dried over anhydrous magnesium sulfate, and filtered. The filtered material is rushed over (flash distilled) to yield 1,338 g of a crude mixture. This crude mixture is then distilled at 103° to 144°C at 0.8 mm Hg pressure. GLC (conditions set forth above) shows three peaks which are identified as three ketones having the generic structure:

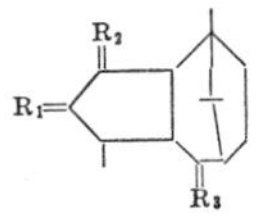

where R_1, R_2 and R_3 are as defined above, the ratio of II:I:III being 70:21:5. The structures are confirmed by nuclear magnetic resonance (NMR) and infrared (IR) analyses. The mixture is separated and isolated via GLC (conditions set forth above). Each of the three isomers possesses strong amber and patchouli fragrance notes, with additional camphoraceous notes. IR analysis of the three mixtures yields the following data.

	Centimeters $^{-1}$		
	II	I	III
5-membered ring carbonyl	1,735	1,730	
Methylene alpha to carbonyl	1,412	1,410	1,410
gem-Dimethyl	1,365, 1,388	1,363, 1,388	1,364, 1,387
Methyl	1,375	1,375	1,375
6-membered ring carbonyl			1,735

Additional studies by *J.D. Grossman, B.D. Mookherjee, R. De Simone and E.T. Theimer; U.S. Patent 3,679,749; July 25, 1972; assigned to International Flavors & Fragrances Inc.* further describe perhydro–1,4,9,9-tetramethyl-4,7-methanoazulenones.

Hexahydro-1,4,9,9-Tetramethyl-4,7-Methanoazulenones

A process described by *B.D. Mookherjee; U.S. Patent 3,679,750; July 25, 1972; assigned to International Flavors & Fragrances Inc.* relates to certain hexahydro-1,4,9,9-tetramethyl-4,7-methanoazulenones and processes for their production. The materials are unsaturated ketones having the structure

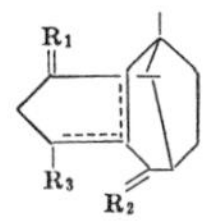

where one of R_1 and R_2 is oxygen and the other represents two hydrogen atoms, R_3 is methyl, or when R_1 is oxygen, methyl or methylene, and one of the dashed lines represents a double bond.

The azulenones provide a superior intense, camphoraceous woody amber fragrance note. The unsaturated ketones of this process are prepared by oxidizing 1,4,9,9-tetramethyl-$\triangle^{3a,8a}$-octahydro-4,7-methanoazulene

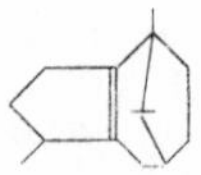

commonly called beta-patchoulene, to provide unsaturated ketones having the structure

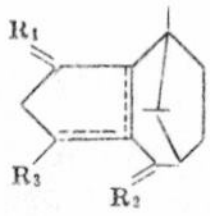

wherein the dashed lines, R_1, R_2 and R_3 are as set forth above. β-patchoulene is readily prepared according to the method of Bates and Slagel, *J.A.C.S.* 84 1307 (1962). The β-patchoulene utilized here as starting material is obtained by treating bulnesol

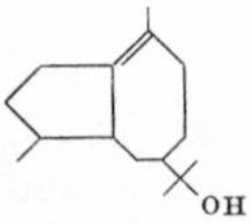

in acid medium to form a methano bridge by cyclization and dehydration. Bulnesol is conveniently obtained from guaiacwood oil. The cyclization is carried out by treating the bulnesol or bulnesol fraction of guaiacwood oil with p-toluene sulfonic acid and formic acid in a vehicle such as toluene. The mixture is heated at reflux till the evolution of water ceases. The reaction mixture is then neutralized with an alkali such as an alkali-metal hydroxide like sodium hydroxide and distilled to obtain the β-patchoulene.

The oxidation reaction of this process is carried out by treating the patchoulene with an agent which will oxidize a methylene group in the position alpha to a carbon-carbon double bond. Suitable agents are metal oxides such as chromium trioxide, selenium dioxide, and the like and alkali-metal dichromates such as sodium dichromate and potassium dichromate.

Pentamethylhexahydroindanones

E.T. Theimer; U.S. Patent 3,681,464; August 1, 1972; assigned to International Flavors & Fragrances Inc. describe saturated indane derivatives having the formula

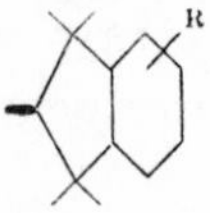

where R is a carbonyl oxygen or a hydroxy, acyloxy, or alkyloxy group. These substances have a persistent strong woody amber fragrance with fruit-like and musk aroma notes. The indanones prepared are 1,1,2,3,3-pentamethylhexahydro-4(5H)-indanone and 1,1,2,3,3-pentamethylhexahydro-5(4H)-indanone having the following formulas.

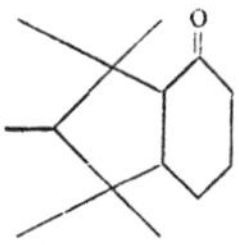

-4(5H)- 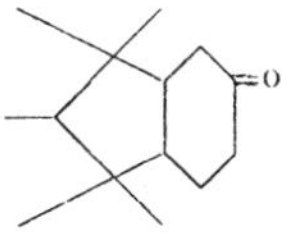   -5(4H)-

The indanols and derivatives contemplated according to this process include 1,1,2,3,3-penta-methylhexahydroindan-4-ol having the formula

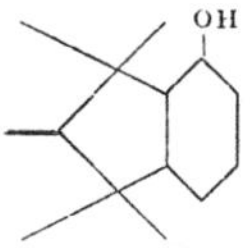

1,1,2,3,3-pentamethylhexahydroindan-5-ol having the formula

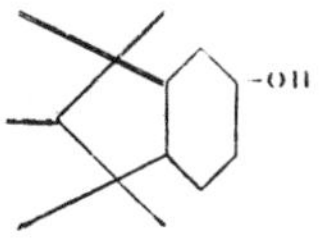

The alcohols can be prepared directly from the corresponding pentamethylindane by sulfonation, alkali fusion, and hydrolysis to provide the pentamethylindanol and then hydrogenation to the hexahydropentamethylindanol. Alternatively, the saturated 3a,7a-epoxy-pentamethylindane can be treated with an aluminum trialkoxide to form the monounsaturated alcohol.

The alcohols can also be produced directly from pentamethylindane by treatment with an acyl halide such as acetyl chloride or the like in the presence of a Friedel-Crafts catalyst followed by oxidation of the indane-alkyl ketone with a peroxygen material such as peracetic acid and the like to provide the indanyl ester.

Hydrolysis of the ester provides the indanol which is then hydrogenated to afford the saturated indanol. A tetrahydroindanol can also be obtained by Birch reduction of 5-indanol as shown in *J. Am. Chem. Soc.*, 89, 1044. The tetrahydroindanols so prepared are then hydrogenated and oxidized to the ketone.

Polyalkylindanylpropanol

C.F. Wight; U.S. Patent 3,660,311; May 2, 1972; assigned to International Flavors & Fragrances Inc. describes a process for imparting fragrances to articles which comprises incorporating with such articles an effective amount of a polyalkylindanylpropanol. The process utilizes 2-(1',1',2',3',3'-pentamethylindane-5'-yl)propanol having the formula

(1)

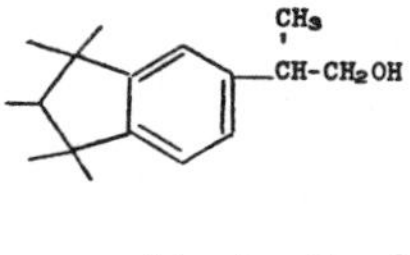

2-(1',1',3',3'-tetramethylindan-5'-yl)propanol having the following formula

(2)

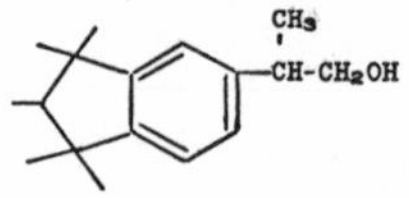

2-(1',1',2',3',3'-pentamethylindan-4'-yl)propanol having the formula

(3)

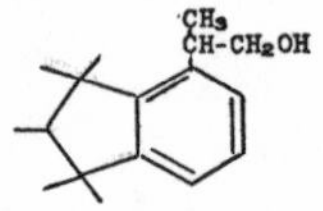

2-(1'-ethyl-1',3',3'-trimethylindan-5'-yl)propanol having the formula

(4)

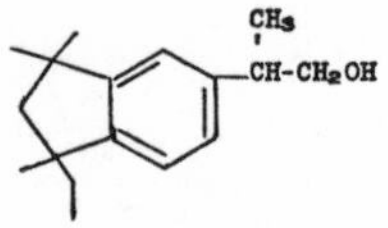

and 2-(1'-ethyl-1',3',3'-trimethylindan-4'-yl)propanol having the formula

(5)

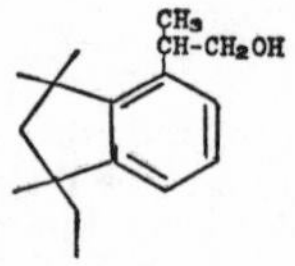

The polyalkylindanylpropanols can be prepared by a number of reaction routes. One desirable route involves the treatment of pentamethylindane with propylene oxide in the presence of a Friedel-Crafts catalyst, desirably an aluminum trihalide such as aluminum chloride. It is desirable to carry out the reaction at temperatures below 10°C to prevent polymerization of the oxide and the formation of unwanted by-products. At extremely low temperatures the reaction velocity becomes low, so it is desirable to carry out the reaction at temperatures not substantially below –20°C. Accordingly, the reaction is desirably carried out at from –20° to 0°C. It is preferred to carry out the reaction at from –15° to –5°C.

The products so obtained are colorless to lightly colored solids having melting points of 50° to 60°C and a very lasting, woody, amber odor character. The individual materials represented by the formulas here can be separated as, and if desired, by conventional methods such as chromatography, distillation, crystallization and like techniques.

The material from Formula (1) generally has a stronger, more persistent aroma than Formula (4) or (5) and is followed in this respect by Formulas (3) and (2). The mixtures produced by the foregoing process generally contain from more than 50% up to 80 or 85% of Formula (1).

Hydrogenated Indane Derivatives

J.B. Hall; U.S. Patents 3,806,472; April 23, 1974; and 3,751,500; August 7, 1973; both assigned to International Flavors & Fragrances Inc. describes a hydrogenated indane derivative, 4,5-dihydro-1,1,2,3,3-pentamethylindane, having the following formula:

This substance has a strong, persistent, woody amber odor with various elegant piney overtones. A convenient starting material according to the process is pentamethylindane. In one aspect, the pentamethylindane is hydrogenated to provide the tetrahydro derivative and/or the hexahydro derivative as the first step in the synthesis. In this synthesis the bridge double bond of the tetrahydro derivative is then oxidized with a suitable agent to obtain the epoxyindane. The hexahydro derivative can be dehydrogenated if desired to obtain the 1,1,2,3,3-pentamethylindane for recycling or for other syntheses. Such dehydrogenation can also provide a useful fragrance material.

The hydrogenation is carried out at substantially superatmospheric pressures of from 50 to 200 atmospheres, and is preferably carried out at 60 to 130 atmospheres. The reaction is desirably carried out at temperatures in excess of 100° up to 225°C, and a preferred range is 150° to 190°C. The hexahydro derivative is obtained under these same conditions through the addition of 3 mols of hydrogen.

In one aspect, the 4,5,6,7-tetrahydropentamethylindane so obtained is oxidized to provide the epoxy oxygen substituent on the 3a,7a bridge carbon atoms. The oxidation is carried out with an oxidizer such as percarboxylic acid. Thus, peracids such as peracetic, perpropionic, perbenzoic, perphthalic, and the like are used. In preferred examples of the process, lower aliphatic percarboxylic acids are used. Thus, peracetic acid can be used, although a combination of acetic anhydride and hydrogen peroxide is equivalent.

The amount of percarboxylic acid used should be about stoichiometric, although slight excesses up to about 10 molar percent can be used. An alkali metal salt of the corresponding carboxylic acid, e.g., sodium acetate for peracetic acid, is desirably used to buffer the reaction mixture. The following examples illustrate the process.

Example 1: The following is a description of the preparation of 4,5,6,7-tetrahydro-1,1,2,3,3-pentamethylindane and hexahydro-1,1,2,3,3-pentamethylindane. 1,800 g (8.14 mols) of 1,1,2,3,3-pentamethylindane (85% pure) and 90 g of Raney nickel are charged into a stainless steel five liter autoclave equipped with a hydrogen gas feed.

Enough hydrogen is fed into the autoclave to raise the pressure to 1,000 psig. The hydrogen feed is continuous until 2 mols of hydrogen are absorbed, and the autoclave is heated to a temperature in the range of 150° to 185°C over a period of about 8 hours until an amount of H_2 equal to 10% in excess of theory is absorbed. During this time the pressure in the autoclave is maintained at 1,500 psig.

The 1,641 g of crude product removed from the autoclave is distilled on a 12 inch Goodloe column after being mixed with 10.0 g of Primol mineral oil. The distillate is recovered in two fractions. Fraction 1 distills at a temperature of 80°C and 4.0 mm Hg to provide 401 g of 4,5,6,7-tetrahydro-1,1,2,3,3-pentamethylindane; and Fraction 2 distills at a temperature range of 86° to 88°C and 3.5 to 3.8 mm Hg to provide 729 g of hexahydro-1,1,2-3,3-pentamethylindane.

A sample of Fraction 1 is further refined on a six foot by three-quarter inch gas liquid chromatographic (GLC) column containing 20% Carbowax polyethylene glycol and operated at 110°C. Analysis by infrared and proton magnetic resonance (PMR) confirms the structure:

Fraction 2 is further refined in a similar manner and analysis confirms the structure.

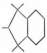

Example 2: (a) Production of 3a,7a-epoxyhexahydro-1,1,2,3,3-pentamethylindane is as follows. Into a 250 ml flask equipped with thermometer, stirrer, reflux condenser and ice bath are introduced 194 g of the tetrahydroindane produced in Example 1 and 15 g of sodium acetate. At 25° to 30°C, 124 g of 40% peracetic acid (0.65 mol) is added during 4 hours. After addition is completed, an equal volume of water is added to the reaction mass.

The aqueous phase is separated from the organic phase and extracted with 150 ml of toluene. The toluene extract is combined with the organic phase and washed with one volume of 5% aqueous sodium hydroxide solution and then with one volume of water. The solvent is stripped off leaving a crude product weighing 208 g. The crude epoxy product is distilled on a 12 inch Goodloe column after addition of 4.0 g of triethanolamine at 72° to 74°C and 1.0 to 1.4 mm Hg. PMR and IR analysis of this material confirm the structure.

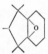

(b) Production of 4,5-dihydro-1,1,2,3,3-pentamethylindane is as follows. Into a 100 ml reaction flask fitted with thermometer and reflux condenser are introduced 10 g of the epoxyhexahydroindane produced above, 50 ml benzene, and 0.5 g of p-toluenesulfonic acid. The reaction mass is stirred for 2 hours at 20° to 30°C and then refluxed for 1 hour.

The reaction mass is subsequently washed with a saturated aqueous sodium bicarbonate solution followed by one volume of a 5% sodium chloride solution and dried over anhydrous sodium sulfate. The resulting product is separated on a gas-liquid chromatographic (GLC) column and the various separated constituents are analyzed by PMR, mass, infrared and UV absorption spectroscopy. These analyses confirm the identity of 4,5-dihydro-1,1,2,3,3-pentamethylindane having the structure.

This material has a fine woody, amber-tobacco aroma with an elegant piney note.

Example 3: The following describes the preparation of soap composition. A total of 100 grams of soap chips (from a toilet soap prepared from tallow and coconut oil) is mixed with 1 g of the perfume composition given below until a substantially homogeneous composition is obtained. The soap composition manifests a characteristic woody-amber odor with piney overtones. The perfume composition comprises the following ingredients.

Ingredient	Parts by Weight	
Vetivert oil	40	
Dihydropentamethylindane produced in Example 2	60	
Sandalwood oil	100	(continued)

Ingredient	Parts by Weight
Rose Geranium oil	200
Musk extract (3%)	25
Civet extract (3%)	25
Benzyl isoeugenol	100
Coumarin	100
Heliotropin	50
Bois de Rose oil	200
Benzoin resin	100
	1,000

In related work *J.B. Hall; U.S. Patent 3,773,836; November 20, 1973; assigned to International Flavors & Fragrances Inc.* describes indanones having the structural formula:

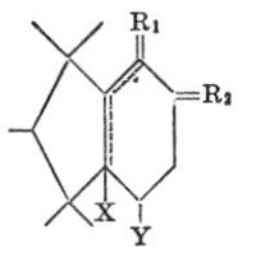

where one of R_1 and R_2 is O and the other is H_2. It will be observed that these compositions also include the 7,7a-epoxy derivative, and the foregoing formula encompasses such monounsaturated and saturated epoxy indanones. Accordingly, Y is H or, taken together with X, an epoxy oxygen, and one of the single dashed lines represents the double bond unless the epoxy oxygen is present. When the double bond is conjugated with R_2 (when this latter is O), then X is H. These substances have strong, persistent, musk woody odors with various rich amber, precious woody, or fine woody overtones.

A convenient starting material according to the process is pentamethylindane. The pentamethylindane is hydrogenated to provide the tetrahydro derivative as the first step in the synthesis of the 4-indanones. The six-membered ring is then oxidized with a suitable agent to obtain a mixture of the monounsaturated indanone and the epoxy indanone. The hydrogenation is carried out under controlled conditions to add 2 mols of hydrogen to each mol of the indane.

A process described by *J.B. Hall; U.S. Patent 3,647,826; March 7, 1972; assigned to International Flavors & Fragrances Inc.* provides epoxyindane derivative, 3a,7a-epoxyhexahydro-1,1,2,3,3-pentamethylindane, having the formula

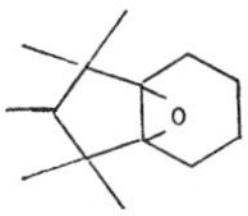

This substance has a good fine-pine woody odor. The process is essentially as described in U.S. Patent 3,806,472.

Substituted 4,7-Methanoindenes

M. Dunkel; U.S. Patent 3,598,745; August 10, 1971; assigned to Universal Oil Products Company describes perfume compositions containing a particularly substituted polyhydro-4,7-methanoindene.

Particularly substituted 4,7-methanoindenes of this process have the following structural formulas.

(1)

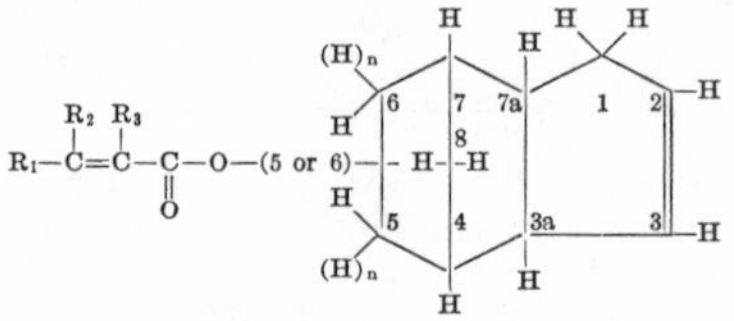

$$R_1-\underset{R_2}{\overset{}{C}}=\underset{R_3}{\overset{}{C}}-\underset{\underset{O}{\parallel}}{C}-O-(5\text{ or }6)-$$

(2)

$$R_1-\underset{R_2}{\overset{}{C}}=\underset{R_3}{\overset{}{C}}-\underset{\underset{O}{\parallel}}{C}-O-$$

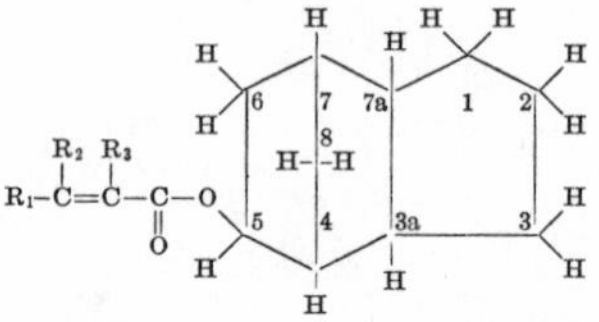

In the above formulas R_1, R_2 and R_3 are taken independently of each other, is a member selected from the group consisting of hydrogen and an alkyl radical and n is an integer of 0 and 1; provided, that for the carbon atom in the 5 or 6 position which is substituted with the substituent

$$R_1-\underset{R_2}{\overset{}{C}}=\underset{R_3}{\overset{}{C}}-\underset{\underset{O}{\parallel}}{C}-O-$$

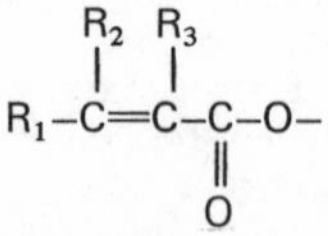

the integer associated therewith is 0 and the other integer is 1. Because of the existence of the double bond in the hexahydromethanoindene illustrated as Formula (1) above, the positions 5 and 6 are not chemically equivalent, and accordingly, when the hexahydro-methanoindene is substituted with the substituent according to this process, different iso-meric compounds result depending upon whether the substituent is on the 5 or 6 positioned carbon atom. The extremely close physical similarity of such isomers, moreover, prevents ready identification and separation of the different isomers from each other.

The 4,7-methanoindenes having the above general structures (1) and (2) are prepared, in general, by reacting the corresponding hydroxy substituted methanoindene with a reactant selected from the group consisting of

(3)

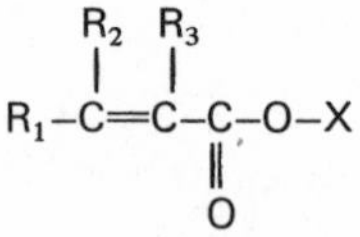

$$R_1-\underset{R_2}{\overset{}{C}}=\underset{R_3}{\overset{}{C}}-\underset{\underset{O}{\parallel}}{C}-O-X$$

and

(4)

$$R_1-\underset{R_2}{\overset{}{C}}=\underset{R_3}{\overset{}{C}}-\underset{\underset{O}{\parallel}}{C}-Y$$

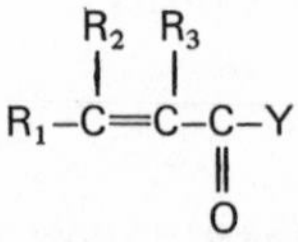

where R_1, R_2 and R_3 have the same meaning as above, Y is a halogen and X is a member selected from the group consisting of hydrogen or an alkyl radical. The following examples illustrate the process.

Example 1: 3a,4,5,6,7,7a-hexahydro-4,7-methanoindene substituted in one of the 5 and 6 positions with senecioyloxy was prepared according to the process by the following pro-cedure. About 50 g (0.5 mol) of senecioic acid, about 130 g of toluene, about 50 g (0.33

mol) of 3a,4,5,6,7,7a-hexahydro-4,7-methanoindene substituted in one of the 5 and 6 positions with hydroxy and about 0.5 ml of concentrated sulfuric acid were charged to a reaction flask equipped with heating and stirring means and an overhead water trap. With stirring the reaction mixture was brought to reflux (120°C) and about 1.5 ml of methane sulfonic acid were added to supplement the sulfuric acid catalyst present. The refluxing was continued for about 13 hours during which time about 6 g of water were collected in the trap.

The reaction mixture was then cooled, washed with a sodium bicarbonate solution followed by several water washings and then dried over sodium sulfate. The toluene solvent was then stripped from the mixture and the remaining mixture was then subjected to vacuum fractionation to recover the product distilling at 130°C at 1.1 mm Hg and having a refractive index of n_D^{20} 1.5148 to 1.5152.

Example 2: 5-senecioyloxy-2,3,3a,4,5,6,7,7a-octahydro-4,7-methanoindene was prepared by the following procedure. About 37 g (0.37 mol) of senecioic acid, about 150 g of toluene, about 51 g (0.33 mol) of 5-hydroxy-2,3,3a,4,5,6,7,7a-octahydromethanoindene and about 1 ml of methane sulfonic acid were charged to a reaction flask equipped with heating and stirring means and an overhead water trap. With stirring the reaction mixture was brought to reflux temperature (120°C) and maintained thereat for about 14.5 hours during which time about 5.4 cc of water were collected in the trap.

The reaction mixture was then cooled, washed with a sodium bicarbonate solution followed by several water washings and then dried over calcium chloride. The toluene solvent was then stripped from the mixture and the remaining mixture was then subjected to vacuum fractionation to recover the product distilling at 117°C at 0.7 mm Hg and having a refractive index of n_D^{20} 1.5050 to 1.5053.

In related work, *M. Dunkel; U.S. Patent 3,558,689; January 26, 1971; assigned to Universal Oil Products Company* describes the preparation of α-(hydroxy or acyloxy 4,7-methanoindenyl) esters or acids useful as perfume ingredients which are prepared basically by a Reformatsky-type reaction of corresponding methanoindenones with α-haloesters.

A number of other processes related to 4,7-methanoindene derivatives which are substituted in the 5- or 6- position have been described by *M. Dunkel; U.S. Patent 3,417,132; Dec. 17, 1968* (alkyl, hydroxy substituted); *U.S. Patent 3,407,225; October 22, 1968* (alkyl, hydroxy substituted); *U.S. Patent 3,445,508; May 20, 1969* (acyl, hydroxy substituted); *U.S. Patent 3,557,188; January 19, 1971* (ester, hydroxy substituted); and *U.S. Patent 3,542,877; November 24, 1970* (acyl, hydroxy substituted); *all assigned to Universal Oil Products Company.*

Ketals from 4,4,10-Trimethyldecahydronaphthalene Derivatives

W. Sandermann and K. Bruns; U.S. Patent 3,427,328; February 11, 1969; assigned to Givaudan Corporation describe chemical compounds having amber-type odors; shown below as Formulas (1) and (2). Other odorants are of the Formulas (3) and (4) below.

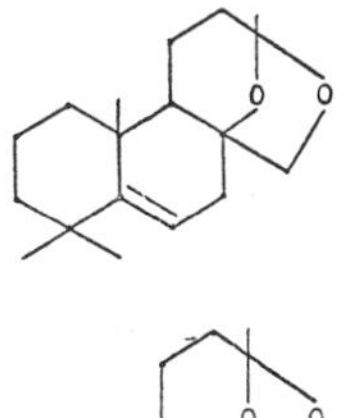

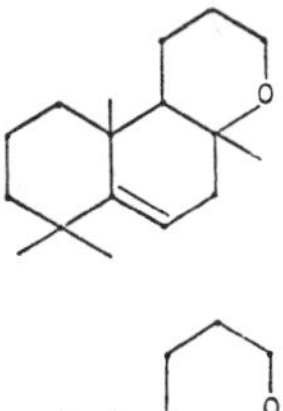

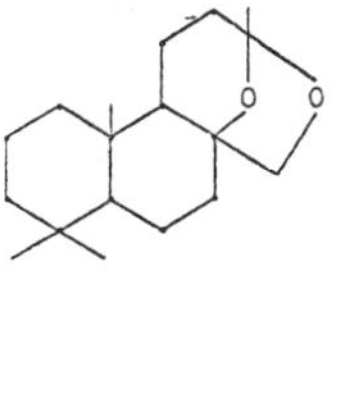

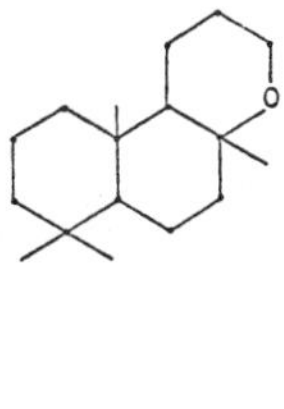

These odorants (3) and (4) are derivable from the odorants (1) and (2), respectively, by hydrogenating the 5,6-double bond of the latter compounds. As far as they are known, these odorants have mainly been obtained starting from the relatively inaccessible, and accordingly costly, manool of the formula

(5)

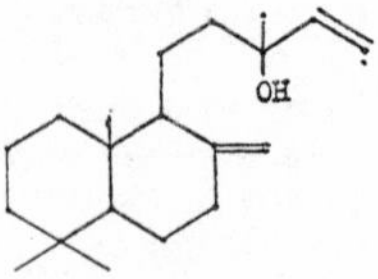

and sklareol of the formula

(6)

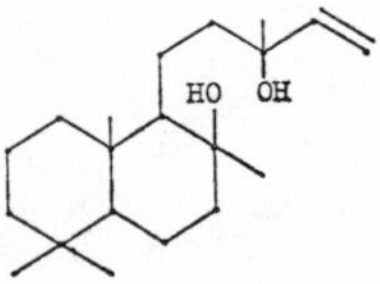

(cf, for example, *Parfumerie und Kosmetik* 1959, 40, 129). According to this process the amber-type odorants (1) and (2) are manufactured by converting the 8-methylidene group and the 9-hydroxyalkenyl group, together with the carbon atoms 8 and 9 to which they are attached, of a 4,4,10-trimethyldecahydronaphthalene derivative of the Formula (7)

(7)

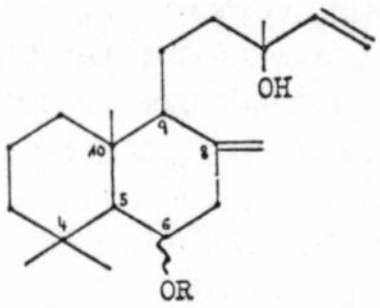

where R represents a hydrogen atom or the acetyl group, according to known methods into one of the odoriphoric groups

(8) 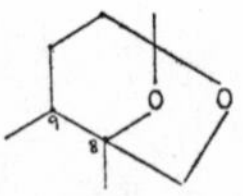   or   (9)

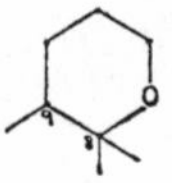

and then removing the hydroxy or acetoxy group OR with concomitant introduction of a 5,6-double bond. The naphthalene derivative of Formula (7), which may be named larixol (R is hydrogen) or larixyl acetate (R is acetyl), can be readily obtained from the resin of larch. Larixol occurs in larch balsam in a percentage of 30% and more (see *Angewandte Chemie*, 1947, 59, 248; *Chemische Berichte*, 1960, 93, 2625; *Bull. Soc. Chim. France* 1961, 1490) and can be readily obtained therefrom in crystalline form.

Alkyl-Substituted Unsaturated Acetals

A.A. Schleppnik and J.B. Wilson; U.S. Patent 3,751,486; August 7, 1973; assigned to Monsanto Company describe alkyl-substituted unsaturated acetals of the formula

$$R_1-CH_2-CH=\underset{\underset{R_2}{|}}{C}-CH+OR)_2$$

where R, R_1 and R_2 represent lower alkyl groups. The compounds are prepared by reacting an alpha, beta-unsaturated aldehyde with a lower alkanol in the presence of the corresponding alkyl ester selected from the group consisting of trialkyl orthoformates, tetraalkyl orthosilicates and dialkyl sulfites and a catalytic amount of ammonium nitrate. The compounds have very pleasant strong green, floral, woody odors and are useful as components in fragrance compositions. The following examples illustrate the process.

Example 1: 1,1-Dimethoxy-2-Ethyl-2-Hexene — To a refluxing solution of 2.0 g of ammonium nitrate in 100 ml of anhydrous methanol were added, with good agitation, a mixture of 63.1 g (0.5 mol) of 2-ethyl-2-hexenal and 63.6 g (0.6 mol) or trimethylorthoformate. The resulting mixture was refluxed for 16 hours.

The reaction mass was allowed to cool to room temperature and was then poured into 250 milliliters of a 2%, by weight, sodium carbonate solution. The resulting solution was extracted twice with benzene. The benzene extract was washed once with water, once with a saturated sodium chloride solution and dried over magnesium sulfate. The benzene was distilled off resulting in a product that had a boiling point of about 36° to 37°C at 0.35 mm Hg, and upon analysis was found to be 1,1-dimethoxy-2-ethyl-2-hexene.

Example 2: 1,1-Dimethoxy-2-n-Butyl-2-Octene — To a mixture of 35.6 g of 2-n-butyloct-2-en-1-al (0.195 mol), 21.2 g (0.20 mol) of trimethylorthoformate and 30 ml of methanol was added a hot solution of 0.8 g ammonium nitrate and 10 ml of methanol. The resulting mixture was heated to reflux for 3 hours. The solution turned greenish and then amber after 3 hours.

Gas-liquid chromatography demonstrated that almost all of the starting material had been consumed. The mixture was allowed to cool to room temperature, treated with 100 ml of 2%, by weight, sodium carbonate solution and the organic material was extracted with benzene. The resulting benzene extract solution was washed with water and concentrated sodium chloride solution followed by drying over sodium sulfate. The solvent was removed by distillation and the residue distilled through a short column. The resulting product had a boiling point of about 77° to 79°C at 0.7 mm Hg. The yield of the product was 36.13 g or about 79%. Upon analysis the product was determined to be 1,1-dimethoxy-2-n-butyl-2-octene.

2-Alkyl-3-(2-Norbornyl)Propanals

A.A. Schleppnik; U.S. Patent 3,780,109; December 18, 1973; assigned to Monsanto Company describes 2-alkyl-3-(2'-norbornyl)propanals which are characterized by the structural formula

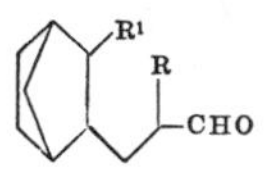

where R^1 represents hydrogen or methyl, and R represents a lower alkyl group. These compounds are prepared by a crossed aldol condensation of 5-norbornene-2-carboxaldehyde or norbornane-2-carboxaldehyde with aliphatic aldehyde in a basic medium. The resulting product is dehydrated to form the 2-alkyl-3-(2'-norbornenyl)prop-2-en-1-als which are subsequently hydrogenated. The compounds have very pleasant, strong and long lasting woody odors and are useful as compounds in fragrance compositions.

Cyclopentadecane Carboxylic Acid Esters

Y. Bonnet and G. Vivant; U.S. Patent 3,330,854; July 11, 1967; assigned to Rhone-Poulenc SA, France describe cycloalkane and cycloalkene carboxylic acids and their esters of the following formula.

(1)

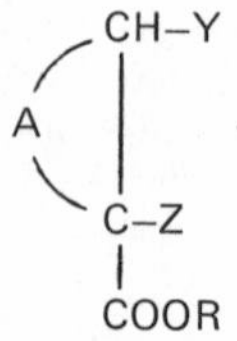

$$A \begin{cases} CH-Y \\ | \\ C-Z \\ | \\ COOR \end{cases}$$

In the above formula Y and Z are each hydrogen or together represent a single bond, R is hydrogen or lower alkyl, and A is an alkylene radical containing more than 3 carbon atoms between the two indicated valence bonds. These compounds are prepared by a process which comprises reacting a sulfonic ester of the formula:

(2)

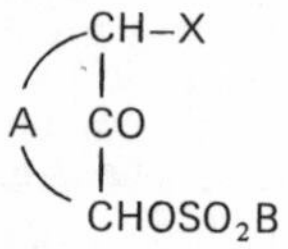

$$A \begin{cases} CH-X \\ | \\ CO \\ | \\ CHOSO_2B \end{cases}$$

where X represents hydrogen or halogen and B represents a hydrocarbon radical, with an alkali metal hydroxide or alkoxide in an organic or aqueous organic medium. Esters such as methyl cyclopentadecane carboxylate and methyl cycloundecane carboxylate possess very characteristic odors and may be used in perfumery. The following examples illustrate the process.

Example 1: In a 500 cc spherical flask provided with a reflux condenser, 20.5 g of 2-oxo-cyclohexadecyl tosylate are dissolved in 50 cc of ethanol, and a solution of 16.8 g of potassium hydroxide in 200 cc of ethanol is added. The mixture is heated under reflux for 5 hours and the ethanol is then driven off and replaced by 200 cc of water. After extraction of neutral products with 2 x 250 cc of diethyl ether, the aqueous fraction is acidified by the addition of 50% hydrochloric acid, and the oily phase formed is extracted with 2 x 250 cc of diethyl ether.

This ethereal fraction leaves, after drying over anhydrous sodium sulfate followed by elimination of the ether, a crystalline residue weighing 10.5 g, MP 52° to 54°C, which is identified by chemical and infrared spectrographical analysis as cyclopentadecane carboxylic acid (yield 84%). On esterification with methanol in the presence of sulfuric acid it gives methyl cyclopentadecane carboxylate, BP 156° to 159°C 1 mm Hg. This ester has a woody odor and can be used in perfumery.

The sulfonic ester employed as starting material was prepared in the following way. Into a 250 cc spherical flask are introduced 25.1 g of cyclohexadecan-2-ol-1-one [prepared by the process described by *Stoll Helv. Chim. Acta* 30, 1820 (1947)] in solution in 15 cc of anhydrous pyridine. There are added 37.7 g of toluene-p-sulfonyl chloride in solution in 75 g of pyridine, and the flask is then purged with nitrogen and left at ambient temperature for 15 hours.

The product is neutralized with 50% hydrochloric acid with cooling. The reaction mass is treated with 3 x 150 cc of benzene and the benzene phase is separated. After elimination of the benzene in vacuo, there is obtained a solid residue which, on recrystallization from 125 cc of petroleum ether and then from 150 cc of methanol and drying at ambient temperature in vacuo (0.5 mm Hg), gives 26.5 g of product melting at 64°C, which is identified by chemical analysis and its infrared spectrum as 2-oxocyclohexadecyl tosylate (yield 65%).

Example 2: 30.2 g of 2-oxocyclododecyl tosylate are dissolved in 100 cc of ethanol, 27 grams of potassium hydroxide in solution in 300 cc of ethanol are added to this solution and the mixture is heated under reflux for 3 hours. After acidification of the reaction mass, followed by extraction with diethyl ether as in the preceding example, there are obtained 10.5 g of cycloundecane carboxylic acid having a boiling point of 118°C 0.06 mm Hg (yield 70%). The sulfonic ester employed as starting material was prepared from 2-hydroxycyclododecanone obtained as by-product, in a yield of 30%, in the preparation of cycloundecane carboxylic acid from 2-bromo-cyclododecanone by the process described in French Patent 1,264,032.

In a 250 cc spherical flask, 19.8 g (0.1 mol) of 2-hydroxycyclododecanone are dissolved in 120 cc of pyridine, 0.2 mol of tosyl chloride is added, and the reaction mass is allowed to stand for 18 hours under a nitrogen atmosphere. By thereafter treating the reaction mass under the same conditions as in the preceding example, there are obtained 30.2 g of 2-oxo-cyclododecyl tosylate, MP 114°C (yield 86%).

Example 3: By proceeding as in Example 2, but replacing tosyl chloride by an equivalent quantity of mesyl chloride, there are obtained from 15 g of 2-hydroxycyclododecanone 13 g of 2-mesyloxycyclododecanone, MP 108°C (yield 62%), which on alkaline treatment gives 6.5 g of cycloundecane carboxylic acid (yield 71%).

Nopyl Phenylacetate

According to a process described by *H.G. Gribou and A.A. Schleppnik; U.S. Patent 3,729,503; April 24, 1973; assigned to Monsanto Company* esters of terpene alcohols with organic acids are prepared in neutral or alkaline medium in order to avoid acid catalyzed dehydration and/or skeletal rearrangements. Organic acid halides, anhydrides or esters are used as acylating agents under the proper conditions. The terpene esters have a characteristic long lasting floral-woody aroma and are useful in the production of perfumes and perfume products. The following examples illustrate the process.

Example 1: A mixture of 450 g of methyl phenylacetate and 500 g of nopol (3 mols each), containing 500 mg of sodium hydride was slowly heated with stirring to a pot temperature of 190°C. Methanol (100 ml) was distilled off through a short, heated, Vigreux-type column. Vacuum was then applied and product, after a small forerun, was collected at 176°C/3 mm, as a colorless liquid. The yield of nopyl phenylacetate was 796.4 g (97.6%). A second run afforded 97% yield of the product, which had a boiling point of 157°C/1.2 mm.

Example 2: A mixture of 162.2 g of methyl cinnamate and 162.2 g of nopol containing 500 mg of sodium methoxide was slowly heated with stirring to a pot temperature of 190°C. Methanol (100 ml) was distilled off through a short, heated, Vigreux-type column. Vacuum was then applied and nopyl cinnamate, after a small forerun, was collected as a liquid, BP 174°C/0.5 mm.

Example 3: A typical rose for perfumes and colognes, comprising nopyl phenylacetate, is set forth below.

Ingredient	Parts by Weight
Nopyl phenylacetate	50
Geraniol	350
Rhodinol	100
Citronellol	100
Ionone alpha	100
Jasmine absolute	100
Nerol	20
Phenyl ethyl alcohol	250
	1,000

The rose has a pleasant long-lasting floral fragrance having a woody note.

Epoxidized Linalyl Esters

A process described by *J.A. Brydon and L.J. Colaianni; U.S. Patent 3,573,331; March 30,*

1971; assigned to Givaudan Corporation relates to the epoxidation of aliphatic and aryl acid esters of 2,6-dimethyl-2,7-octadien-6-ol, hereinafter referred to as linalyl esters. The epoxides are useful in perfumery, for example, as odorants in the compounding of perfumes and other scented compositions by virtue of their fine fragrances. More particularly, the process comprises preparing a compound of the formula

(1)
$$\underset{CH_3\quad O}{\overset{R_1\qquad R_2\qquad\qquad OOCR}{C\text{---}C\text{-}CH_2\text{-}CH_2\text{-}C\text{-}CH\text{=}CH_2}}$$

where R is H, lower alkyl or aryl, R_1 is lower alkyl and R_2 is hydrogen or methyl, by treating a compound of the formula

(2)
$$\underset{CH_3}{\overset{R_1\qquad R_2\qquad\qquad OOCR}{C\text{=}C\text{-}CH_2\text{-}CH_2\text{-}C\text{-}CH\text{=}CH_2}}$$

where R, R_1 and R_2 have the same significance as above with an aqueous preparation of perphthalic acid, containing sufficient water to act as an aqueous, solvent, reaction medium for the epoxidation reaction. The following examples illustrate the process. Temperatures are stated in degrees Centigrade.

Example 1: A 12 liter three neck, round bottom flask, equipped with agitator and thermometer, containing 4,500 cc water was cooled to 0°C with an external bath and 527 g sodium perborate (3.42 mols) and 520 g phthalic anhydride (3.54 mols) were added. Stirring was continued for 2 hours at 0°C. Then 250 cc aqueous sulfuric acid 30% w/w and 500 g ice were added. Then 517 g linalyl acetate (2.63 mols) was added rapidly while cooling with an external ice bath to keep the temperature below +10°C.

Stirring was continued for 1 hour. The contents of the flask were transferred to a large agitated separating funnel and solid sodium carbonate was added until the pH of the solution was alkaline. 300 cc of toluene was added and the water layer extracted. The water layer was separated and extracted with 2 x 200 cc of toluene. The toluene layers were combined and washed with 2 x 100 cc of 10% salt water. The toluene fractions were concentrated and distilled to give 3-acetoxy-3,7-dimethyl-6,7-epoxy-1-octene (linalyl acetate epoxide).

Example 2: A 5 liter, three neck flask with agitator and thermometer containing 2,500 cc of water was cooled to 0°C with a Dry Ice bath and 527 g of sodium perborate and 535 g of phthalic anhydride were added. The mixture was stirred at 0°C for 3 hours. The aqueous sulfuric acid (30%) was added until the mixture became strongly acid. 1 liter of ether was added to the aqueous acid solution and the mixture stirred for 1 hour at 0°C. To the stirring acid mixture there was added 517 g of linalyl acetate (1.96 mol) and stirring was continued for 1 hour without cooling.

The entire aqueous mixture was transferred to a large open separatory funnel containing 2.5 liters of water. Sufficient sodium carbonate monohydrate powder was added to bring the mixture to alkaline pH. The water and ether were separated. The water layer was extracted with 3 x 200 cc of ether.

The ether layers were combined and washed with 100 cc of sodium thiosulfate solution 1% and washed neutral with 2 x 100 cc of salt water (10%). The ether solution was concentrated and distilled under vacuum to give 3-acetoxy-3,7-dimethyl-6,7-epoxy-1-octene (linalyl acetate epoxide). This procedure can also be employed to produce the corresponding compounds in which R is ethyl, propyl, caproic, salicylic, cinnamic or phenyl, by use of corresponding linalyl ester starting materials.

Bicyclo[10.1.0] Tridec-1-yl Alkyl Ethers

P. Nageli; U.S. Patent 3,754,039; August 21, 1973; assigned to Givaudan Corporation describes bicyclo[10.1.0] tridec-1-yl alkyl ethers which possess woody amber-like odors. Certain derivatives of cyclododecane are known to have odorant properties. Ethyl 4,8-cyclo-dodecadiene-1-carboxylate has a woody, vetiver oil-like odor. Ketals of cyclododecanone possess odors reminiscent of cedar and sandalwood with musk and ambrette notes and certain ethers of cyclododecanol possess cedar and musk odors. While bicyclo[10.1.0] tridecane derivatives have been prepared, the 13-alkyl-1-ether derivatives have not been prepared previously. This process is concerned with bicyclic ethers of the cyclododecane series of the general formula

(I)

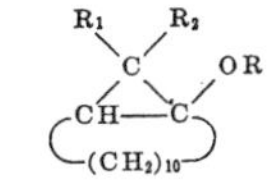

where R signifies an alkyl group containing 1 to 4 carbon atoms (such as methyl, ethyl, propyl, isopropyl, normal or branched butyl) and R_1 as well as R_2 independently of each other signify hydrogen, methyl or ethyl. The compounds of general Formula (I) are distinguished by particular odor properties (warm-woody, amber to musk-like notes with good adhesion) on the basis of which they can be used for perfumery purposes such as manufacture of perfumes or for perfuming products of all kinds such as cosmetic articles (soaps, powders, creams, lotions, etc.). The compounds of Formula (I) can be obtained by:
(a) adding to the olefinic double bond of a compound of the general formula

(II)

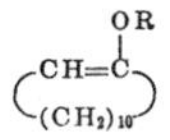

where R signifies the same as above, a group of the general formula

(III)

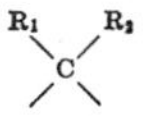

where R_1 and R_2 signify the same as above; or by:
(b) replacing the halogen atoms of a compound of the general formula

(IV)

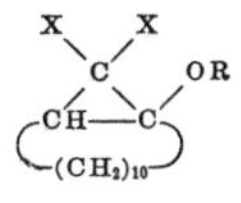

where R has the above significance and X signifies a halogen atom (especially chlorine or bromine), by hydrogen, methyl or ethyl. The processes may be schematically summarized as follows:

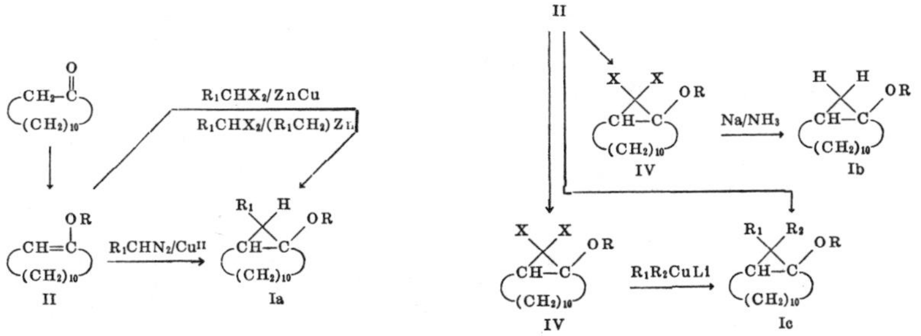

The following examples illustrate the process. In the examples all temperatures are in degrees centigrade.

Example 1: (a) 9.8 g of zinc copper alloy are stirred with a few crystals of iodine for about 15 minutes in 100 ml of absolute ether until the iodine color disappears. 9.86 g of 1-methoxy-1-cyclododecene and 40.2 g of freshly distilled methylene iodide are thereupon rapidly added. The mixture is heated under reflux in nitrogen atmosphere with good stirring for 48 hours.

Filtration from the residue, rinsing thereof with a large amount of ether, thereupon washing of the combined ether phases three times with saturated ammonium chloride solution and subsequently with saturated bicarbonate solution give, after drying and concentration, 11 g of a product which is distilled at 80°C/0.001 mm Hg. The bicyclo[10.1.0] tridec-1-yl methyl ether thus obtained [Formula (I): R = CH_3, R_1 = H, R_2 = H] is distinguished by a woody, warm, amber-like odor note.

(b) The 1-methoxy-1-cyclododecene used as the starting material can be manufactured as follows. 182 g of cyclododecanone and 117 g of orthoformic acid trimethyl ester are heated with stirring to 40°C until a clear yellowish solution exists. 1 ml of concentrated sulfuric acid is added dropwise and the mixture is immediately cooled to 20°C. The solution is subsequently stirred at room temperature for a further 15 to 20 hours. After the addition of 3 ml of triethylamine, the product is fractionated in vacuum. Yield of 1-methoxy-1-cyclododecene was over 90%.

Example 2: According to the process described in Example 1 or in the following Example 3, but using 1-ethoxy-1-cyclododecene as the starting material, there is obtained bicyclo-[10.1.0] tridec-1-yl ethyl ether. The odor of this product displays the woody, amber-like note of the methyl ether described in Example 1, but is somewhat weaker.

Example 3: 400 ml of an ethereal diazoethane solution are added dropwise within 30 min with ice-cooling and stirring to 16.6 g of 1-methoxy-1-cyclododecene and 1 g of anhydrous $CuSO_4$. Overnight, the mixture is further stirred at room temperature. The ethereal solution is then dried with a little anhydrous magnesium sulfate, filtered and evaporated. The resulting oily crude product (17.9 g) is chromatographed on the 50 fold amount by weight of silica gel. The desired product is eluted with benzene and further purified by preparative gas chromatography. The odor of the 13-methyl-bicyclo[10.1.0] tridec-1-yl methyl ether [Formula (I): R = CH_3, R_1 = H, R_2 = CH_3] thus obtained is weakly woody, musk-like.

3,3-Trimethylcyclohexane Methyl Alkanoates

J.H. Blumenthal; U.S. Patent 3,487,102; December 30, 1969; assigned to International Flavors & Fragrances Inc. describes a number of compounds represented by the formulas

where R is H or an acyl group containing no more than 4 carbon atoms. These compounds are formed by treating dihydromyrcene (3,7-dimethyl-1,6-octadiene) with formic acid alone or with a lower carboxylic acid or water in the presence of an acid catalyst, such as sulfuric acid, phosphoric acid, polyphosphoric acid, a Lewis acid, or a sulfonic acid resin.

A rearrangement occurs to yield the compounds, namely esters of α,3,3-trimethylcyclohexane methanol and the alcohol itself. Compound (II) above is formed by oxidation of the alcohol α,3,3-trimethylcyclohexane methanol. In carrying out the above process for producing compound (I) where water is present, more or less alcohol is formed.

The course of the reaction is shown as follows.

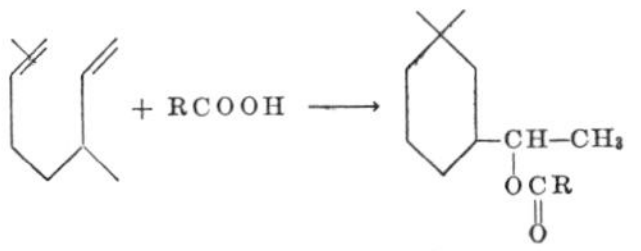

Any water present can either form the alcohol directly or can hydrolyze the ester formed to produce quantities of the corresponding alcohol. Although the reaction may be performed in aqueous solution, higher conversions are obtained in refluxing formic acid or by the use of the catalysts mentioned above in formic or other carboxylic acids. The following examples illustrate the process.

Example 1: To a stirred mixture of 422 g of dihydromyrcene (94%) and 307 g of 90% formic acid was added 44 g of BF_3-etherate over a period of 10 minutes. The mixture was stirred at 50°C for 4 hours. The heat was then removed and stirring continued for another 30 minutes. An equal volume of water was added and the oil layer separated.

The oil layer contained the formate ester. The water layer was extracted with benzene and the combined organic layers washed neutral. After the solvent was stripped off, the residue weighed 490 g and tested 66.6% as the formate ester. Fractionation yielded $\alpha,3,3$-trimethylcyclohexane methyl formate, BP 70°C/3 mm. The formate had a woody, minty, rosy odor. It is represented by the formula:

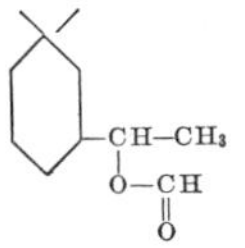

Example 2: The crude ester (500 g) prepared as in Example 1, was refluxed with a solution of 500 g of methanol, 200 g of sodium hydroxide 50%, and 58 g of water for 1.5 hours. Another 100 g of water was added to the reaction mixture and the methanol was stripped off to 90°C at atmospheric pressure. The residue was washed with water, 1% acetic acid and water. The dried residue weighed 355 g and tested 76% as the alcohol. Fractionation yielded $\alpha,3,3$-trimethylcyclohexane methanol, BP 100°C/10 mm. The product had a sweet, pungent, minty, camphoraceous odor. It is represented by the formula:

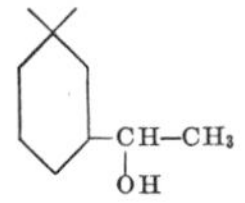

Formate Esters from Cyclooctene and Cyclooctadiene

A process described by *B.J. Heywood and O. Meresz; U.S. Patent 3,652,656; March 28, 1972; assigned to May & Baker Limited, England* relates to formate esters, to processes for their preparation and to their use in perfumery.

The Prins reaction, i.e., the acid catalyzed reaction of aldehydes such as formaldehyde and acetaldehyde with olefins, has previously been used to prepare many different types of organic compounds including alcohols, diols, monoesters, diesters, m-dioxans and cyclic ethers. A typical example is the application of the Prins reaction to cyclohexene utilizing formaldehyde and acetic acid to give 2-acetoxymethylcyclohexyl acetate originally studied by S. Olsen and H. Padberg, *Naturforsch.* I 448 to 458 (1946) and subsequently by other workers.

This diester does not possess properties useful in perfumery products. It has been found that the Prins reaction is applied to an eight membered monocyclic hydrocarbon containing one or two olefinic linkages (i.e., cyclooctene or a cyclooctadiene), optionally carrying one or two methyl groups, utilizing formaldehyde and formic acid, a reaction which has not previously been described, a transannular reaction occurs and diformate esters are produced which are useful in perfumery.

Thus, there are provided new diformates which are obtained by reacting an unsaturated hydrocarbon selected from cyclooctene and cyclooctadiene, optionally carrying one or two methyl groups on carbon atoms not forming part of an olefinic linkage, with formaldehyde, or a compound which liberates formaldehyde (for example, paraformaldehyde or methylal), in the presence of formic acid, and separating from the reaction mixture the diformate or diformates so produced.

The diformates possess very interesting odors and have proved to be very versatile and extremely useful in the formulation of various types of perfumery products. For example, they may be used in formulations in place of orris concrete, an expensive natural perfumery material. Preferred products of the process are those obtained from cyclooctene and cyclooctadiene unsubstituted by methyl groups. Individual products of particular value are:

(a) 4-formoxymethylcyclooctyl formate, the single diformate ester which can be isolated from the reaction of cyclooctene with formaldehyde and formic acid;

(b) the diformate fraction $C_{11}H_{16}O_4$ isolated from the reaction of cycloocta-1,5-diene with formaldehyde and formic acid, BP 90° to 110°C/0.05 to 0.2 millimeters Hg. The fraction is a complex mixture of diformates, two of which, 3-formoxymethylcyclooct-5-enyl formate and 6-formoxymethylcyclooct-3-enyl formate, are particularly important in producing the valuable properties of the mixture; and

(c) the diformate fraction $C_{11}H_{16}O_4$ isolated from the reaction of cycloocta-1,3-diene with formaldehyde and formic acid, BP 170° to 178°C/22 mm Hg. The fraction is a mixture of two diformates, 4-formoxymethylcyclooct-2-enyl formate and 2-formoxymethylcyclooct-7-enyl formate.

The following examples illustrate the preparation of the products of the process.

Example 1: Paraformaldehyde (93.8 g) and formic acid (90% w/w aqueous solution, 350 milliliters) were stirred and heated just to reflux. The heating was stopped and cis,cis-cycloocta-1,5-diene (220 g) was added with vigorous stirring over 6 minutes. The resulting exothermic reaction caused spontaneous refluxing to occur. On complete addition the mixture was refluxed for 4 hours, during which time it darkened and the paraformaldehyde dissolved.

After cooling, the mixture was diluted with water (1.75 liters), and extracted with methylene chloride (700 ml). The organic phase was separated, washed sequentially with water (250 ml) and saturated sodium bicarbonate solution (250 ml), then dried over magnesium sulfate. The desiccant was removed by filtration, and the filtrate evaporated in vacuo. The residue was distilled through a 6 inch Vigreux column under vacuum to give the following fractions:

Fraction A-1: BP 55° to 142°C at 17 mm Hg, 67 g
Fraction A-2: BP 142° to 197°C at 17 mm Hg, 200 g
Fraction B-1: BP 75° to 95°C at 0.06 mm Hg, 21 g
Fraction B-2: BP 95° to 100°C at 0.06 mm Hg, 141 g (33% calculated as $C_{11}H_{16}O_4$).

Fraction A-2 was redistilled under high vacuum through a 6 inch Vigreux column to give Fraction B-1 and B-2. Fraction B-2 was a colorless liquid possessing a persistent orris odor with a suggestion of methyl heptine carbonate, density d_4^{22} 1.148 g/ml, refractive index n_D^{21} 1.4865. The corresponding diol mixture was prepared by hydrolysis of Fraction B-2 using potassium hydroxide in methanol. Examination of this diol mixture by gas-liquid chromatography (0.5% diethylene glycol succinate polymer stationary phase on Chromosorb G 70-80 mesh support; column temperature 150°C) revealed that it consisted of seven main components.

The structure, physical data and method of separation of the diformate components are given in the table below. Phenylurethane derivatives were prepared by known methods from the separated diols, themselves prepared either by hydrolysis of the diformate mixture and separation from the mixture of the diols obtained, or by hydrolysis of the separated diformates obtained from the diformate mixture.

Hydrolysis in either case is effected with potassium hydroxide in methanol. The structural formulas of the components were elucidated by nuclear magnetic resonance spectroscopy and mass spectroscopy. Olfactory examination of the various components of Fraction B-2 indicated that the components 6 and 7 imparted on the mixture the valuable orris-like odor.

Component	Structure	Diformate component	Approx. percent-age in mixture	Melting point of phenyl-urethane deriva-tive, °C.	Method of separation
1	CH_2OCOH / $HOCO-$ bicyclic structure	Endo-4-formoxy-1-formoxy-methyl-cis-bicyclo-[3.3.0.]-octane.	6	....	Counter-current distributions on low boiling fractions from distillation of ester mixture, followed by repeated chromatography on Florisil.
2	CH_2OCOH / $-OCOH$ cyclooctenyl structure	Trans-2-formoxy-methyl-cy-clooct-5-enyl formate.	3	168.5–170	Chromatography of a main distillation fraction from efficient fractionation of the mixture, using $AgNO_3$ impregnated silica gel column.
3	$HOCO$ / CH_2OCOH bicyclic structure	Endo-2-formoxy-exo-6-formoxy-methyl-cis-bicyclo-[3.3.0.]octane.	14	168–169	Counter-current distributions on certain hydrolysed high-boiling fractions from the distillation of the ester mixture, followed by column chromatography on silica gel.
4	$HOCO$ / CH_2OCOH bicyclic structure	Exo-2-formoxy-endo-6-formoxy-methyl-cis-bicyclo[3.3.0.]octane.	22	175–176	Counter-current distributions on diol mixture.
5	$HOCO \!-\!H$ / CH_2OCOH bicyclo structure	Endo-8-formoxy-endo-2-formoxy-methyl-bicyclo [3.2.1.]octane.	18	178–179	Counter-current distributions and column chromatographies on a hydrolysed main distillation fraction from efficient fractionation of ester mixture.
6	CH_2OCOH / $-OCOH$ cyclooctenyl structure	3-formoxymethyl cyclooct-5-enyl formate (main component).	14	....	Chromatography on $AgNO_3$ impregnated silica-gel column from a high-boiling fraction from efficient fractionation of ester mixture.
7	CH_2OCOH / $OCOH$ cyclooctenyl structure	6-formoxymethyl cyclooct-3-enyl formate.	12	193	Alternate counter-current distributions and column chromatographies on hydrolysed residue from efficient fractionation of ester mixture.

Example 2: Paraformaldehyde (451 g) and formic acid (98 to 100% w/w; 2,500 ml) were heated together under reflux until all solid had dissolved. The solution was cooled to room temperature and cis,cis-cycloocta-1,5-diene (1,080 g) was added. The mixture was stirred vigorously for 3 days at room temperature, during which time the heterogeneous mixture became homogeneous. Excess formic acid was removed in vacuo keeping the temperature below 40°C and the residue distilled to give the following fractions.

Fraction A-1: BP below 90°C at 0.5 mm Hg, 720 g
Fraction A-2: BP 90° to 126°C at 0.5 mm Hg, 1,070 g
Fraction B-1: BP below 102°C at 0.2 mm Hg, 90 g
Fraction B-2: BP 102° to 109°C at 0.2 mm Hg, 787 g; 37% yield,
     calculated as $C_{11}H_{16}O_4$.

Fraction A-2 was redistilled through a 35 cm vacuum jacketed Widmer column to give Fractions B-1 and B-2. Fraction B-2 had an identical odor to that of Fraction B-2 in Example 1.

Myrcene Sulfone Hydrate

J.H. Blumenthal; U.S. Patent 3,176,022; March 30, 1965; assigned to International Flavors & Fragrances Inc. describes a process which involves the reaction product of myrcene with sulfur dioxide to produce myrcene sulfone, and then hydration of the myrcene sulfone with an aqueous mineral acid to produce myrcene sulfone hydrate.

This myrcene sulfone hydrate is then decomposed by heating it to liberate sulfur dioxide, and thereby to produce the compound 2-methyl-6-methylene-7-octene-2-ol in pure form. The sulfur dioxide is the usual product which is substantially anhydrous. The myrcene is a commercial product ordinarily found on the market containing approximately 75% myrcene together with other terpenes, notably dipentene, as impurities. The reaction occurring as above indicated is as follows.

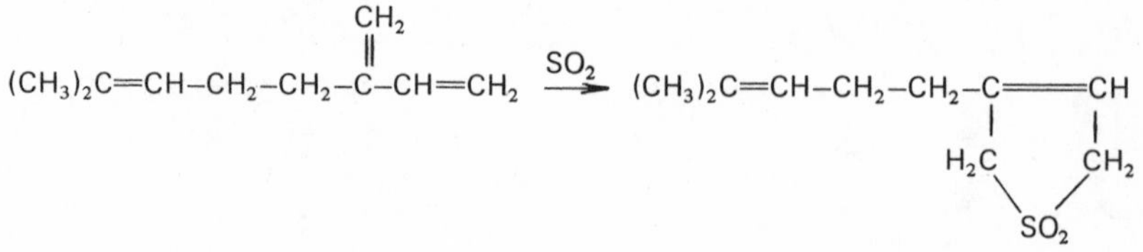

Myrcene   Myrcene Sulfone

The crude sulfone is then hydrated at the isopropylidene double bond. The reaction mixture is then separated into an oil layer and water layer. The oil layer is separated with the aid of a solvent such as benzene, and the solvent removed under vacuum. The reaction occurring here is:

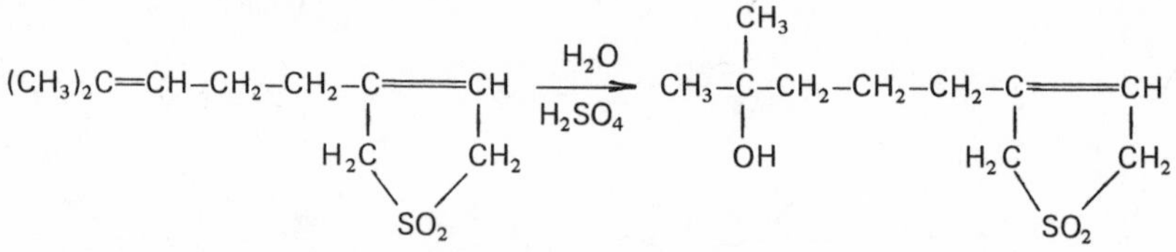

Myrcene Sulfone   Myrcene Sulfone Hydrate

The crude sulfone hydrate is then decomposed by heating under vacuum at 120° to 170°C to obtain the desired hydrate, 2-methyl-6-methylene-7-octene-2-ol. The following examples illustrate the process. The myrcene used (approximately 75% myrcene) in the examples is the usual product of commerce obtained from the pyrolysis of β-pinene, and contains other terpenes, notably dipentene, as impurities.

Example 1: *(A) Preparation of Myrcene Sulfone –* 1,200 g of commercial myrcene (75% myrcene) and 1,200 g of anhydrous sulfur dioxide and 10 g of Ionol (2,6-ditertiary butyl-p-cresol) were placed in a 4 liter stainless steel autoclave and stirred at 70°C for 2 hours. The reaction mass was cooled and the excess sulfur dioxide vented.

The residue was stripped of any unreacted materials by distillation at 5 mm to a liquid (pot) temperature of 82°C. The weight of the residue was 1,322 g and by analysis, consisted of 95% myrcene sulfone. Yield: 94.5% of theory (based on myrcene content of commercial myrcene). The crude sulfone was fractionated in a wiping still with final pressure and temperature at 20 to 30 microns vacuum and at 80° to 90°C. Characteristics of the distilled myrcene sulfone, at least 99% pure, are as follows: very pale yellow heavy oil n_D^{20} 1.5069, water-insoluble, generally soluble in usual organic solvents; limited solubility in hydrocarbon solvents, sulfur 15.9% obtained, theoretical 16.0%.

(B) Hydration of Myrcene Sulfone — 400 g of crude myrcene sulfone as prepared in Example 1 (A) was stirred vigorously with 1,200 g of 50% (by weight) sulfuric acid for a period of one-half hour at 20°C. The reaction mass was added to 2,400 cc of cold water and some polymeric material was separated and discarded. The acid was carefully neutralized to pH 8 with sodium hydroxide while keeping the temperature below 50°C, with cooling and good stirring. The oil layer which formed was separated with the aid of some benzene and the water layer was extracted with additional benzene. The benzene solutions were combined and the benzene plus traces of water were removed under a vacuum of 5 mm to a liquid temperature of 70°C.

The weight of the residue (crude sulfone hydrate) was 384 g, and by analysis consisted of 93% of the sulfone hydrate. Yield 86% of theory (based on myrcene sulfone used). The crude myrcene sulfone hydrate was distilled in the wiping still with final pressure and temperature at 20 microns vacuum and 90° to 95°C and the distilled myrcene sulfone hydrate was at least 98.5% pure. Its characteristics are as follows: pale yellow viscous oil n_D^{20} 1.5020, partially soluble in water at 25°C; soluble in ether and in benzene; insoluble in hexane; sulfur 14.5% obtained, theoretical 14.68%.

(C) Decomposition of Myrcene Sulfone Hydrate and Production of 2-Methyl-6-Methylene-7-Octen-2-ol — 96 g of the sulfone hydrate prepared as in Example 1 (B) was placed in a 200 ml flask fitted with a short column and a water condenser. The liquid temperature was brought to 140° to 160°C, and the myrcene hydrate distilled over at 85° to 100°C at a vacuum of 2 to 4 mm. The distillate weighed 57 g, and after being freed of traces of sulfur dioxide by purging with nitrogen had a refractive index of n_D^{20} 1.4729.

The gas-liquid partition chromatogram (GLPC) showed a purity of over 98%. Yield 88.5% of theory, based on myrcene sulfone hydrate used. The 2% impurity was mainly myrcene with no other alcohol present. Redistillation gave a pure water-white liquid product (as shown by the GLPC) BP 78°C (5 mm). The product has a fresh, slightly limey, flowery odor. The product is 2-methyl-6-methylene-7-octen-2-ol.

Since 2-methyl-6-methylene-7-octen-2-ol polymerizes readily, it should be protected at all times with an inhibitor such as hydroquinone, Ionol, phenyl-β-naphthylamine, etc. When working on a larger scale a continuous thin film evaporator is preferred for the decomposition to minimize the formation of by-odors. A dilute caustic wash, followed by a water wash, is also effective for the same purpose.

Example 2: Preparation of Acetate of Myrcene Hydrate — 750 g of acetic anhydride and 5.0 g of 85% phosphoric acid are placed in a suitable flask and heated to 40°C. To this solution at 40°C there is added over a period of 1 to 2 hours, 500 g of 2-methyl-6-methylene-7-octen-2-ol (containing 1% Ionol). After stirring for one additional hour after the completion of addition, sodium bicarbonate is added to neutralize the phosphoric acid, and stirring is continued for 1 hour.

The mass is then treated with two volumes of water with stirring for 30 minutes, and the oil which separates is washed neutral with sodium bicarbonate solution. Fractionation of this washed oil at 0.5 mm yields 450 g of the acetate of 2-methyl-6-methylene-7-octen-2-ol, a water-white liquid boiling at 53°C. The ester tests 99.4% by saponification. It should be protected with one of the usual polymerization inhibitors, as mentioned in Example 1 (C). The odor is an individual fresh, woody cologne odor, with a mossy undertone.

Further examples for the preparation of myrcene sulfone and myrcene sulfone hydrate are given below.

Example 3: (A) Preparation of Myrcene Sulfone — To 5,100 g of 76% myrcene and 20 g of Ionol (2,6-ditertiary butyl-p-cresol) in a 4 liter stainless steel autoclave was added, with stirring, 2,000 g of sulfur dioxide at 70° to 80°C over a 3 hour period. The reaction mixture was stirred at 80°C for another three hours, then cooled and the autoclave vented. The product was distilled (topped) at 5 mm to a liquid temperature of 70°C to remove unreacted terpenes to give a crude myrcene sulfone. The residue weighed 6,250 g and tested 88% as myrcene sulfone by infrared analysis.

(B) Hydration of Myrcene Sulfone — To 1,800 g of 50% sulfuric acid was added rapidly at 18°C 4.17 mols of topped myrcene sulfone (88% by IR analysis) prepared as in Example 3 (A). The reaction mixture was stirred at 20° to 22°C for 4 hours and then was added to a mixture of 2,500 g of 15% Na_2SO_4 solution and 400 g of benzene.

After stirring for 30 minutes, the layers were separated and the aqueous layer extracted three times with benzene. The combined organic layer was washed neutral with sodium bicarbonate solution (saturated with myrcene sulfone hydrate) and the solvent stripped off at 5 mm to a liquid temperature of 70°C. The residue weighed 1,070 g and contained 73.8% myrcene sulfone hydrate (87% of theory).

MUSK FRAGRANCES

NAPHTHALENE AND INDENE DERIVATIVES

Alkylmercapto Derivatives of Polyalkyltetrahydronaphthalenes

A process described by *R. Lusskin and J. Levy; U.S. Patent 3,297,764; January 10, 1967; assigned to Universal Oil Products Company* relates to alkylmercapto substituted acylated polyalkyltetrahydronaphthalenes. The alkylmercapto substituted, acylated polyalkyltetrahydronaphthalenes have many valuable properties, one of which is a musk-like odor making these compounds extremely useful in the perfume industry.

Compounds having musk-like odors are valuable in perfumery because in addition to their odor, they generally have fixative and blending properties useful in perfume formulating. The most valuable of these compounds are the macrocyclic musks which are organic compounds having 15 to 18 carbon atoms in an alicyclic ring such as muskone, civetone, pentadecanolide or ethylene brassylate.

These macrocyclic compounds, however, are not readily available because they either have to be extracted from not readily available natural sources or must be synthesized by difficult and complicated chemical processes. Accordingly, many types of compounds have been prepared which have musk-like odors as substitutes for the macrocyclic musks. One class of these compounds is known as nitro musks which are relatively easy to prepare and inexpensive, but generally have harsh odors.

Another class of these compounds are acylated polyalkyltetrahydronaphthalenes which possess extremely fine musk-like odors. The numerous compounds included within both of these classes generally do not contain sulfur substituents and it is, therefore, quite surprising that members of the class of compounds of this process which contain a sulfur substituent have musk-like odors. Examples of these compounds include 1,1,4,4-tetramethyl-6-acetyl-7-methylmercapto-1,2,3,4-tetrahydronaphthalene; 1,1,2,4,4-pentamethyl-6-acetyl-7-methylmercapto-1,2,3,4-tetrahydronaphthalene; and 1,1,2,3,4,4-hexamethyl-6-acetyl-7-methylmercapto-1,2,3,4-tetrahydronaphthalene.

The compositions can be prepared by reacting a dialkyldisulfide with a polyalkyltetrahydronaphthalene in the presence of a catalyst followed by acylation of the alkylmercapto substituted polyalkyltetrahydronaphthalene thus obtained with a acyl halide in the presence of a catalyst. The following examples illustrate the process.

Example 1: 1,1,4,4-tetramethyl-6-acetyl-7-methylmercapto-1,2,3,4-tetrahydronaphthalene was prepared according to the process by charging 37.6 g (0.2 mol) of 1,1,4,4-tetramethyl-1,2,3,4-tetrahydronaphthalene, 4.7 g (0.05 mol) of dimethyldisulfide and 13.3 g (0.1 mol) of aluminum chloride to a reaction flask equipped with a thermometer and stirring means. The mixture was stirred at about 25°C for about 23 hr, at which time the mixture was poured with stirring onto about 200 g of ice.

As the ice melted, an aqueous layer and an organic layer formed and the aqueous layer was separated and any soluble organic material contained therein extracted with about 90 grams of benzene. The benzene extract was then combined with the organic layer and distilled to remove the benzene. The residue was fractionated to recover 7.0 g of 1,1,4,4-tetramethyl-7-methylmercapto-1,2,3,4-tetrahydronaphthalene.

A 4.68 g (0.02 mol) sample of the methylmercapto substituted polyalkyltetrahydronaphthalene thus prepared was acetylated by adding it to a reaction flask containing 2.26 g (0.029 mol) of acetyl chloride and 31 g of ethylene dichloride. The flask was cooled in an ice bath and 5.32 g (0.04 mol) of aluminum chloride were added over a period of about 5 minutes. The resultant mixture was stirred for about 1.5 hr during which time the temperature rose to about 25°C. The entire contents of the flask were then poured with stirring onto about 150 g of ice.

As the ice melted, an aqueous layer and an organic layer formed and the aqueous layer was separated and any soluble organic material contained therein extracted with about 50 g of ethylene dichloride. The ethylene dichloride extract was then combined with the organic layer and washed with about 50 g of water. The resultant, washed organic mixture was filtered and evaporated to obtain 5.0 g of a heavy oil which solidified upon cooling. The solids were recrystallized twice from methanol to give 1.8 g of 1,1,4,4-tetramethyl-6-acetyl-7-methylmercapto-1,2,3,4-tetrahydronaphthalene having a melting point of 94.4° to 97.0°C. This material had a musk-like odor.

Example 2: 1,1,2,4,4-pentamethyl-6-acetyl-7-methylmercapto-1,2,3,4-tetrahydronaphthalene is prepared according to the process by charging 39.8 g (0.2 mol) of 1,1,2,4,4-pentamethyl-1,2,3,4-tetrahydronaphthalene, 4.7 g (0.05 mol) of dimethyldisulfide and 13.3 g (0.1 mol) of aluminum chloride to a reaction flask equipped with a thermometer and stirring means. The mixture is stirred at about 25°C for about 23 hr, at which time the mixture is poured with stirring onto about 200 g of ice.

As the ice melts, an aqueous layer and an organic layer form and the aqueous layer is separated and any soluble organic material contained therein extracted with about 90 g of benzene. The benzene extract is then combined with the organic layer and distilled to remove the benzene. The residue is fractionated to recover the 1,1,2,4,4-pentamethyl-7-methylmercapto-1,2,3,4-tetrahydronaphthalene.

Four and ninety-six hundreths grams (0.02 mol) of the methylmercapto substituted polyalkyltetrahydronaphthalene thus prepared is then acetylated by adding it to a reaction flask containing 2.26 g (0.029 mol) of acetyl chloride and 31 g of ethylene dichloride. The flask is cooled in an ice bath and 5.32 g (0.04 mol) of aluminum chloride are added over a period of about 5 minutes. The resultant mixture is stirred for about 1.5 hr during which time the temperature rises to about 25°C.

The entire contents of the flask are then poured with stirring onto about 150 g of ice. As the ice melts, an aqueous layer and an organic layer form and the aqueous layer is separated and any soluble organic material contained therein extracted with ethylene dichloride. The ethylene dichloride extract is then combined with the organic layer and washed with about 50 g of water. The resultant, washed organic mixture is filtered and evaporated to obtain a heavy oil which solidifies upon cooling. The solids are recrystallized twice from methanol to obtain the 1,1,2,4,4-pentamethyl-6-acetyl-7-methylmercapto-1,2,3,4-tetrahydronaphthalene product.

In related work R. Lusskin and J. Levy; U.S. Patent 3,320,323; May 16, 1967; assigned to

Universal Oil Products Company describe alkyl sulfur derivatives of polyalkyltetrahydro-naphthalenes which have the following structural formula:

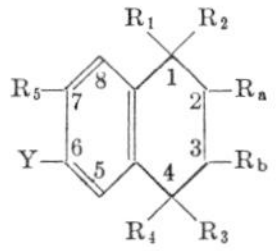

in which R_1, R_2, R_3, R_4 and R_5 are alkyl radicals selected from the group consisting of methyl and ethyl; R_a and R_b are selected from the group consisting of hydrogen, methyl and ethyl; and Y is selected from the group consisting of methyl and ethyl-mercapto, -sulfinyl and -sulfonyl radicals.

The alkylsulfinyl and alkylsulfonyl substituted polyalkyltetrahydronaphthalenes, besides being useful as intermediates in the preparation of other compounds, have a musk-like odor which makes these compounds extremely useful in the perfume industry.

The compositions can be prepared by first forming an alkylmercapto substituted polyalkyl-tetrahydronaphthalene by reacting a dialkyldisulfide with a polyalkyltetrahydronaphthalene in the presence of a catalyst followed by reacting the alkylmercapto substituted polyalkyl-tetrahydronaphthalene thus obtained with the oxidizing agent to prepare the alkylsulfinyl or alkylsulfonyl substituted polyalkyltetrahydronaphthalenes.

7-Acetyl-2a,3,4,5-Tetrahydro-1,1,5,5–Tetramethylacenaphthene

E.T. Theimer and J.H. Blumenthal; U.S. Patent 3,400,159; September 3, 1968; assigned to International Flavors & Fragrances Inc. describe acenaphthenes and tetrahydronaphthalenes having a musk-like odor and intermediates for producing same, including 7-acetyl-2a,3,4,5-tetrahydro-1,1,5,5-tetramethylacenaphthene.

The process for making the acenaphthene is a four step process. The known compound 1,1-dimethyl-1,2,3,4-tetrahydronaphthalene is initially halogenated at the 4 position to provide a 1,1-dimethyl-4-halo-1,2,3,4-tetrahydronaphthalene, for example, 1,1-dimethyl-4-chloro-1,2,3,4-tetrahydronaphthalene. The halo compound is then reacted with a methallyl magnesium halide to produce the intermediate 1,1-dimethyl-4-methallyl-1,2,3,4-tetrahydro-naphthalene which is then cyclized to form 2a,3,4,5-tetrahydro-1,1,5,5-tetramethylacenaph-thene. This compound is acylated at the 7 position to produce the final product.

4-Acetyl-Tetramethyl Hydrindacenes

E.T. Theimer and J.H. Blumenthal; U.S. Patent 3,244,751; April 5, 1966; assigned to International Flavors & Fragrances Inc. describe the compound 4-acetyl-1,1,6,6-tetramethyl-as-hydrindacene (I) and the compound 4-acetyl-1,1,7,7-tetramethyl-s-hydrindacene (V), both of which are perfumes.

In carrying out the process for making these compounds, α,α'-dichloro-m-xylene is reacted with the Grignard reagent formed from methallyl chloride to produce m-bis-(3-methyl-3-butenyl)-benzene (II).

Upon cyclizing this latter compound a mixture of two hydrindacenes, namely 1,1,6,6-tetramethyl-as-hydrindacene (III) and 1,1,7,7-tetramethyl-s-hydrindacene (IV), which are isomers, are formed and may be separated by fractional distillation. The asymmetrical isomer is acetylated to form the ketone (I), which is a strong musk. The reaction is shown on the following page.

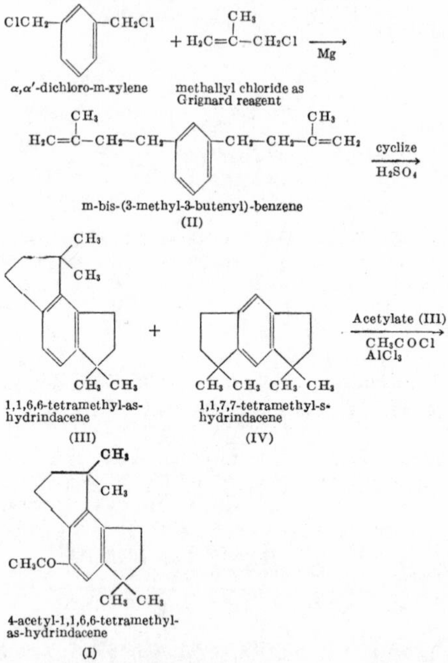

α,α'-dichloro-m-xylene

methallyl chloride as Grignard reagent

m-bis-(3-methyl-3-butenyl)-benzene
(II)

1,1,6,6-tetramethyl-as-hydrindacene
(III)

1,1,7,7-tetramethyl-s-hydrindacene
(IV)

Acetylate (III)
$\xrightarrow{\begin{array}{c} CH_3COCl \\ AlCl_3 \end{array}}$

4-acetyl-1,1,6,6-tetramethyl-as-hydrindacene
(I)

Conversely the mixture of the two hydrindacenes may be acetylated and the resulting ketones separated by fractional crystallization. Ketone V derived from the symmetrical hydrindacene (IV) by acetylation is also a musk, but weaker than I. The reaction is:

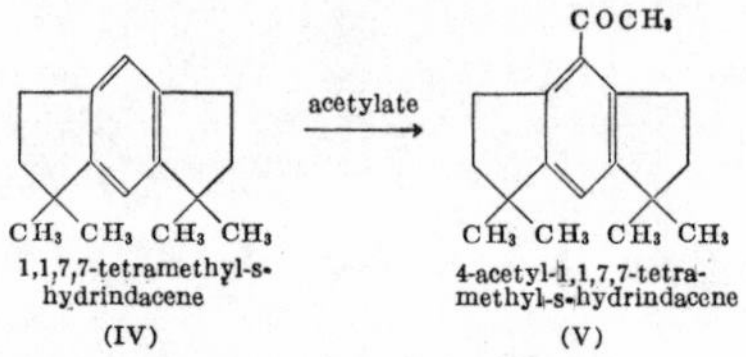

1,1,7,7-tetramethyl-s-hydrindacene
(IV)

4-acetyl-1,1,7,7-tetra-methyl-s-hydrindacene
(V)

5,7-Diisopropyl-1,1-Dimethyl-6-Hydroxyindan

A process described by *T.F. Wood and G.H. Goodwin; U.S. Patent 3,644,540; February 22, 1972; assigned to Givaudan Corporation* provides 5,7-diisopropyl-1,1-dimethyl-6-hydroxyindan which is made by reacting 2,6-diisopropylphenol and isoprene, in the presence of a protonic acid catalyst, at temperatures from about –20° to about 150°C. The compound of this process may be represented by its skeletal structural formula as follows.

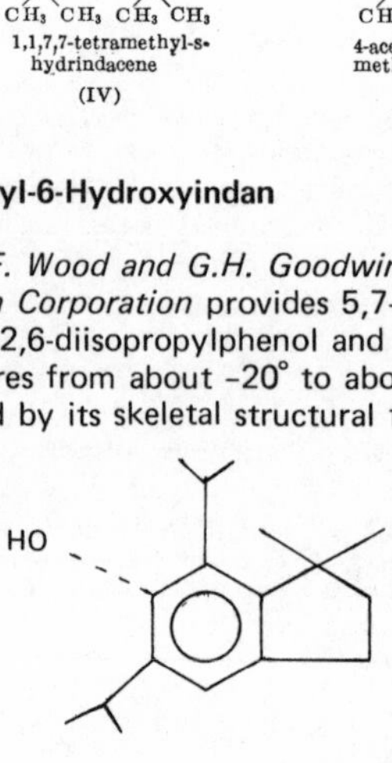

The following examples illustrate the process. The parts or percentages are by weight, the temperatures are in degrees centigrade, and all melting points and boiling points are uncorrected unless otherwise specified.

Example 1: 5,7-Diisopropyl-1,1-Dimethyl-6-Hydroxyindan (Using 93% H_2SO_4) — A solution of 68 g (1 mol) of isoprene in 100 g of 2,6-diisopropylphenol was fed over a 3 hr period into a rapidly stirred mixture of 240 g of 2,6-diisopropylphenol and 120 g of 93% sulfuric acid while the reaction temperature was maintained at 25° to 30°C. The resulting thick reaction mixture was stirred 10 min longer and quenched by addition of 300 g of ice water. Two hundred milliliters of benzene was stirred in to facilitate separation. After settling, the lower acid layer was withdrawn and discarded.

The remaining benzene solution was washed successively with water and 10% sodium bicarbonate solution and distilled for removal of the benzene solvent. The residual liquid was vacuum distilled and the fraction boiling from 127° to 132°C at 2 mm collected as a colorless solid amounting to 46 g. After crystallization, first from petroleum ether and then from 90% aqueous ethanol, the product was obtained as colorless crystals, melting point 99° to 100°C, having a strong and pleasant musk odor. Analysis: calculated for $C_{17}H_{26}O$ (percent) — C, 82.87; H, 10.64. Found (percent): C, 82.81; H, 10.75.

Example 2: 5,7-Diisopropyl-1,1-Dimethyl-6-Hydroxyindan (Using 95% H_3PO_4) — A solution of 68 g of isoprene in 178 g of 2,6-diisopropylphenol was added dropwise over a 4 hr period to a rapidly stirred mixture of 356 g (2 mols) of 2,6-diisopropylphenol and 50 g of 95% phosphoric acid at 81° to 82°C. The mixture was stirred 60 min longer at this temperature and allowed to settle. The lower phosphoric acid layer was discarded. The oil layer was washed with 150 ml of 10% sodium bicarbonate solution and vacuum distilled.

After recovery of 370 g of 2,6-diisopropylphenol, the desired product was obtained as a fraction, boiling point 115° to 122°C (1 mm), amounting to 164 g. This material rapidly crystallized in the receiver as it distilled. After being crystallized, first from petroleum ether, then from methanol, and finally once from 90% isopropanol, the product was obtained as a colorless solid, melting point 98.5° to 99°C, having a musk-like odor.

A mixed melting point run with the product of Example 1 above was 98.5° to 99.0°C. The identity was further established by comparison of the infrared spectra. The spectrum of this compound shows the following characteristic bands: 2.80 m, 3.45 to 3.55 s, 6.88 s, 7.01 s, 7.27 m, 7.36 ms, 7.80 s, 7.97 m, 8.28 s, 8.40 s, 8.82 s, 9.08 m, 9.31 s, 10.07 mw, 10.55 mw, 11.18 m, 11.50 s, 11.98 mw, 12.38 s and 12.75 w microns. The structure of this compound was further confirmed by NMR and mass spectra determination. The NMR spectrum shows the following:

> Two isopropyl groups (quartet centered at 1.33 ppm)
> One ethylene group, $-CH_2CH_2-$
> One $-OH$ group (4.75 ppm)
> One aromatic proton (6.88 ppm)
> Two equivalent CH_3 groups on a quaternary carbon (gem-dimethyl
> grouping, 1.37 ppm)

Example 3: 1,1-Dimethyl-5,7-Diisopropyl-6-Hydroxyindan in a Rose Perfume — 1,1-Dimethyl-5,7-diisopropyl-6-hydroxyindan, DDHI, has a clean musk odor with a slight ambrette seed note. The following Rose perfume composition demonstrates its fixative value.

	Parts by Weight
Citronellol	243
β-Phenylethyl alcohol	116
Geraniol	254
Rhodinol	96
Laurine	126
Guaiacwood concrete	13
Eugenol	6

(continued)

	Parts by Weight
Irisone	58
Cinnamic alcohol	5
Phenylacetic acid	1
Undecylenic aldehyde	1
2-Trichloromethyl benzyl acetate	46
Citral	24
Folione, 10% in diethylphathalate	1
DDHI	10
	1,000

Laurine is the registered trademark of Givaudan Corporation for its brand of hydroxycitronellal. Irisone is the registered trademark of Givaudan Corporation for its brand of alpha-ionone. Folione is the registered trademark of Givaudan Corporation for its brand of methyl heptine carbonate.

The formulation was tested with and without the musk compound from concentrations of 0.1 to 5% by weight. The preferred 1% concentration of DDHI enhanced the floral character of the composition giving sweetness, warmth and body to the fragrance. A marked improvement was noted over the composition with DDHI both in terms of odor quality and stability after several months storage.

1,4,6,6,7,9,9-Heptamethyl-1,2,6,7,8,9-Hexahydro-3H-Benz(e)inden-3-one

T.F. Wood and E. Heilweil; U.S. Patent 3,769,348; October 30, 1973; assigned to Givaudan Corporation describe tricyclic carbocyclic compounds containing a total of 20 carbon atoms which are odorants of the musk type. These compounds possess all of the desirable properties of natural musks while possessing greater tenacity. The compounds of the process have the following structure:

(I)

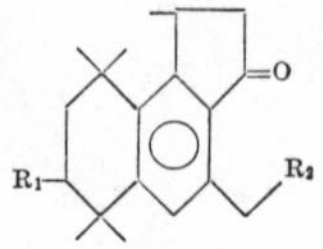

where R_1 and R_2 are hydrogen or methyl, provided that when R_1 is hydrogen, R_2 is methyl and when R_1 is methyl, R_2 is hydrogen. The compounds are produced in two steps.

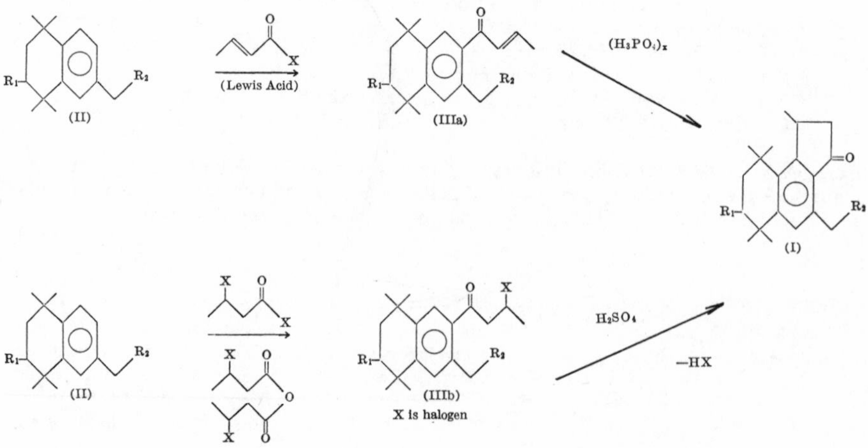

The first step involves acylation of the corresponding tetrahydronaphthalene with a crotonylating agent or its equivalent in the presence of a Lewis acid in a suitable solvent; the second step involves cyclization, as shown in the above sequence. In the first sequence shown above a crotonyl halide is employed as the acylating agent while in the second its equivalents, a β-halobutyryl halide or a β-halobutyryl anhydride, are shown leading to the respective intermediates (IIIa) and (IIIb). Either of the intermediates (IIIa) or (IIIb) will yield the desired product (I) when cyclized by treatment with concentrated sulfuric acid, polyphosphoric acid, or other suitable cyclizing agent.

The compounds of the process were found to exhibit three times the tenacity of a synthetic musk well-known in the art, namely 7-acetyl-1,1,3,4,4,6-hexamethyl-1,2,3,4-tetrahydronaph-thalene. 15 μl of solutions containing 3.0% of the musk odorants were allowed to evaporate on smelling blotters at room temperature for 6 weeks. After 2 weeks the prior art synthetic musk had disappeared while the compounds of the process were detectable for 6 weeks.

This desirable property of tenacity has the effect of maintaining a desired odor for three times as long as was possible using prior art musks in say, sachets, area odorants and soaps. The odorant formulation base employed in the tenacity tests had the following composition.

	Parts by Weight
1,4,6,6,7,9,9-Heptamethyl-1,2,6,7,8,9-hexahydro-3H-benz(e)inden-3-one, or 4-ethyl-1,6,6,9,9-pentamethyl-1,2,6,7,8,9-hexahydro-3H-benz(e)inden-3-one	543
P-cresylphenyl acetate	403
Castorium liquid	27
Tobacco absolute	18
Costus oil	9
	1,000

As used in the tests, the resulting composition was diluted by mixing 5 parts of it with 95 parts of ethanol. The following examples illustrate the process.

Example 1: 1,4,6,6,7,9,9-Heptamethyl-1,2,6,7,8,9-Hexahydro-3H-Benz(e)inden-3-one —
(a) 126 g of crotonyl chloride (1.2 mol) is added over a period of 15 minutes to a suspension of 140 g (1.05 mol) of anhydrous aluminum chloride in 450 ml of ethylene chloride at 0°C. Then 216 g (1 mol) of 1,1,3,4,4,6-hexamethyl-1,2,3,4-tetrahydronaphthalene in 250 ml of ethylene dichloride is added during the course of 1.5 hours at 0° to –5°C.

Stirring is continued for 2 hours after the addition. The solution is quenched on ice and hydrochloric acid solution and the resulting ethylene dichloride solution separated and washed with water and sodium bicarbonate solution until neutrality. The extract is filtered and distilled. After removal of solvent the residual oil is vacuum distilled to yield an oil (166.5 g), BP 147° to 152°C (1 mm), n_D^{20} 1.5462. Recrystallization from ethanol gave 7-crotonyl-1,1,3,4,4,6-hexamethyl-1,2,3,4-tetrahydronaphthalene (114 g), MP 53° to 54.5°C. Calculated for $C_{20}H_{28}O$: C, 84.45; H, 9.92. Found: C, 85.09; H, 9.85.

(b) 73 g of the above product are cyclized by heating in the presence of 800 g of polyphosphoric acid first at 70°C and finally at 105°C over a 30 minute period. The batch is stirred and allowed to cool to 80°C over a period of 20 minutes. After quenching in ice, the product is extracted with toluene. The solution is washed to neutrality sequentially with water and with 10% $NaHCO_3$ solution.

The solvent is removed by distillation and the residual oil vacuum distilled (BP 169° to 175°C at 1.5 mm) to yield an oil (56 g). This oil is crystallized from ethanol to yield the desired 1,4,6,6,7,9,9-heptamethyl-1,2,6,7,8,9-hexahydro-3H-benz(e)inden-3-one (20.5 g), double MP 98.5° to 99°C/103° to 104.5°C, having a strong musk-like odor.

Calculated for $C_{20}H_{28}O$: C, 84.45; H, 9.92. Found: C, 84.66; H, 10.00. Mass spec MW: 284 (parent peak). NMR analysis shows the following peaks:

	Tau Values
Multiplicity:	
Doublet CH_3CHCH_2	9.00
Doublet $CH_3-C-\phi$	8.70
4-Singlets (methyls)	8.82, 8.70, 8.65. 8.45
Broad multiplet	8.15
Singlet CH_3	7.40
Doublet	7.70
Multiplet (doublet of doublets) $CH_2C=O$	7.20
Multiplet $HC-CH_3$	6.20
Singlet $\phi-H$	2.82

The infrared spectrum shows the following characteristic bands (KBr pellet, ca 0.1 mm): 3.26 mw, 3.34 s, 3.38 s, 3.44 s, 3.46 s, 3.53 s, 5.88 s, 5.92 s, 6.08 m, 6.39 s, 6.27 m, 6.85 s, 6.95 ms, 7.22 m, 7.30 s, 7.35 s, 7.65 ms, 7.70 ms, 7.88 ms, 7.95 ms, 8.00 s, 8.12 s, 8.55 mw, 8.78 ms, 8.92 s, 9.25 ms, 9.35 m, 9.45 m, 9.65 m, 9.90 ms, 10.00 m, 10.20 m, 10.60 w, 10.95 m, 11.05 m, 11.42 ms, 11.60 mw, 12.64 mw, 13.55 w, 14.50 m, 14.75 mw, 15.65 m, 16.30 w, 17.40 w, 18.00 w, 18.55 mw, 19.00 mw, 20.00 w microns.

Example 2: 4-Ethyl-1,6,6,9,9-Pentamethyl-1,2,6,7,8,9-Hexahydro-3H-Benz(e)inden-3-one — (a) 1.2 mol (126 g) of crotonyl chloride is added over a period of 15 minutes to a suspension of 140 g (1.05 mol) of anhydrous aluminum chloride in 450 ml of ethylene chloride at 0°C. Then 216 g (1 mol) of 6-ethyl-1,1,4,4-tetramethyl-1,2,3,4-tetrahydronaphthalene in 250 ml of ethylene dichloride is added during the course of 1.5 hours at 0° to 5°C. Stirring is continued for 2 hours after the addition. The solution is quenched on ice and hydrochloric acid solution and the resulting ethylene dichloride solution separated and washed with water and sodium bicarbonate solution until neutrality.

The extract is filtered and distilled. After removal of solvent the residual oil is vacuum distilled to yield an oil (150.5 g), BP 155° to 163°C (1 mm), n_D^{20} 1.5394. Recrystallization from ethanol gave 7-crotonyl-6-ethyl-1,1,4,4-tetramethyl-1,2,3,4-tetrahydronaphthalene (114 g) MP 37° to 38.5°C. Calculated for $C_{20}H_{28}O$: C, 84.45; H, 9.92. Found: C, 85.45; H, 10.10.

(b) A portion (64 g) of the above product is cyclized by heating in the presence of 800 g of polyphosphoric acid first at 70°C and finally at 105°C over a 30 minute period. The batch is stirred and allowed to cool to 80°C over a period of 20 minutes. After quenching in ice the product is extracted with toluene. The solution is washed to neutrality sequentially with water and with 10% $NaHCO_3$ solution.

The solvent is removed by distillation and the residual oil vacuum distilled (BP 148° to 155°C at 1 mm) to yield an oil (52 g). The oil is crystallized from ethanol to yield the desired 4-ethyl-1,6,6,9,9-pentamethyl-1,2,6,7,8,9-hexahydro-3H-benz(e)inden-3-one (25.5 g) having a strong musk-like odor, MP 96° to 97°C. Calculated for $C_{20}H_{28}O$: C, 84.45; H, 9.92. Found: C, 84.49; H, 9.96; mass spec MW 284 (parent peak). NMR analysis shows the following peaks:

	Tau Values
Multiplicity:	
Triplet CH_3CH_2	8.80
Doublet CH_3CH	8.70
Multiplet 4 t-methyls	8.28, 8.39, 8.67
Singlet $-(CH_2)_2-$	8.28
Doublet	7.72
Multiplet (doublet of doublets) $CH_2C=O$	7.18

(continued)

	Tau Values
Quartet ϕ CH$_2$CH$_3$	6.98
Multiplet H–C–CH$_3$	6.18
Singlet ϕ H	2.82

Example 3: Cologne Base Formulation — A compound of Formula (1) was formulated to make a cologne base having the following composition.

	Parts by Weight
1,4,6,6,7,9,9-Heptamethyl-1,2,6,7,8,9-hexahydro-3H-benz(e)inden-3-one	20
Benzyl isoeugenol	27
Bergamot oil	291
Geranium oil	10
Lavender oil	32
Lemon oil	283
Lime oil	54
Neroli oil	10
Orange oil, bitter	140
Orange oil, sweet	75
Rosemary oil	32
Sage clary oil	21
Thyme oil, white	5
	1,000

Tricyclic Isochromans

L.G. Heeringa and M.G.J. Beets; U.S. Patent 3,591,528; July 6, 1971; assigned to International Flavors & Fragrances Inc. describe compositions containing as a musk odorant, including a tricyclic isochroman having the structural formula:

(I)

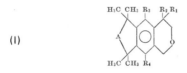

where R$_1$, R$_2$, R$_3$, and R$_4$ are methyl or hydrogen and where either R$_3$ or R$_4$ is methyl, the other is hydrogen, and A is methylene, ethylene, ethylidene, 1,2-propylene, or 2,3-butylene. In many preparations in which the compounds of type (I) are obtained as the main products, angular tricyclic isomers are obtained in minor quantities. Some of the strongest of this series are 2-oxa-4,5,5,8,8-pentamethyl-1,2,3,4,5,6,7,8-octahydroanthracene; 6-oxa-1,1,2,3,3,8-hexamethyl-2,3,5,6,7,8-hexahydro-1H-benz(f)-inden; and 6-oxa-1,1,2,3,3-pentamethyl-2,3,5,6,7,8-hexahydro-1H-benz(f)-inden. The following examples illustrate the process.

Example 1: 2-Oxa-5,5,8,8-Tetramethyl-1,2,3,4,5,6,7,8-Octahydroanthracene — A suspension of 1,000 g of aluminum chloride in 2 liters of dry CCl$_4$ was cooled to −10°C. In the course of 1½ hours there was added with vigorous stirring a solution of 402 g of isochroman and 549 g of 2,5-dichloro-2,5-dimethylhexane in 1,250 ml of dry CCl$_4$.

During the addition, the temperature was maintained at −5° to −10°C by using an ice-salt bath while a vigorous stream of nitrogen was bubbled through the reaction mixture. After an additional stirring period of half an hour at 0°C the reaction product was poured onto a mixture of 5 kg ice and 600 ml of concentrated HCl. The oil layer was separated and stirred 2 hours at 50°C with 600 ml of a 50% alcoholic KOH solution. The solution was then poured into 6 liters of water and the oil layer was separated.

The solvent was distilled off and the crude product, 720 g was distilled at 3 mm Hg in a nitrogen atmosphere to separate residue, yielding the following fractions: (1) BP 60° to 123°C 180 g; (2) BP 130° to 170°C 356 g; and (3) BP 170° to 180°C 17 g; and a residue 166 g.

The crude musk from fractions (2) and (3) was purified by crystallization from an equal volume of ethanol, yielding 260.5 g of virtually pure product, white crystals with a strong musk odor; MP 65.5° to 66.2°C, i.e., 35.6% of theory of the title compound. Recrystallization of 10 g of this material from 10 ml of ethanol gave 8.5 g with MP 65.5° to 66.3°C.

Column chromatography of the product on Al_2O_3 with benzene as eluent, and gas chromatography on a 1.20 m glass column packed with 30% Reoplex-400, which is a commercially available stationary phase for GLPC, and is a polyester, on Embacel, which is a commercially available support material, essentially SiO_2, at 155°C, demonstrated that the product was pure. This was confirmed by CH analysis ($C_{17}H_{24}O$). Found: C, 83.57, 83.61; H, 9.94, 9.87. Calculated: C, 83.55; H, 9.90. The linear structure was confirmed by mass spectrometry, NMR and IR.

Example 2: 2-Oxa-5,5,8,8-Tetramethyl-1,2,3,4,5,6,7,8-Octahydroanthracene — According to the same procedure as in Example 1 the cycloalkylation was carried out in 1,2-dichloroethane at 25° to 30°C under a nitrogen blanket, using a suspension of 305 g (2.28 mols) of aluminum chloride in 305 ml of redistilled dichloroethane and a solution of 122 g (0.91 mol) of isochroman, and 167 g (0.91 mol) of dichlorodimethylhexane in 320 ml of redistilled dichloroethane. The reaction mixture was worked up as described in Example 1.

Upon flash distillation of the crude product there were obtained 124 g of distillate, BP 120° to 250°C at 4 mm Hg and 67 g of residue. Fractionation of the distillate through a 12 plate Vigreux column yielded 62.53 g of a colorless viscous liquid with a strong musk odor, which was shown by gas liquid partition chromatography to contain about 92% of the title compound. Crystallization from an equal volume of ethanol yielded the nearly pure crystalline musk with MP 64.0° to 65.8°C.

Example 3: 2-Oxa-5,5,8,8-Tetramethyl-1,2,3,4,5,6,7,8-Octahydroanthracene — By the same procedure as in Example 2, using dichloromethane as a solvent, and starting from a suspension of 333.5 g (2.5 mols) of aluminum chloride in 334 ml of redistilled dichloromethane and a solution of 134 g (1 mol) of isochroman, and 183 g (1 mol) of dichlorodimethylhexane in 350 ml of dichloromethane there were obtained after fractionation through a 12 plate Vigreux column: 68.37 g of a colorless semicrystalline product with a strong musk odor. Gas chromatography on Reoplex-400 as mentioned in Example 1, proved the presence of about 92% of the linear isomer mentioned in the title.

Additional studies with tricyclic isochromans are described by *L.G. Heeringa and M.G.J. Beets; U.S. Patent 3,360,530; December 26, 1967; assigned to International Flavors & Fragrances Inc.*

Aromatic Hydrocarbon-Alkylene Oxide Reaction Products

E.T. Theimer; U.S. Patent 3,532,719; October 6, 1970; assigned to International Flavors & Fragrances Inc. describes a process for producing isochromans by reaction of aromatic hydrocarbons with an alkylene oxide in the presence of aluminum chloride to produce an aryl alkanol-aluminum chloride complex, partially deactivating the aluminum chloride, and treating the aryl alkanol-aluminum chloride complex with formaldehyde to produce an isochroman. The following examples illustrate the process.

Example 1: Preparation of 6-Oxa-1,1,2,3,3,8-Hexamethyl-2,3,5,6,7,8-Hexahydro-1H-Benz(f)indene — A 5 liter reaction flash fitted with a stirrer, reflux condenser, dropping funnel, and a subsurface addition tube is immersed in a Dry Ice-isopropanol bath and charged with 665 g of aluminum chloride, 487.5 g of monochlorobenzene and 940 g of 1,1,2,3,3-pentamethyl indane.

No exotherm is observed as the contents are cooled to -20°C. An additional 487.5 g of monochlorobenzene is mixed with 290 g of propylene oxide and half of this mixture is charged to the flask through the addition tube during 40 minutes. A strong exothermic action occurs, and the addition is carried out so that the temperature of the flask contents is about -190°C.

The remaining monochlorobenzene and propylene oxide mixture is added during the next 45 minutes while the temperature is maintained at -18° to -20°C. After addition is completed, the flask contents are stirred for an additional 15 minutes and a 5 cc sample is withdrawn. Then, 135 g of water is slowly added during one-half hour and the temperature of the flask contents is permitted to rise to 1° to 2°C so that ice does not form. After completion of the water addition 126 g of paraformaldehyde is added, and stirring is continued for 5 hours while the temperature is maintained at 0° to 5°C.

The reaction mass is then poured over a mixture of 1 kg of ice and 1 kg of water, whereupon the temperature rises to 32°C. The mixture is stirred 10 minutes, and the lower layer is drained from the mass. 500 g of 50% aqueous sodium hydroxide and 1,240 g of water are added to the remaining upper layer, and this is permitted to stand overnight.

700 additional grams of water is added and then 500 g of concentrated hydrochloric acid is used to acidify the mixture. An additional kilogram of water is added and the aqueous phase is separated from the upper organic phase. The organic material is then washed with 1 kg of 10% aqueous sodium chloride twice and 975 g of organic material is obtained. The monochlorobenzene and any remaining water are stripped off under vacuum, and the organic material is flash distilled to obtain 881 g of product.

The product is washed with 580 g of 50% aqueous sodium hydroxide diluted to 1,740 g with water, then twice with 1 kg of water and once with 1 kg of hot (55°C) water. The remaining 880 g of organic material is drained into a 2 liter distillation flask and distilled at 89° to 139°C at 0.9 mm Hg to obtain 812 g of product. Based upon the amount of pentamethyl indane starting material the overall yield of the title compound is 65.5%.

Example 2: A 5 liter reaction flask fitted out as in Example 1 is charged with 532.5 g of 85% pentamethyl indane and 71.4 g of anhydrous aluminum chloride. The mixture is cooled to -15°C and 29.1 g of propylene oxide in 185.2 g of 85% pentamethyl indane is slowly charged to the flask below the surface of the liquid. The temperature is maintained between -10° and -15°C, and the reaction mixture is held at that temperature for about 1 hour with stirring.

Then 25.5 g of methanol is slowly added during one-half hour. The methanol partially deactivates the aluminum chloride in the aryl alkanol-aluminum chloride complex, and 7 g of paraformaldehyde is slowly added with continued stirring while the temperature rises to 35°C. The stirring is continued for 1 hour after addition of the paraformaldehyde.

The reaction mass is then quenched in ice water, treated with sodium hydroxide, esterified, and washed as in Example 1. The organic layer so obtained is stripped to remove 660 g of unreacted pentamethyl indane. This pentamethyl indane can be used as the starting material for the production of more aryl alkanol and isochroman. About 41 g of the benz(f)-indene is obtained. This is about a 60% yield, based upon pentamethyl indane consumption.

Acetyl Derivatives of Chromans

H.S. Bloch; U.S. Patent 3,551,456; December 29, 1970; assigned to Universal Oil Products Company describes acetyl derivatives of substituted chromans and coumarans which are prepared by condensing a phenolic compound with a dienic hydrocarbon and then acetylating the resultant compound. The following examples illustrate the process.

Example 1: In this example 100 cc of a solid phosphoric acid catalyst was placed in a stainless steel tube surrounded by an electrically heated furnace containing an aluminum block. 1,400 g of phenol were melted and poured into a 3 liter charger; and after resealing the charger, 762 g of butadiene were charged thereto from a small pressure vessel. After being shaken and allowed to stand for a period of 16 hours, the mixture was considered homogeneous. The reactor was then heated to a temperature of about 130°C while the phenol-butadiene mixture was charged thereto at a space velocity of 7.4.

In addition, the reactor was maintained at 100 psi of pressure during the reaction period, which took approximately 3 hours. During this time the reaction product was discharged from the bottom of the catalyst tube into a 3 liter flask, which served also as a separator, with the gaseous products passing on to gas traps which were cooled in a Dry Ice-acetone mixture.

The liquid product was vacuum distilled to remove the dissolved unreacted butadiene and phenol. The liquid fractions were extracted with a 10% aqueous sodium hydroxide solution and thereafter with Claisen's alkali solution. The alkali-insoluble portion was distilled under reduced pressure whereby the desired product comprising 2-methylchroman and isomers thereof, including 3-methylchroman, 2,3-dimethylcoumaran and 3-ethylcoumaran, were recovered.

The methylchromans and alkylcoumarans which were prepared according to the above description are then acetylated by placing one molar proportion of the methylchromans and alkylcoumarans with one molar proportion of acetyl chloride in a reaction flask which contains 67 g of aluminum chloride. The reaction mixture is stirred constantly for a period of about 4 hours while maintaining the reaction flask at ambient temperature and atmospheric pressure.

Upon completion of the abovementioned residence time, the catalyst is removed by water-washing and the reaction mixture is then subjected to fractional distillation under reduced pressure whereby the unreacted chromans and coumarans are separated from the desired products which comprise 6-acetylmethylchromans and 5-acetylalkylcoumarans, which have a musk-like scent.

Example 2: In this example 324 g (3.0 mols) of m-cresol is stirred and admixed with 2,3-dimethyl-1,3-butadiene. The resulting mixture is charged to a reaction vessel which contains 50 cc of solid phosphoric acid catalyst at a liquid hourly space velocity of about 4.5. The reaction vessel during the addition of the charge is maintained at a temperature of about 150°C and a pressure of 100 psi.

The reaction mixture is recovered and treated in a manner similar to that set forth in Example 1, that is, by being distilled under vacuum to remove the unreacted cresol and 2,3-dimethyl-1,3-butadiene. Following this, the liquid fractions are extracted with an aqueous alkali solution and the alkali-insoluble portion is recovered. This portion is then subjected to fractional distillation under reduced pressure whereby the desired products comprising 2,2,3,7-tetramethylchroman and 2,2,3,3,6-pentamethylcoumaran are recovered.

The polymethyl substituted chromans and polymethyl substituted coumarans which are prepared according to the above, are then placed in a flask along with an equimolar proportion of acetyl chloride. In addition, the flask contains a catalytic amount of aluminum chloride as the acetylation catalyst. The reaction is continuously agitated by means of a mechanical stirrer for a period of about 4 hours while maintaining the operating conditions at slightly above ambient temperature and atmospheric pressure.

At the end of this reaction time, the mixture is recovered, the catalyst removed, and the products subjected to fractional distillation under reduced pressure. From the distillation, the desired products are recovered, comprising 2,2,3,7-tetramethyl-6-acetylchroman and 2,2,3,3,6-pentamethyl-5-acetylcoumaran.

DIHYDROCOUMARINS

Propylene Reaction Products

J. King; U.S. Patent 3,437,670; April 8, 1969; assigned to Universal Oil Products Company describes a process for preparing diisopropyl-3,4-dihydrocoumarins and, more particularly to a process for preparing these compounds by condensing propylene with 3,4-dihydro-coumarin in the presence of a modified orthophosphoric acid catalyst.

Polyalkylated 3,4-dihydrocoumarins are valuable compounds having many industrial applications. Certain of these dihydrocoumarins, and particularly diisopropyl substituted dihy-drocoumarins, have unique odor properties which render them particularly valuable in per-fumery. For example, 5,7-diisopropyl-3,4-dihydrocoumarin possesses odor and fixative properties similar to the highly valuable, naturally occurring macrocyclic musks such as muskone or civitone. The following examples illustrate the process.

Example 1: Diisopropyl-3,4-dihydrocoumarin was prepared by the following procedure. The catalyst mixture for the reaction was prepared by charging 500 g of 85 weight percent orthophosphoric acid to a stirred reactor equipped with heating/cooling means and a gas inlet port. With stirring, the temperature was adjusted to about 100°C and while maintain-ing such temperature, 247.5 g of phosphorus pentoxide were added over about ¼ hour. The stirring was continued for about ½ hour more to obtain a catalyst mixture of about 747.5 g of substantially anhydrous orthophosphoric acid containing about 6.7 weight per-cent of phosphorus pentoxide.

About 370 g (2.5 mols) of 3,4-dihydrocoumarin were then charged to the reactor and into contact with the catalyst mixture with the temperature being raised to about 155° to 165°C. While maintaining the temperature, propylene gas was then charged to the reactor until about 6 mols of propylene had been absorbed, a period requiring about 14 hours. The reaction mixture was then cooled to about 60°C and 235 g of hexane were added followed by 375 g of water.

The resultant organic layer was separated and washed first with water and then with aqueous sodium bicarbonate and finally with salt water. The washed mixture was then distilled to recover 561.3 g of an isomeric product mixture of diisopropyl-3,4-dihydrocoumarin. The yield was 97% of theory based upon charged dihydrocoumarin. The isomeric product was further treated by vacuum fractionation to separate the isomer, believed to be the 5,7-iso-mer having the valuable musk-like odor. This isomer fraction weighed 299.6 g and had a boiling point of from 159° to 161°C at 3 mm Hg pressure and a refractive index n_D^{20} of 1.5284 to 1.5287.

Example 2: The following two experiments, (A) and (B) were conducted using different types of phosphoric acid catalysts for the condensation of propylene and dihydrocoumarin. In both instances the desired reactions did not take place.

(A) Aqueous Orthophosphoric Acid Containing 85 Weight Percent Acid — About 100 g of the acid and 74 g (½ mol) of 3,4-dihydrocoumarin were charged to a stirred reactor equipped with heating/cooling means and a gas inlet port. With stirring, the mixture was heated to about 140°C and propylene was charged to the reactor. No reaction occurred as indicated by an absence of any absorption of the propylene.

(B) Substantially Anhydrous Orthophosphoric Acid — The catalyst was prepared by charg-ing 100 g of aqueous orthophosphoric acid (85 weight percent acid) to a stirred reactor equipped with heating/cooling means and an inlet port. With stirring, the temperature was adjusted to about 100°C and, while maintaining such temperature, 39.5 g of phosphorus pentoxide were added to convert all of the water present to orthophosphoric acid. While the stirring was continued, 74 g (0.5 mol) of 3,4-dihydrocoumarin were added and the temperature was raised to 110° to 120°C. Propylene was charged to the reactor but the reaction as indicated by the absorption of propylene (¹⁄₁₀ of a mol in 2 hours) was so slow

that the reaction was terminated with negligible product formation.

W.J. Houlihan; U.S. Patent 3,144,467; August 11, 1964; assigned to Universal Oil Products Company describes additional studies to prepare polyalkylated dihydrocoumarins by condensing an alkylating agent with a dihydrocoumarin in the presence of an acid catalyst.

Conversion to Odorous Isomer

J. King; U.S. Patent 3,437,669; April 8, 1969; assigned to Universal Oil Products Company describes a process for preparing an odorous isomer of diisopropyl-3,4-dihydrocoumarin and more particularly, to a process for preparing such isomer by treating substantially odorless diisopropyl dihydrocoumarin isomers with an isomerization catalyst comprising a modified orthophosphoric acid.

Diisopropyl-3,4-dihydrocoumarin is a highly valuable perfumery material characterized by a very fine musk-like odor similar to the naturally occurring macrocyclic musks such as muskone or civitone. While this material usually exists as a mixture of isomers, actually only one of the isomers, believed to be the 5,7-isomer, possesses the desirable odor properties with the other isomers being substantially odorless.

In preparing diisopropyl-3,4-dihydrocoumarin, such as by the condensation of 3,4-dihydrocoumarin with propylene in the presence of an acid catalyst, the diisopropyl dihydrocoumarin product of the reaction usually is treated, such as by distillation, to separate the valuable odor isomer from the odorless isomers. This, of course, leaves a substantial amount of diisopropyl dihydrocoumarin isomers which have little practical value. It has now been discovered, however, that these odorless and valueless diisopropyl dihydrocoumarin isomers may be readily and simply converted to the highly valuable odorous isomer by treating with a modified orthophosphoric acid isomerization catalyst.

The odorless diisopropyl-3,4-dihydrocoumarin isomers which may be treated according to this process by contacting with the isomerization catalyst mixture to form the highly valuable odorous isomers comprise any of the five possible odorless isomers. The odorous isomer is believed to be the 5,7-isomer it may also be defined as the isomer having a fine musk-like odor which boils at about 159° to 161°C at 3 mm Hg pressure and has a refractive index of n_D^{20} of 1.5284 to 1.5287.

While any of the odorless isomers such as the 6,8 or 6,7-isomers may be treated individually, it usually is more convenient to simply treat a mixture of isomers without separating any of the particular isomers. The isomer mixture subject to treatment may also contain other isopropyl substituted 3,4-dihydrocoumarins such as mono- or tri-substituted compounds inasmuch as these do not interfere with the treatment.

Example: An isomeric mixture of diisopropyl-3,4-dihydrocoumarin was treated according to the process to prepare an odorous isomer according to the following procedure. The catalyst mixture for the treatment was prepared by charging 500 g of 85 weight percent orthophosphoric acid to a stirred reactor equipped with heating/cooling means. With stirring, the temperature was adjusted to about 100°C and, while maintaining such temperature, 247.5 g of phosphorus pentoxide were added over about ¼ hour. The stirring was continued for about ½ hour more to obtain a catalyst mixture of about 747.5 g of substantially anhydrous orthophosphoric acid containing about 6.7 weight percent of phosphorus pentoxide.

About 15 g of the catalyst mixture were charged to a reactor and then about 7.4 g of an isomeric diisopropyl-3,4-dihydrocoumarin mixture containing a small amount of a triisopropyl dihydrocoumarin were added to the reactor. This isomeric diisopropyl-3,4-dihydrocoumarin mixture was substantially odorless and had a boiling range of from about 165° to 187°C at 2 mm Hg. With stirring, the reaction mixture was heated to about 150° to 160°C and maintained thereat for about 1½ hours. The organic, diisopropyl dihydrocoumarin phase of the reaction mixture now had a fine musk-like odor.

The reaction mixture was cooled and diethyl ether was added to extract the organic phase. The extract was washed with water, dried and then analyzed by gas liquid chromatography. This analysis, as compared to the analysis of the starting material, is summarized in the following table.

Isomer fraction	Weight percent	
	Before treatment	After treatment
A (odor fraction)	0	18
B	14.2	18.4
C	25.7	4.3
D	8.6	10.3
E	18.3	17.7
F (tri-isopropyl dihydrocoumarin fraction)	33.2	31.2

As indicated in the above table, the odor fraction (A), believed to be the 5,7-isomer, increased from 0 to 18% in the final mixture. This odor fraction boils within the range of 159° to 161°C at 3 mm Hg and, if desired, may be readily separated from the substantially odorless isomers by distillation.

5,7-Diisopropyl-3,4-Dihydrocoumarin

W.J. Houlihan; U.S. Patent 3,258,400; June 28, 1966; assigned to Universal Oil Products Company describes the preparation and use of 5,7-diisopropyl-3,4-dihydrocoumarin which has the following structure.

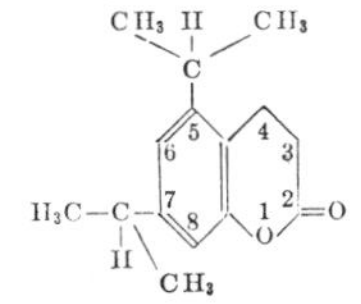

This compound may be prepared according to the procedure described in U.S. Patent 3,144,467 by alkylating 3,4-dihydrocoumarin with isopropyl alcohol in the presence of an acid catalyst such as relatively anhydrous sulfuric or polyphosphoric acids. The alkylation is usually effected with stoichiometric quantities of reactants at a temperature in the range of from 0° to about 80°C, under atmospheric pressures.

In preparing 5,7-diisopropyl-3,4-dihydrocoumarin by alkylation of 3,4-dihydrocoumarin, the alkylation product obtained frequently also contained in admixture with the 5,7-diisopropyl compound small amounts of the 6,8-diisopropyl isomer as well as mono substituted isopropyl dihydrocoumarins such as 6 or 8 isopropyl-3,4-dihydrocoumarins. These other isopropyl isomers may, if desired, be separated from the 5,7-diisopropyl-3,4-dihydrocoumarin prior to its use in perfumery.

However, since the other isopropyl isomers do not detract from the remarkable odor and fixative properties of the 5,7-diisopropyl-3,4-dihydrocoumarin, small quantities of these isomers may be present in admixture with the 5,7-diisopropyl compound without substantially lowering its perfumery value. 5,7-diisopropyl-3,4-dihydrocoumarin has a powerful long-lasting musk odor and a highly effective fixative property which renders the compound of great value in giving perfumes increased lasting quality, and pleasantly sweetened and richly enhanced fragrance. The following examples illustrate the process.

Example 1: About 960 g of concentrated sulfuric acid were added to an alkylation flask provided with stirring means and immersed in an ice bath. The acid was stirred and cooled to an internal temperature of 15°C. A solution of 180 g (3.0 mol) of isopropyl alcohol and 222 g (1.5 mol) of 3,4-dihydrocoumarin was added dropwise with continuous stirring at such a rate so that the internal temperature did not exceed 15°C.

During the addition period the acid fraction changed from colorless to yellow. Upon completion of the addition the ice cooling bath was removed and the reaction was stirred for an additional 9 hours. The reaction mixture was then allowed to stand at room temperature for a period of about 48 hours, following which the orange-red solution was slowly poured onto 1.5 kg of ice and water and then stirred for about 0.25 hour. The organic material was separated from the water, extracted with benzene, washed with a 10% sodium carbonate solution and dried with magnesium sulfate.

The mixture was filtered and the filtrate subjected to removal of the benzene in vacuum on a rotary evaporator. The residue which remained was subjected to fractional distillation under reduced pressure through a 36 inch spinning band column to recover 5,7-diisopropyl-3,4-dihydrocoumarin mixed with 8-isopropyl-2,4-dihydrocoumarin having a boiling point in the range of 147° to 150°C at 2 mm Hg pressure and a refractive index of n_D^{20} 1.5272 to 1.5281. The desired product was subjected to infrared analysis which disclosed a characteristic unconjugated lactone carbonyl band at 5.63 to 5.73μ and isopropyl bands at 7.23 and 7.33μ.

Example 2: A modern floral blend perfume backed up by a woody-ionone combination was made using the compound of this process as an olfactory and fixative ingredient. The perfume contained the following ingredients.

	Parts by Weight
5,7-Diisopropyl-3,4-dihydrocoumarin	5
Vetivert acetate	3
Linalyl acetate	3
Hydroxycitronellal	12
Phenylethyl alcohol	2
Citronellol	3
Linalool	2
Methyl gamma-ionone	10
Benzyl alcohol	5
Guaiac acetate	1
α-Amylcinnamic aldehyde	1

Example 3: A perfume having a muguet character was made using the compound of this process as an olfactory and fixative ingredient. The perfume contained the following ingredients.

	Parts by Weight
5,7-Diisopropyl-3,4-dihydrocoumarin	2
Hydroxylcitronellal	45
p-Tertiary-α-methyl dihydrocinnamic aldehyde	5
Citronellol	15
Oil Cananga	5
Linalool	5
Heliotropine	2
Aubepine	3
Isoeugenol 10%	1
Oil Cardamom 10%	1
Citronellyl formate	6
Ionone white	3
Tepyl acetate	1
Amyl phenyl acetate	3
Benzyl salicylate	5
Oil cade 10%	1

CEDARWOOD OIL DERIVATIVES

N.B. The numbering and lettering scheme used to describe the compounds in the second patent in this section is the same as that used in the first patent.

Chamigrenes and Tricyclic Olefins

G.C. Kitchens, A.R. Hochstetler and K. Kaiser; U.S. Patent 3,681,470; August 1, 1972; assigned to Givaudan Corporation have found that when thujopsene and thujopsene isomers derived from hibawood oil and American cedarwood oil are treated with substantially anhydrous protonating acids, suitably in the presence of an alkanoic acid containing from 2 to 6 carbon atoms, they are isomerized to give a mixture of hydrocarbons including substantial amounts of alpha- and beta-chamigrenes and $C_{15}H_{24}$ olefinic hydrocarbons rich in 6,8a-ethano-1,1,6-trimethyl-1,2,3,5,6,7,8,8a-octahydronaphthalene.

Perfume materials derived by the acetylation of the hydrocarbon fractions of cedarwood oil have been manufactured for over 15 years and sold under various trade names. The earlier products were derived by acetylating the hydrocarbons with acetic anhydride or acetyl chloride and catalysts such as aluminum chloride, zinc chloride or boron trifluorode.

These products were essentially derived from the more stable α-cedrene (I) in the hydrocarbon fractions and were essentially acetylcedrene (II). A perfume product has been manufactured by applying an acetylation procedure employing acetic anhydride and polyphosphoric acid to the hydrocarbon functions of American cedarwood oil containing 40 to 50% α-cedrene (I), 5 to 10% β-cedrene (III), 40 to 50% cis-thujopsene (IV) and 5 to 10% thujopsene isomers.

The known procedures for the isomerization of thujopsene (IV) with aqueous sulfuric acid, aqueous perchloric acid and dioxane have been shown to yield mainly a hydrocarbon, 1,4,11,11-tetramethylbicyclo[5.4.0]undeca-3,7-diene (X) which can be further isomerized with a catalytic amount of perchloric acid in acetic acid to the tricyclic hydrocarbon, 2,2,3,7-tetramethyltricyclo[5.2.2.0^{1,6}]undec-3-ene (XI).

It has been stated that β-chamigrene (VII) was isolated as one of the major products from the hydrocarbon mixture either by the isomerization with oxalic acid or by the acid-catalyzed dehydration of widdrol. The formation of β-chamigrene (VII) by the isomerization of thujopsene (IV) was not revealed. The process described here involves a method for isomerizing thujopsene and thujopsene isomers derived from hibawood oil and American cedarwood oil, to give chamigrenes and tricyclic $C_{15}H_{24}$ olefinic hydrocarbons.

It has been established that the acetylated product derived from cedarwood oil hydrocarbons contains principally 40 to 55% acetylcedrene (II) derived from α- and β-cedrene and 40 to 50% acetylated $C_{15}H_{24}$ hydrocarbons derived from thujopsene and thujopsene isomers. It has been further established that the portion of the product derived from the thujopsene-thujopsene isomers contains 7 isomeric $C_{15}H_{24}COCH_3$ ketones. Six (22 to 26%) of these ketones, designated as isomers A, B, C, D, E, F, possess very weak woody odors while the seventh ketone (18 to 24%), 4-aceto-6,8a-ethano-1,1,6-trimethyl-1,2,3,5,6,7,8,8a-octahydronaphthalene (V) designated as isomer G, is a compound possessing a powerful and valuable musk odor.

The structure of isomer D (shown on the following page) was established as 4-aceto-2,2,3,7-tetramethyltricyclo[5.2.2.0^{1,6}]undec-3-ene (VI) by comparison with an authentic sample prepared from the hydrocarbon 2,2,3,7-tetramethyltricyclo[5.2.2.0^{1,6}]undec-3-ene (XI).

A schematic representation of the various reactions is given on the following page.

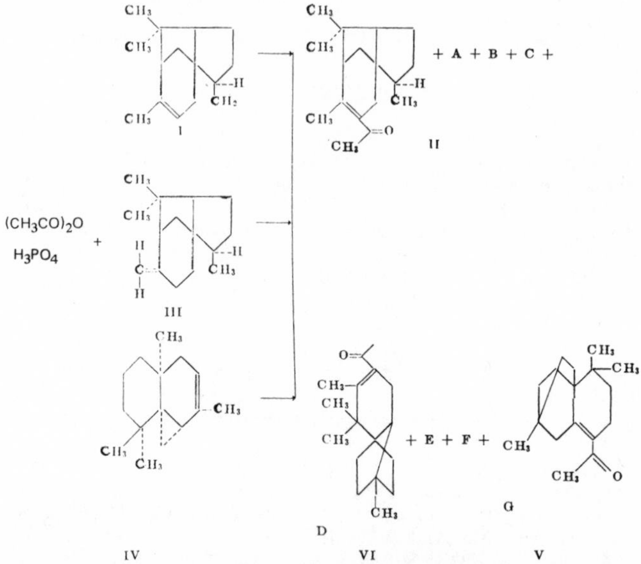

The process is also concerned with a method for the preparation of pure 4-aceto-6,8a-ethano-1,1,6-trimethyl-1,2,3,5,6,7,8,8a-octahydronaphthalene (V, isomer G) and mixtures, rich in this ketone (V) and free of acetylcedrene (II) and mixtures with acetylcedrene (II) containing 40% of more of the desired ketone (V) from thujopsene (IV) derived from naturally occurring essential oils as hibawood and cedarwood oils, β-chamigrene (VII), α-chamigrene (VIII) and thujopsene isomers rich in the hydrocarbon, 6,8a-ethano-1,1,6-trimethyl-1,2,3,5,6,7,8,8a-octahydronaphthalene (IX). The ketones derived by the acetylation of thujopsene (IV), chamigrenes (VII and VIII) or the tricyclic hydrocarbons (IX) are seven isomeric $C_{17}H_{26}O$ ketones and are designated again as isomers A to G.

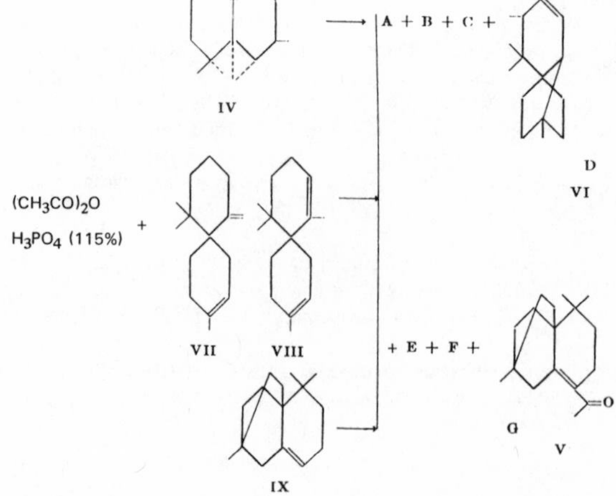

This process involves isomerization procedures utilizing protonating acids whereby thujopsene (IV) can be isomerized to β-chamigrene (VII) and α-chamigrene (VIII) or to a new series of tricyclic $C_{15}H_{24}$ olefinic hydrocarbons rich in the hydrocarbon 6,8a-ethano-1,1,6-trimethyl-1,2,3,5,6,7,8,8a-octahydronaphthalene (IX). The chamigrenes (VII) and (VIII) also can be isomerized by these procedures to a series of tricyclic $C_{15}H_{24}$ olefinic hydrocarbons (IX).

It has been found that strong acids isomerize thujopsene (V, IV) by Path A to α- and β-chamigrenes (VII and VIII) which in turn can be isomerized to a series of tricyclic $C_{15}H_{24}$ olefinic hydrocarbons, rich in the hydrocarbon 6,8a-ethano-1,1,6-trimethyl-1,2,3,5,6,7,8,8a-octahydronaphthalene (IX hydrocarbons A and B) while weak or dilute aqueous acids follow a different isomerization (Path B) to yield the hydrocarbon 1,4,11,11-tetramethyl-bicyclo[5.4.0]undeca-3,7-diene (X) which can be further isomerized to the hydrocarbon 2,2,3,7-tetramethyltricyclo[5.2.2.0^{1,6}] undec-3-ene (XI).

Path A

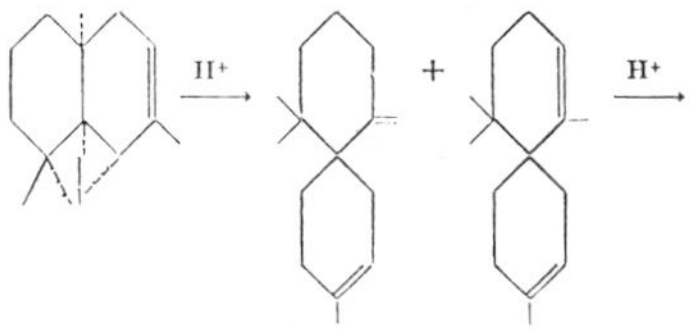

IV   VII   VIII

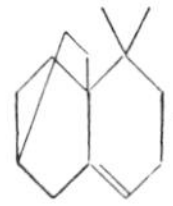

IX   + other $C_{15}H_{24}$ tricyclic hydrocarbons

Path B (hydrocarbons A and B)

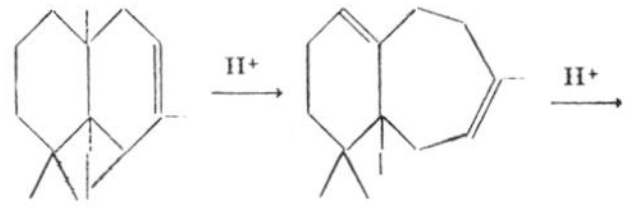

IV   X

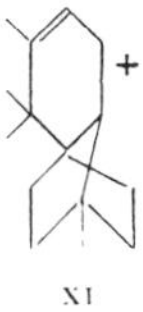

XI   + minor $C_{15}H_{24}$ tricyclic hydrocarbons

Example 1: Tricyclic $C_{15}H_{24}$ hydrocarbons rich in 6,8a-ethano-1,1,6-trimethyl-1,2,3,5,6,7-8,8a-octahydronaphthalene (IX) is prepared as follows. Into a reaction flask, equipped with an agitator, thermometer, feeding funnel and a condenser, is charged 500 g glacial acetic acid and 200 g polyphosphoric acid (115%).

The mixture is agitated and 500 g thujopsene (IV) is fed in at 40°C over a 5 minute period. The batch is agitated at 40°C for 3 hours and poured onto 1,000 g water. The oil layer is separated and the aqueous layer extracted 2 x 100 ml benzene. The combined oil and benzene extracts are washed 2 x 50 ml water, made alkaline with 10% sodium carbonate and washed neutral with salt water. The benzene is distilled off under reduced pressure leaving 505 g crude hydrocarbons.

Vapor phase chromatography (vpc) of the crude shows eight components: (1) 0.4%, (2) 1.3%, (3) 4.7%, (4) 4.9%, (5) 9.3%, (6) 27.3%, (7) 44.5%, (8) 7.5%. Components (1) through (4) are tricyclic $C_{15}H_{24}$ hydrocarbons of unknown structure. Component (5) is 2,2,3,7-tetramethyltricyclo[5.2.2.0^{1,6}] undec-3-ene (XI). Components (6) and (7) are the desired tricyclic $C_{15}H_{24}$ hydrocarbons and are referred to as hydrocarbons A and hydrocarbons B (IX). Component (8) is chamigrenes (VII and VIII), principally α-chamigrene (VIII).

Example 2: β- and α-Chamigrenes (VII and VIII) — Into a reaction flask, equipped with an agitator, thermometer and a condenser, is charged 200 g thujopsene (IV) and 20 g of 90% formic acid. The batch is heated to 100°C and agitated at 100°C for 1 hr. 100 ml of water is added and the oil layer is separated. The aqueous layer is extracted 2 x 50 ml of benzene. The combined oil and benzene extracts are washed 2 x 50 ml of water, neutralized with 10% sodium bicarbonate and washed with 50 ml of water. The benzene is distilled off under reduced pressure leaving 200 g of crude hydrocarbons.

Vapor phase chromatography of the crude shows seven components: (1) 0.7%, (2) 2.8%, (3) 2.8%, (4) 1.9%, (5) 4.7%, (6) 25.1%, (7) 62.0%. Components (1) and (2) are hydrocarbons of unknown structures, component (3) is 2,2,3,7-tetramethyltricyclo[5.2.2.0^{1,6}]-undec-3-ene (XI). Components (4) and (5) are the tricyclic hydrocarbons A and B (IX) of Example 1. Components (6) and (7) are the desired β- and α-chamigrenes (VII and VIII).

In related work *G.C. Kitchens, A.R. Hochstetler and K. Kaiser; U.S. Patent 3,678,119; July 18, 1972; assigned to Givaudan Corporation* have found that when α- and β-chamigrenes are treated with substantially anhydrous strong acids, suitably in the presence of an alkanoic acid they are isomerized to give a mixture of tricyclic $C_{15}H_{24}$ olefinic hydrocarbons rich in 6,8a-ethano-1,1,6-trimethyl-1,2,3,5,6,7,8,8a-octahydronaphthalene. This compound is useful as an intermediate in the preparation of compounds in perfume compounding.

4-Aceto-6,8a-Ethano-1,1,6-Trimethyloctahydronaphthalene

G.C. Kitchens, A.R. Hochstetler and K. Kaiser; U.S. Patent 3,799,987; March 26, 1974; assigned to Givaudan Corporation have found that thujopsene and thujopsene isomers, when treated with acetic anhydride in the presence of polyphosphoric acid yields 4-aceto-6,8a-ethano-1,1,6-trimethyl-1,2,3,5,6,7,8,8a-octahydronaphthalene.

This compound may also be obtained by the acetylation of 6,8a-ethano-1,1,6-trimethyl-1,2,3,5,6,7,8,8a-octahydronaphthalene in which case boron trifluoride may also be used as a catalyst. The compound of the process is extremely useful as an odorant and fixative in perfume compounding when employed per se or in a mixture containing ketones derived from thujopsene and at least 40% by weight of the compound.

It has been established that the acetylated product derived from cedarwood oil hydrocarbons contains principally 40 to 55% acetylcedrene (II) derived from α- and β-cedrene and 40 to 50% acetylated $C_{15}H_{24}$ hydrocarbons derived from thujopsene and thujopsene isomers.

It has been further established by use that the portion of the product derived from the thujopsene-thujopsene isomers contains seven isomeric $C_{15}H_{24}COCH_3$ ketones. Six (22 to 26%) of these ketones, designated as isomers A, B, C, D, E, F, possess very weak woody odors and are not of practical interest in perfumery while the seventh ketone (18 to 24%), 4-aceto-6,8a-ethano-1,1,6-trimethyl-1,2,3,5,6,7,8,8a-octahydronaphthalene (V) designated as isomer G, is a compound possessing a powerful and valuable musk odor.

AMBRETTE OIL

Ambrettolide from 1,9-Cyclohexadecadiene

B.D. Mookherjee and W.I. Taylor; U.S. Patent 3,681,395; August 1, 1972; assigned to

International Flavors & Fragrances Inc. describe a process for the preparation of ambrettolide and isomers from 1,9-cyclohexadecadiene. Diepoxidized 1,9-cyclohexadecadiene is reduced to a mixture of cyclohexadecadiols and oxidized to the corresponding hydroxy ketones. These, upon oxidation in the presence of a boron trifluoride etherate catalyst, are converted into hydroxy cyclohexadecanolides which are dehydrated to form a mixture of isomers of ambrettolide which can be separated by conventional means, if desired.

Ambrettolide naturally occurs in musk ambrette seed oil and is a valuable perfume base because of its desirable odor. Ruzicka and Stoll [*Helv. Chem. Acta,* 17, 1609 (1928)] show a method for preparing macrocyclic lactones involving the oxidation of macrocyclic ketones with Caro's acid (persulfuric acid) to the corresponding lactones. Ambrettolide is said to be prepared by this method. U.S. Patent 2,417,151 describes a process for the preparation of ambrettolide involving intramolecular esterification.

In this process sodium 6,16-dihydroxypalmitate is condensed with 1-chloropropanediol-2,3 to form the glycerol monoester which is treated with sodium acid sulfate to produce a mixture of unsaturated isomeric glycerol monoesters. This mixture is then distilled and worked up to yield a mixture of unsaturated isomeric large ringed cyclic lactones including ambrettolide which can be separated out, if desired. The following examples illustrate the process.

Example 1: Preparation of Ambrettolide and Isomers — The following is the preparation of 1,2,9,10-diepoxycyclohexadecane from 1,9-cyclohexadecadiene. An apparatus consisting of a 100 ml reaction flask fitted with a thermometer, mechanical stirrer, addition funnel and ice bath is charged with 5.0 g (0.023 mol) of 1,9-cyclohexadecadiene; 7.0 g of sodium acetate; and 30 ml of methylene chloride and cooled to 0°C. A solution containing 9.4 g (0.046 mol) 40% peracetic acid and 20 ml of methylene chloride is prepared and is then added slowly to the flask during a one-half hour period while the temperature is maintained at 0°C.

The mixture is then stirred for 3 hours at 0° to 5°C and is then permitted to return to room temperature. The mixture is then poured into a separatory funnel containing 40 ml of water. The aqueous layer is extracted three times with 30 ml portions of methylene chloride. The combined organic layer is then washed with a saturated sodium chloride solution until it tests neutral and then is dried over anhydrous sodium sulfate. The solvent is removed by means of a rotary evaporator yielding 6.16 g of crude material which is then chromatographed to obtain 5.15 g (90% yield) of 1,2,9,10-diepoxycyclohexadecane.

The following is a preparation of a mixture of 1,9- and 1,8-cyclohexadecadiols from 1,2,9,10-diepoxycyclohexadecane. An apparatus consisting of a 1 liter reaction flask fitted with an addition funnel, thermometer, mechanical stirrer, condenser, heating mantle and nitrogen purge is charged with 12.14 g (0.32 mol) of lithium aluminum hydride and 300 ml of anhydrous ether. A solution containing 20.0 g (0.079 mol) of 1,2,9,10-diepoxycyclohexadecane and 200 ml of anhydrous ether is then added slowly over a one hour period.

After the addition is completed the mixture is refluxed for four hours and then cooled down to 4°C. The reaction mixture is then decomposed with 40 ml of cold water and the lithium hydroxide salt is extracted and washed with carbon tetrachloride until neutral and the ether extract is washed three times with 50 ml portions of a 50% sodium chloride solution until neutral. The solvent is then removed yielding 15.6 g of a crude cyclohexadecadiol mixture.

The preparation of a mixture of 9-hydroxy-1-cyclohexadecanone and 8-hydroxy-1-cyclohexadecanone from 1,9- and 1,8-cyclohexadecadiols is as follows. An apparatus consisting of a 1 liter reaction flask fitted with an addition funnel, reflux condenser, thermometer, mechanical stirrer and Dry Ice bath is charged with 14.0 g (0.956 mol) of a mixture of 1,9- and 1,8-cyclohexadecadiol and 550 ml of acetone and cooled to 0°C. A solution containing 5.6 g (0.056 mol) of chromic oxide, 4.2 g of concentrated sulfuric acid and 28 ml of water is prepared and added dropwise over a 2 hour period.

After the addition is completed the reaction mixture is stirred for 1 hour at 0°C and then the acetone is removed by vacuum and replaced with 400 ml of water. The aqueous solution is then transferred to a separatory funnel and saturated with sodium chloride and then extracted five times with 100 ml portions of carbon tetrachloride. It is then washed three times with a 50% sodium chloride solution until neutral and then dried over sodium sulfate yielding 12.6 g of crude material. This crude material is then chromatographed to obtain 5.2 g (41% yield) of hydroxy cyclohexadecanones.

The following is a description of the preparation of a mixture of 9-hydroxy-1-cyclohexadecanolide, 8-hydroxy-1-cyclohexadecanolide and 10-hydroxyl-1-cyclohexadecanolide from 9-hydroxy-1-cyclohexadecanone and 8-hydroxy-1-cyclohexadecanone. An apparatus consisting of a 100 ml reaction flask fitted with an addition funnel, mechanical stirrer, thermometer, reflux condenser, heating mantle and thermo watch is charged with 2.0 g (0.0078 mol) of a mixture of hydroxy cyclohexadecanones, 40 ml of chloroform and 0.6 g of boron trifluoride etherate and the mixture is stirred.

Over a 15 minute period, 5 g (0.028 mol) of 40% peracetic acid is added and the resulting reaction mixture is then stirred for 12 hours at 50 ± 5°C and then for 24 hours at room temperature. The chloroform layer is then washed three times with 20 ml portions of a 50% sodium chloride solution and twice with cold water until neutral and then dried over sodium sulfate yielding 2.0 g of crude material. This crude material is then chromatographed to obtain 0.35 g (30% yield) of hydroxy cyclohexadecanolides.

The preparation of ambrettolide from hydroxy cyclohexadecanolides is as follows. An apparatus consisting of a 15 ml receiver fitted with an addition funnel, glass stopper and magnetic stirrer is charged with 100 mg of a mixture of hydroxy cyclohexadecanolides, 1 ml of anhydrous benzene and 30 mg of p-toluene sulfonic acid and the mixture is stirred for one hour at room temperature.

The reaction mixture is then injected into a pyrolytic glass column packed with 5 g of Anakrom coated with 10% silicone rubber (SE 30 Gum Rubber) and 1 g stainless steel turnings at a temperature of 310°C and the distillate is collected in a cooled vial, and purged of the solvent leaving 50 mg of a mixture of ambrettolide and isomers thereof.

This mixture is separated by gas-liquid chromatography using helium as the gas and a 25 foot, one-quarter inch inside diameter stainless steel column at 100°C and with a flow rate of 80 ml/min and packed with 5% polyethylene glycol (Carbowax 20M) supported on Anakrom ABS (a treated diatomaceous earth composition). The analysis shows the presence of ambrettolide as well as the other isomers.

Example 2: A perfume composition is prepared by admixing the following ingredients in the indicated proportions.

Ingredient	Parts by Weight
Geranium, Algerian	100
Clove	100
Cassin	30
Labdanum resin	60
Castoreum absolute	10
Sandal	50
Cedarwood	150
Ionone residues	30
Vetivert	20
Benzyl benzoate	150
Terpineol	150
Ambrettolide from Example 1	150
	1,000

This perfume composition is found to have a desirable musk fragrance quality.

Purification of Seed Oil

P.D. Thomas and C.R. Stephens, Jr.; U.S. Patent 3,415,813; December 10, 1968; assigned to Chas. Pfizer & Co., Inc. describe a method which comprises deodorizing and decolorizing impure musk by treating such musk at an elevated temperature in an inert solvent with a minor amount of Raney nickel. The following examples illustrate the process.

Example 1: In a 1 liter, 3-necked flask fitted with a mechanical stirrer, thermometer, nitrogen inlet tube and reflux condenser with drying tube, was placed 20 g of Raney nickel that had been previously washed three times with dry ethanol then three times with purified hexane. A gentle flow of nitrogen gas was started before the addition of catalyst to minimize combustion hazards.

One hundred grams of freshly distilled ambrette seed oil, obtained by the distillation of whole, uncrushed seeds, and dissolved in 300 ml of purified hexane, was added. The resulting mixture was stirred at reflux for 2 hours. The mixture was cooled to room temperature and filtered under a nitrogen atmosphere through a sintered glass funnel. The filtrate was concentrated to dryness on a rotary evaporator and then held at 70°C (0.5 mm Hg) for about 1 hour and finally allowed to cool to room temperature.

The resulting ambrette seed oil (95 g) could not be distinguished from commercial ambrette seed oil which had been stored for several months to subdue its initial fatty odor and to develop its distinctive rich, floral-musky odor. Similar results are obtained when the ambrette seed oil is treated with 5% Raney nickel and with 10% Raney nickel.

Example 2: One hundred grams of distilled cyclopentadecanolide prepared by the method of Beets and Van Essen, German Patent 1,025,861, was treated by the method of Example 1 except that 5 g of Raney nickel were used. The resulting musk had a strong floral-musky bouquet and no longer possessed the sour, sulfur-like odor it had prior to the Raney nickel treatment.

Vapor phase chromatography on samples before and after treatment indicated that trace impurities with retention times up to 6 minutes had been almost completely removed.

OTHER PROCESSES

Civetone by Reduction of Cyclic Diacetylenes

A process described by *C.G. Parsons and W.H. Pittman; U.S. Patent 3,235,601; February 15, 1966; assigned to Diamond Alkali Company* relates to trans-olefinic compounds represented by the structure:

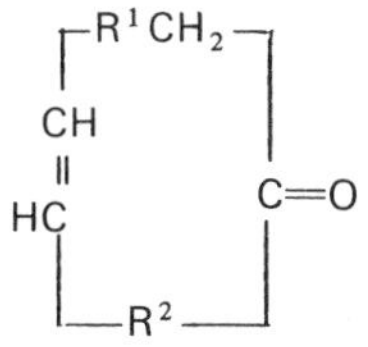

$$
\begin{array}{c}
\lceil\text{—} R^1 CH_2 \text{—}\rceil \\
CH \\
\parallel \qquad\qquad C{=}O \\
HC \\
\lfloor \text{—} R^2 \text{—}\rfloor
\end{array}
$$

where R^1 and R^2 are divalent hydrocarbon radicals containing straight chains of from 4 to 10 carbon atoms. Civetone, a constituent of an oil secreted by the civet cat, is a valuable perfume base. The determination of the gross structure of civetone was accomplished by Ruzicka and coworkers [*Helv. Chim. Acta.* 9, 230 (1926); ibid, 10, 695 (1927)], who identified it as 9-cycloheptadecene-1-one. In 1948, Stoll and coworkers [*Helv. Chim. Acta* 31, 543 (1948)] proved, by an elegant sequence of reactions, that naturally occurring civetone has the cis configuration. The high demand and short supply of civetone and of muscone (3-methylcyclopentadecanone), a secretion of the musk deer which is also a valuable perfume base, have encouraged attempts to prepare synthetic products which may be substituted for natural civetone and muscone. Thus, Blomquist and coworkers [*J. Am. Chem. Soc.*, 77, 1804 (1955)] synthesized cyclic monoketones which possessed strong musk odors.

The synthesis of civetone, both the cis and trans forms, and homologs thereof, has also been the subject of much investigation. In U.S. Patent 1,720,748, there is described a process for preparing civetone by oxidation of civetol, another constituent of civet oil. In effect, this increases the yield of natural civetone, but it does not dispense with the necessity of reverting to natural sources.

Preparation of civetone by pyrolysis of the thorium salt of 9-octadecene-1,18-dioic acid (Swiss Patent 136,543) or the yttrium salt of the same acid (U.S. Patent 1,873,154) has been successfully attempted. The expense of this method is prohibitive, since thorium and yttrium salts are not readily available and yields are rather low.

Hunsdiecker [*Ber.,* 76B, 142 (1943); ibid, 77B, 185 (1944)] has prepared civetone by a rather long series of reactions from aleuritic acid (1,10,16-trihydroxyhexadecanoic acid), a constituent of shellac. However, the number of reactions required and the necessity for isolation of the starting material from natural sources make this process commercially unattractive.

Blomquist et al (U.S. Patent 2,790,005) have prepared civetone analogs by partial reduction of macrocyclic diketones, followed by dehydration. This process, however, apparently gives a mixture of cis and trans isomers (judging from the reported melting point of the product), rather than pure cis or trans material.

In this process, civetone homologs of the structure

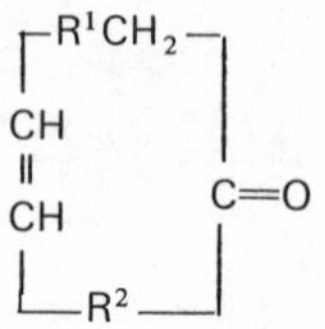

$$\begin{array}{c} \lceil R^1CH_2 \rceil \\ CH \qquad \qquad | \\ \parallel \qquad \qquad C{=}O \\ CH \\ \lfloor R^2 \rfloor \end{array}$$

where R^1 and R^2 are divalent hydrocarbon radicals containing straight chains of from 4 to 10 carbon atoms, are prepared by a method which comprises the steps of (a) partially reducing a cyclic diacetylene of the structure

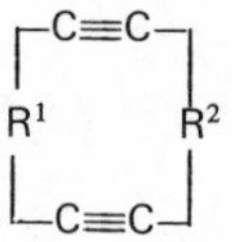

$$\begin{array}{c} \lceil C{\equiv}C \rceil \\ R^1 \qquad R^2 \\ \lfloor C{\equiv}C \rfloor \end{array}$$

thereby producing an enyne of the structure

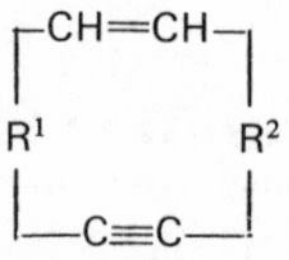

$$\begin{array}{c} \lceil CH{=}CH \rceil \\ R^1 \qquad R^2 \\ \lfloor C{\equiv}C \rfloor \end{array}$$

and (b) hydrating the enyne in the presence of a mercury-containing catalyst. The method to be employed for the reduction of the cyclic diacetylene to the corresponding enyne will depend on whether a cis or trans product is desired.

In the preferred case the reduction is carried out by means of sodium in liquid ammonia, and the products are the trans olefinic ketones. In the reduction of cyclic diacetylenes by sodium in liquid ammonia, a molar ratio of sodium to diacetylene of between about 3:1 and 5:1 is used. Owing to the fact that the reaction does not go to completion, this amount of sodium is satisfactory for selective reduction of one triple bond. (The theoretical ratio is 2:1.) The preferred means of addition is to add the sodium in small quantities to the diacetylene in liquid ammonia, thus avoiding a large excess of sodium which would promote indiscriminate reduction of both triple bonds. The following examples illustrate the process.

Example 1: Preparation of 1,8-Cyclotetradecadiyne — Two and one-half liters of liquid ammonia is placed in a flask, followed by the addition of 1.35 g of ferric nitrate hydrate (0.3 g for each gram atom of sodium employed). Two grams of sodium metal is then added and activated by bubbling dry air into the mixture. Sodium metal, 103.5 g (4.4 mols), is added in small portions and 54.3 liters (2.22 mols) of acetylene gas at 28°C and 747 mm Hg is bubbled into the suspension of the sodium amide. 1,5-dibromopentane, 500 g (2.2 mols) is added at a fast dropwise rate sufficient to retain gentle refluxing of the ammonia.

Upon completion of addition of the dibromopentane, agitation of the mixture is increased to wash down the splattered material on the sides of the reaction flask. The reaction is then stopped and the openings of the reaction vessel covered with polyvinyl chloride film, the reaction mixture being allowed to stand overnight. The reaction mixture is then agitated while water is added slowly with caution. The pressure is vented by loosening the plastic sheets covering the reaction vessel opening.

Upon addition of about 400 ml of water, the reaction vessel walls are washed by increasing the agitation. The resultant gummy solid is found to be soluble in organic solvents, i.e., pentane and ether. Isolation of the desired acetylenic cyclic hydrocarbon is accomplished by recrystallization from ether, yielding not only the cyclic hydrocarbon but also the respective linear triyne and tetrayne as by-products.

The crude product is further vacuum distilled and recrystallized from ether, yielding the desired product, melting at 99° to 100°C. The isolation of the desired 1,8-cyclotetradecadiyne, $C_{14}H_{20}$, having a molecular weight of 188.3, is indicated by the following elemental analytical data.

Element	Actual Percent by Weight	Calculated Percent by Weight
Carbon	89.6	89.3
Hydrogen	10.6	10.7

Infrared spectra indicate the presence of internal acetylenic linkage and the absence of terminal acetylenic linkage.

Example 2: Preparation of Trans-7-Cyclotetradecen-1-one — Part A describes the reduction of 1,8-cyclotetradecadiyne. To a stirred suspension of 138.7 g (0.74 mol) of 1,8-cyclotetradecadiyne in 1,500 ml of liquid ammonia is added 51 g (2.22 gram atoms) of freshly cut sodium metal and 50 ml of anhydrous ether. The mixture is stirred for several hours, after which the openings in the reaction flask are sealed with plastic film (cellophane) to retard the evaporation of ammonia and the flask is allowed to stand overnight.

When nearly all of the ammonia has evaporated, about 200 ml of water is cautiously added dropwise with stirring. The solid product is removed by filtration and freed of inorganic impurities by dissolving in a mixture of acetone and ether, filtering and evaporating the solvent. There is obtained 109.9 g of solid product which is analyzed by vapor phase chromatography and by comparison with known compounds, found to have the following composition.

	Percent
Trans,trans-1,8-cyclotetradecadiene	13.9
1,8-Cyclotetradecadiyne	72.7
Trans-1-cyclotetradecen-8-yne	13.4

Part B is a description of the hydration. The material hydrated is a mixture of reduction products, prepared as in Part A and having the following composition.

	Percent
Trans,trans-1,8-cyclotetradecadiene	23.2
1,8-Cyclotetradecadiyne	52.5
Trans-1-cyclotetradecen-8-yne	24.3

To a solution of 94.7 g of this mixture in 400 ml of methanol is added, with stirring, a warm solution of 6 g of red mercuric oxide, 4 ml of boron trifluoride etherate and 10 g of trichloroacetic acid in 175 ml of methanol. The temperature rises to 62°C as the catalyst solution is added. The solution is heated under reflux for 2 hours.

The solvent is removed by vacuum evaporation and the residue is treated with about 200 milliliters of 5% aqueous sodium bicarbonate, followed by an equal volume of 1:1 hydrochloric acid. It is then dissolved in a boiling mixture of acetone and ether, filtered and cooled. The precipitated solids weigh 104.4 g. Of this crude product, 90 g is subjected to absorption chromatography on a column 2 ft long by 25 mm i.d., packed with 200 g of alumina.

Upon elution of n-pentane, benzene, ether and methanol, the components of the mixture are recovered in the following order: trans,trans-1,8-cyclotetradecadiene; trans-7-cyclotetradecen-1-one; 1,7-cyclotetradecanedione; 1,8-cyclotetradecanedione. Separation of diene from enone is not complete.

The mixture of diene and enone is again chromatographed on a column 4 ft long by 18 mm i.d., packed with 250 g of alumina. Upon elution with n-pentane, there is first obtained 18.7 g of trans,trans-1,8-cyclotetradecadiene, and then 18.3 g (76.2% of the theoretical amount, based on the percentage of enyne in the reduction product) of trans-7-cyclotetradecen-1-one, $C_{14}H_{24}O$, MP 23°C. The structure is confirmed by comparison of its infrared spectrum with those of known compounds, and by the following analytical results.

	Actual Percent by Weight	Calculated Percent by Weight
Carbon	80.5	80.7
Hydrogen	11.7	11.6
Molecular weight	206	208

The purity of the civetone homolog, as determined by vapor phase chromatographic analysis, is 98%.

Muscone from Epoxidized 1,9-Cyclohexadecadiene

B.D. Mookherjee and E.T. Theimer; U.S. Patent 3,718,696; February 27, 1973; assigned to International Flavors & Fragrances Inc. describe a process for preparing muscone from 1,9-cyclohexadecadiene involving a number of steps. Monoepoxidized 1,9-cyclohexadecadiene upon treatment with alkyl lithium is converted into an α,β-unsaturated alcohol and oxidized into the corresponding α,β-unsaturated ketone.

This compound, upon treatment with alkyl magnesium halide in the presence of cuprous chloride, is converted to β-methylcyclohexadecenone and then hydrogenated to homomuscone (β-methylcyclohexadecanone). Homomuscone dibromide undergoes a Favorski rearrangement to produce a mixture of β- and γ-methylcyclopentadecenecarboxylates (3:7) which on treatment with hydrazoic acid is converted into α-methylcyclopentadecanone and muscone, respectively. The following examples illustrate the process. All percentages and ratios are by weight, unless otherwise indicated. Temperatures are expressed in degrees centigrade and room temperature is 25° to 30°C.

Example 1: Preparation of Muscone and α-Methylcyclopentadecanone –(A) The following is the preparation of 1,2-epoxy-9-cyclohexadecene from 1,9-cyclohexadecadiene. An apparatus consisting of a 100 ml reaction flask fitted with a thermometer, mechanical stirrer, addition funnel and ice bath is charged with 5.0 g (0.023 mol) of 1,9-cyclohexadecadiene, 7.0 g of sodium acetate and 30 ml of methylene chloride and cooled to 0°C. A solution containing 4.7 g (0.023 mol) 40% peracetic acid and 10 ml of methylene chloride is prepared and added slowly to the flask during a one-half hour period while the temperature is maintained at 0°C.

The mixture is then stirred for 3 hours at 0° to 5°C and allowed to return to room temperature. The mixture is poured into a 125 ml separatory funnel containing 40 ml of water and the layers are separated. The aqueous layer is extracted three times with 30 ml portions of methylene chloride. The combined organic layer is then washed with a saturated sodium chloride solution until it tests neutral and then is dried over anhydrous sodium sulfate. The solvent is removed by means of a rotary evaporator yielding 5.58 g of crude product which is then chromatographed to obtain a yield of 4.5 g (90% yield) of 1,2-epoxy-9-cyclohexadecene.

(B) The following is a description of the preparation of α,β-unsaturated cyclohexadecenol from 1,2-epoxy-9-cyclohexadecene. An apparatus consisting of a 500 ml reaction flask fitted with an addition funnel, stirrer, thermometer, ice bath and reflux condenser with drying tube is flushed with nitrogen. 80 ml (0.13 mol) of 15% butyl lithium in hexane is added to the reaction flask and cooled to 0°C.

A solution containing 100 ml of hexane and 30 g of the crude nonchromatographed material from Part A of this example (out of which 7.5 g was 1,9-cyclohexadecadiene) is prepared and added slowly dropwise to the butyl lithium for ½ hour, with stirring and maintenance of the temperature at 0°C. After the addition is completed, the mixture is stirred for an additional one-half hour. The temperature is then slowly raised to 65°C and the mixture is refluxed for 3 hours.

The reaction mixture is cooled to 5°C and 30 ml of water are added to this cooled mixture. The mixture is poured into a separatory funnel and the layers are separated. The organic layer is washed with water until it tests neutral and is dried. The solvent is removed by means of a rotary evaporator yielding 33 g of crude product which is then chromatographed to obtain a 54% yield of α,β-unsaturated cyclohexadecenol.

(C) The following describes the preparation of α,β-unsaturated cyclohexadecenone from α,β-unsaturated cyclohexadecenol. A chromic acid solution is prepared by cautiously adding 11 ml of concentrated sulfuric acid to a 500 ml flask containing 10 g of chromic oxide. The mixture is cooled in an ice bath and 50 ml of water are slowly added, resulting in the formation of a chromic acid solution.

An apparatus consisting of a 1 liter reaction flask fitted with an addition funnel, thermometer, mechanical stirrer, Dry Ice bath and reflux condenser is charged with 12 g of α,β-unsaturated cyclohexadecenol and 300 ml of acetone and cooled to 0°C. The chromic acid, as prepared above, is added dropwise with stirring until an orange-yellow color persists.

The solution is stirred for 3 hours at 0°C and allowed to return to room temperature. 150 milliliters of the acetone solvent is removed in vacuo without any heat. 200 ml of water are added and the solution is extracted five times with 200 ml portions of methylene chloride. The combined extracts are washed three times with 50 ml portions of a saturated sodium chloride solution until it tests neutral and dried over anhydrous sodium sulfate. The remaining solvent is removed in vacuo yielding 10 g of crude product which is chromatographed to obtain 8.3 g of (70% yield) α,β-unsaturated cyclohexadecenone.

(D) The following describes the preparation of β-methylcyclohexadecenone from α,β-unsaturated cyclohexadecenone. An apparatus consisting of a 250 ml reaction flask fitted with an adaptor, thermometer, mechanical stirrer, addition funnel, nitrogen purge, reflux condenser equipped with drying tube and Dry Ice bath is charged with 10 ml (0.03 mol) of methylmagnesium bromide, 50 ml of anhydrous ether and 0.15 g of cuprous chloride and cooled to 10°C. A solution of 5.5 g (0.024 mol) of α,β-unsaturated cyclohexadecenone and 40 ml of anhydrous ether is prepared and slowly added to the flask over a period of ½ hour.

The reaction mixture is stirred for 1 hour at 10°C decomposed by adding 25 ml of a cold 10% hydrochloric acid solution. The ether layer is separated and washed three times with 20 ml portions of a cold 10% bicarbonate solution and two times with 20 ml portions of water until it tests neutral and is dried. The solvent is removed, yielding 5.7 g of crude material which is chromatographed to obtain 4.9 g (90% yield) of β-methylcyclohexadecenone.

(E) The following describes the preparation of homomuscone from β-methylcyclohexadecenone. An apparatus consisting of a 500 ml reaction flask fitted with a Brown's hydrogenation apparatus connected to a hydrogen cylinder is charged with 10 g of β-methylcyclohexadecenone, 1.5 g of a 10% palladium on carbon catalyst and 200 ml of methanol.

Hydrogen is passed from the cylinder into the apparatus until no more is absorbed (940 milliliters) at which point the reduction is complete. The catalyst is removed by vacuum filtration through a glass sintered funnel covered with celite and upon evaporation of the solvent in vacuo, 10 g (100% yield) of the saturated ketone, homomuscone (β-methylcyclohexadecenone) is obtained.

(F) The following is the preparation of dibromohomomuscone from homomuscone. An apparatus consisting of a 500 ml reaction flask equipped with an addition funnel, mechanical stirrer, heating bath and connected to a vacuum system is charged with 15 g (0.06 mol) of homomuscone, 200 ml of anhydrous benzene and 20 ml of anhydrous ether. 19.2 g (0.12 mol) of bromine is added dropwise, at room temperature, over a period of one-half hour to the reaction flask.

The hydrogen bromide liberated by the reaction is removed by turning on the vacuum system while simultaneously heating the flask to 50°C. This operation is continued until the solution in the flask tests neutral. Analysis of the product confirmed the formation of the desired dibromohomomuscone (3-methyl-2,16-dibromocyclohexadecanone).

(G) The following describes the preparation of a mixture of β-methylcyclopentadecenecarboxylate and γ-methylcyclopentadecenecarboxylate from dibromohomomuscone. The same apparatus is utilized as in (F) above, except that the heating bath is replaced with a cooling bath. Over a 1 hour period, 7.6 g (0.14 mol) of sodium methoxide is added to the reaction flask containing the dibromohomomuscone prepared above.

The temperature is maintained at room temperature by means of an ice bath. The mixture is stirred for an additional one-half hour at room temperature, and then is cooled to 5°C by means of an ice bath. 200 ml of cold water are added and the solution is permitted to return to room temperature. The organic layer is separated, washed twice with 50 ml portions of 5% hydrochloric acid and twice with 50 ml portions of 50% sodium chloride until it tests neutral and it is then dried. After the solvent is removed, 19.0 g (90% yield) of a mixture of β-methylcyclopentadecenecarboxylate and γ-methylcyclopentadecenecarboxylate remains.

(H) The following describes the preparation of a mixture of muscone and α-methylcyclopentadecanone from β-methylcyclopentadecenecarboxylate and γ-methylcyclopentadecenecarboxylate. An apparatus consisting of a 250 ml flask equipped with an addition funnel, mechanical stirrer, thermometer, ice bath and nitrogen purge is charged with 42 ml of concentrated sulfuric acid and cooled to 5°C. 19.0 g of the mixture of β-methylcyclopentadecenecarboxylate and γ-methylcyclopentadecenecarboxylate are added over a period of one-half hour while maintaining the temperature at 5°C. 50 ml of chloroform are then added, and the mixture warmed to 40°C and at this temperature 6.2 g of sodium azide are added over a period of 1 hour. The resultant mixture is stirred for 15 minutes at 40°C and cooled to 5°C and the mixture is poured into 200 ml of wet ice.

This entire mixture is then transferred into a microsteam distillation apparatus and steam distilled at steam temperatures of 100° to 160° to 200°C and the distillate is collected. The distillate is saturated with solid sodium chloride and extracted four times with 50 ml portions of ether. The ether extract is then washed with 50 ml of a saturated sodium chloride solution and dried. The solvent is removed yielding 12.0 g of crude material which is chromatographed to obtain 10.5 g of a mixture of muscone and α-methylcyclopentadecanone. NMR analysis showed 70% muscone and 30% α-methylcyclopentadecanone.

Example 2: A perfume composition is prepared by admixing the following ingredients in the indicated proportions.

Ingredient	Parts by Weight
Geranium, Algerian	100
Clove	100
Cassin	30
Labdanum resin	60
Castoreum absolute	10
Sandal	50
Cedarwood	150
Ionone residues	30
Vetwert	20
Benzyl benzoate	150
Terpineol	150
Mixture of muscone and β-methylcyclopentadecanone from Example 1	150
	1,000

This perfume composition is found to have a desirable musk fragrance quality.

1-Hydroxy-9-Cyclohexadecanolide

According to a process described by *B.D. Mookherjee and W.I. Taylor; U.S. Patent 3,728,358; April 17, 1973; assigned to International Flavors & Fragrances* macrocyclic ketones are converted into the corresponding lactones with a peracid in the presence of a boron trifluoride etherate catalyst and an inert solvent to form a reaction mixture. This mixture is heated until the conversion is complete and the desired lactones can be recovered by conventional means. The lactone obtained, 1-hydroxy-9-cyclohexadecanolide, is useful as a fragrance ingredient. The general reaction of the process is illustrated by the equation below.

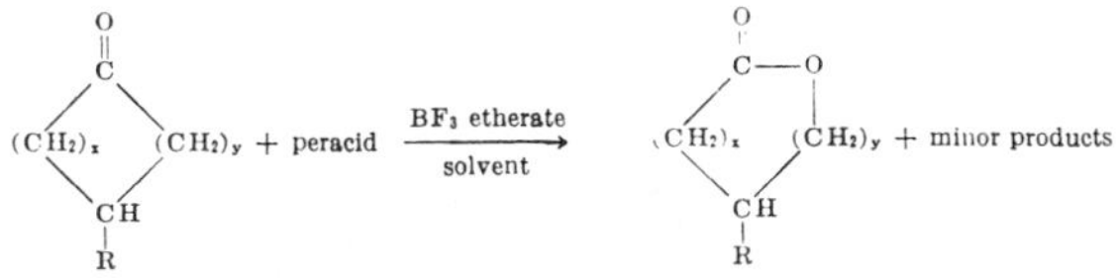

The principal product is the macrocyclic lactone corresponding to the macrocyclic ketone starting material. The macrocyclic lactone product can be recovered by conventional means from the reaction mixture of the above general equation. These lactones have a highly desirable and useful odor characterized as a musk odor.

Example 1: Preparation of Cyclohexadecanolide from Cyclohexadecanone — An apparatus consisting of a 100 ml reaction flask equipped with an addition funnel, magnetic stirrer, thermometer and reflux condenser fitted with drying tube is charged with 2.15 g (0.009 mol) of cyclohexadecanone and 18 ml of chloroform. 0.45 ml of freshly distilled 98% boron trifluoride etherate is then added over a period of 5 minutes and the temperature rises from 25° to 29°C and the solution assumes an orange color. 5.13 g (0.027 mol) of 40% peracetic acid is then added over a period of 15 minutes and the temperature rises to 33°C and the solution becomes pale yellow.

The temperature is then raised to 45°C and the contents are stirred for 11½ hours. The solution is then cooled and 20 ml of water are added and the organic layer is then extracted twice with 50 ml portions of hexane, washed three times with 50 ml portions of a saturated sodium chloride solution and dried over anhydrous sodium sulfate. The solvent is then removed in vacuo yielding 2.65 g of crude material which is then chromatographed to obtain 0.963 g of cyclohexadecanolide.

Example 2: Preparation of 1-Hydroxy-9-Cyclohexadecanolide from 1-Hydroxy-9-Cyclohexadecanone — An apparatus consisting of a 100 ml reaction flask fitted with an addition funnel, mechanical stirrer, thermometer, reflux condenser, heating mantle and thermo watch is charged with 2.0 g (0.0078 mol) of 1-hydroxy-9-cyclohexadecanone, 40 ml of chloroform and 6.0 g of boron trifluoride etherate and the mixture is stirred.

Over a fifteen minute period, 5.0 g (0.028 mol) of 40% peracetic acid are added and the resulting reaction mixture is then stirred for 12 hours at 50 ± 5°C. The chloroform layer is then washed three times with 20 ml portions of a 50% sodium chloride solution and twice with cold water until neutral and then dried over sodium sulfate yielding 2.0 g of crude material. This crude material is then chromatographed to obtain 0.35 g (30% yield) of 1-hydroxy-9-cyclohexadecanolide.

When the procedures set forth in Examples 1 and 2 are duplicated using stannous chloride, aluminum chloride and zinc chloride in place of boron trifluoride etherate as the catalyst, no significant yields of lactone are obtained.

Example 3: A perfume composition is prepared by mixing the following ingredients in the indicated proportions.

Ingredient	Parts by Weight
Geranium, Algerian	100
Clove	100
Cassia	30
Labdanum resin	60
Castoreum absolute	10
Sandal	50
Cedarwood	150
Ionone residues	30
Vetivert	20
Benzyl benzoate	150
Terpineol	150
Cyclohexadecanolide from Example 1	150
	1,000

This perfume composition is found to have a desirable musk fragrance quality.

In related work *B.D. Mookherjee and W.I. Taylor; U.S. Patent 3,681,396; August 1, 1972; assigned to International Flavors & Fragrances* describe a process for preparing cyclohexadecanolide from 1,9-cyclohexadecadiene involving a number of steps. Monoepoxidized 1,9-cyclohexadecadiene is reduced to 9-cyclohexadecene-1-ol and oxidized to the corresponding unsaturated ketone and then hydrogenated to cyclohexadecanone.

This upon oxidation in the presence of a boron trifluoride catalyst is converted into cyclo-hexadecanolide.

4-Ethoxybutyrate from Butyrolactone and Triethyl Borate

According to a process described by *R.A. Dombro; U.S. Patent 3,639,456; February 1, 1972; assigned to Universal Oil Products Company* ether esters of carboxylic acids are prepared by treating a lactone with a borate ester in the presence of an acidic catalyst to prepare the desired ether ester of the carboxylic acid.

The compounds which result from the esterification of butyrolactone with triethyl borate, namely, ethyl 4-ethoxybutyrate, possess a musk-like odor and will be utilized in the formulation of fragrances and aromas, these compounds then being compounded with other compositions of matter to prepare the final fragrance or aroma compositions of matter which are used in the preparation of soaps, detergents, shaving creams, colognes, perfumes, etc.

A specific example is found in the process for the preparation of an ether ester of a carboxylic acid which comprises treating butyrolactone with triethyl borate in the presence of methanesulfonic acid at a temperature in the range of from about 20° to about 200°C and a pressure in the range of from about atmospheric to about 100 atmospheres, and recovering the resultant ethyl 4-ethoxybutyrate.

2,3-Decamethylenecyclopentanone

According to a process described by *H.Nozaki, R. Noyori and T. Mori; U.S. Patent 3,465,040; September 2, 1969; assigned to Chugai Seiyaku KK, Japan* the compound 2,3-decamethylene-cyclopentanone, having a musk-like and white sandalwood-like odor is useful for perfume. The compound is prepared by reducing 2,3-decamethylene-2-cyclopentenone and the reaction is shown as follows.

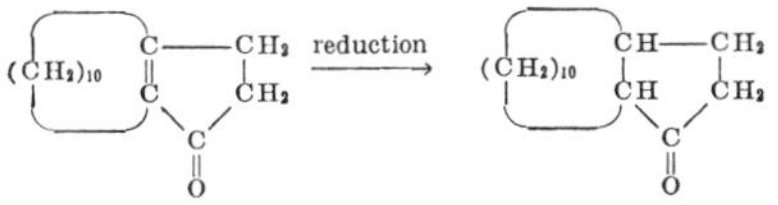

Catalytic reduction is the preferred method of carrying out the above reduction. However, the other reduction method using a reducing agent may be used as well. The following examples illustrate the process.

Example 1: To a solution of 5 g of 2,3-decamethylene-2-cyclopentenone in 20 ml of ethanol was added 5 ml of 10% palladium on carbon. The mixture was shaken vigorously under atmospheric pressure of hydrogen for 20 hours. After the reaction was completed, the catalyst was removed by filtration and the filtrate was concentrated. Distillation under reduced pressure gave 5 g of oily 2,3-decamethylenecyclopentanone; MP 150°C/0.1 mm Hg. The following is the elemental analysis. Calculated for $C_{15}H_{26}O$: C, 81.02%; H, 11.78%. Found: C, 80.95%; H, 11.70%. The compound was converted to 2,4-dinitrophenylhydrazone; MP 147.5° to 148°C.

Example 2: To a solution of 4 g of 2,3-decamethylene-2-cyclopentenone in 20 ml of dioxane was added 3 ml of Raney nickel (W-2). The mixture was shaken under hydrogen at normal pressure for 20 hours. After absorption of hydrogen gas had ceased, the catalyst was removed by filtration and the filtrate was concentrated. Distillation under reduced pressure gave 3.6 g of oily 2,3-decamethylenecyclopentanone; MP 147° to 150°C/0.1 mm Hg.

Example 3: A solution of 1 g of 2,3-decamethylene-2-cyclopentenone in 10 ml of anhydrous ether was added to 50 ml of liquid ammonia containing 0.5 g of metallic lithium in the course of 15 minutes and kept overnight. Resulting mixture was decomposed by aqueous ammonium chloride and extracted with ether. Removal of the solvent followed by distillation under reduced pressure gave 0.7 g of oily 2,3-decamethylenecyclopentanone; MP 145° to 150°C/0.1 mm Hg.

Haloundecyl Alkyl Ketones

P. Lafont and Y. Bonnet; U.S. Patent 3,240,812; March 15, 1966; assigned to Societe des Usines Chimiques Rhone-Poulenc, France describe omega-haloketones of the Formula (1):

$$(1) \qquad\qquad R-CO-(CH_2)_{10}-CH_2X$$

where R represents an alkyl group containing from 1 to 5 carbon atoms and X represents a chlorine or bromine atom. The omega-haloundecyl alkyl ketones are valuable intermediate products for use in organic synthesis. Furthermore, they are of value in the preparation of artificial musks, which are valuable in perfumery.

For example, it is possible, by condensing these haloketones with a malonic diester and then saponifying and decarboxylating them by known methods, to obtain ketonic acids of the type: $HOOC-(CH_2)_{12}-CO-R$ which, after reduction to alcohol acids and cyclization by conventional methods, can be used in the preparation of macrocyclic lactones having a strong musky odor. The following examples illustrate the process.

Example 1: Into a 1 liter spherical flask provided with a reflux condenser, a dropping funnel, a stirrer and a gas bubbler are introduced 150 cc of carbon tetrachloride and then 19.8 g (0.1 mol) of 1-methylcyclododecanol. After dissolution, there are introduced 200 cubic centimeters of an aqueous sodium hypochlorite solution, representing 0.03 mol of NaOCl. The flask is kept in darkness and a current of carbon dioxide is bubbled through it for 4 hours with vigorous stirring.

There is thus passed a total quantity of carbon dioxide corresponding to an excess of about 100% in relation to the quantity of sodium hypochlorite. The stirring is continued for 2 days in darkness, and the reaction mass is then decanted and the organic layer extracted and then washed with water and dried over calcium chloride. Infrared spectroscopy of the liquid obtained does not reveal the characteristic band of the hypochlorite, but it shows the characteristic band of the ketone grouping $>C=O$.

The carbon tetrachloride is evaporated and the residual oil, amounting to 23.75 g is distilled under a pressure of 0.25 mm Hg. There is thus obtained a middle fraction of 20.95 grams, which is a colorless liquid boiling between 120° and 125°C under the indicated pressure, and analysis of which corresponds to the formula $C_{13}H_{25}OCl$.

When treated with sodium acetate in acetic acid and then saponified, this compound yields 1-hydroxy-12-tridecanone, of which the melting point, 56°C, corresponds to that indicated in the literature for this hydroxyketone prepared by an entirely different method [M. Stoll, *Helv. Chim. Acta* 34, 1817 (1951)]. It is thus confirmed that the middle fraction consists of 1-chloro-12-tridecanone.

The 1-methylcyclododecanol employed as starting material was prepared in the following manner. Into a spherical flask of the same type as that previously described, are introduced 16 g of magnesium and 200 cc of dry diethyl ether. There are then gradually added, in half an hour, 94 g of methyl iodide in solution in 200 cc of dry ether.

After complete dissolution of the magnesium there is introduced, in 1 hour, a solution of 91 g of cyclododecanone in 200 cc of dry diethyl ether. The mixture is then heated under reflux for 15 hours. The complex magnesium compound precipitates. It is hydrolyzed at 0°C by treatment with 2 N hydrochloric acid at a pH of 5 and then decanted. The ethereal layer is washed with water and then with an aqueous sodium thiosulfate solution and again with water. It is dried over anhydrous calcium chloride and the ether is then evaporated.

The residue, when twice recrystallized from a 50/50 mixture of ether and petroleum ether (35° to 50°C fraction), gives 85 g of 1-methylcyclododecanol, MP 94° to 95°C.

Example 2: By proceding in the same way as before, but using only 110 cc of Javelle water of 47 to 50 chlorometric degrees, representing about 0.2 mol of NaOCl, and bubbling the carbon dioxide through for 22 hours, there are obtained 23.6 g of 1-chloro-12-tridecanone.

2,4-Dialkoxy-5,6-Hydrocarbylene-3-Nitropyridines

A process described by *A. Grüssner and O. Schnider; U.S. Patent 3,271,403; September 6, 1966; assigned to Hoffmann-La Roche Inc.* relates to pyridine derivatives having the general formula:

(1)

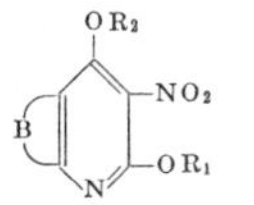

in which R_1 is a lower alkyl group; R_2 is a lower alkyl group; and B is a $-(CR_3=CR_4)_2$ group or a $-(CR_3H)_x$ group, in which groups R_3 is hydrogen or a lower alkyl group, R_4 is hydrogen or a lower alkyl group and x is the integer 4 or 5.

The following are examples of certain of the compounds produced in the process: 2,4-dimethoxy-3-nitro-5,6,7,8-tetrahydroquinoline; 2,4-diethoxy-3-nitro-5,6,7,8-tetrahydroquinoline; 2,4-dimethoxy-3-nitroquinoline; and 2,4-dimethoxy-3-nitro-5,6-cyclopentamethylene pyridine.

In general, these compounds are, because of their fragrance and fixative properties, useful as odorants and as fixatives in the preparation of perfumes and other scented preparations. The compounds can be prepared quite readily. In general, the method of preparation involves the reaction of a 2,4-dihalogeno-3-nitropyridine compound having the formula:

(2)

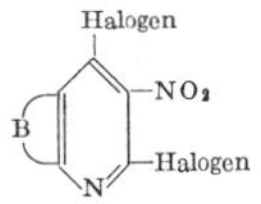

in which the symbol B has the same meaning as in Formula (1) and in which the word Halogen represents a halogen atom, preferably a chlorine or bromine atom with an alkali alcoholate of a lower alcohol. In such reaction there is employed, preferably, an alkali alcoholate of an alcohol having a carbon chain length of from 1 to 3 carbon atoms, such as methanol and ethanol.

The reaction of the halogen substituted compound of Formula (2) with the alkali alcoholate brings about the replacement of the halogen substituents of the first named compound by alkoxy groups. Such result can be accomplished, conveniently, by reacting the halogen compound with an alcoholic solution of the alkali alcoholate. The latter solution can be obtained by dissolving an alkali metal, an alkali hydroxide or an alkali metal alcoholate in an alcohol.

It has been observed that 2,4-dimethoxy-3-nitro-5,6,7,8-tetrahydroquinoline is most suitable for use where an intense musk-like odor is desired. In contrast, 2,4-diethoxy-3-nitro-5,6,7,8-tetrahydroquinoline; 2,4-dimethoxy-3-nitroquinoline and 2,4-dimethoxy-3-nitro-5,6-cyclopentamethylene pyridine are characterized by an odor which is fainter and less intense than that of 2,4-dimethoxy-3-nitro-5,6,7,8-tetrahydroquinoline. However, the odor of 2,4-dimethoxy-3-nitro-5,6-cyclopentamethylene pyridine is considered to be the closest to the natural musk.

Example 1: To a solution of 5.6 grams of potassium hydroxide in 40 milliliters of methanol there was added 4.94 grams of 2,4-dichloro-3-nitro-5,6,7,8-tetrahydroquinoline. The mixture was heated at its reflux temperature for 2 hours while nitrogen was passed through it. After cooling, the reaction mixture was made slightly congo acid with concentrated hydrochloric acid, filtered with suction to remove the potassium chloride present and, thereafter, concentrated.

By this procedure there was obtained 2,4-dimethoxy-3-nitro-5,6,7,8-tetrahydroquinoline. That compound was dissolved in ether and washed with water. Subsequently, ether was evaporated off and the product was allowed to crystallize from dilute methanol. The crystalline product which was thus obtained exhibited a faint yellow coloration and had a melting point of 36° to 38°C. The product was obtained in a yield of 70% of theory.

Example 2: By the procedure described in Example 1, using ethanol instead of methanol, there was obtained 2,4-diethoxy-3-nitro-5,6,7,8-tetrahydroquinoline. That product precipitated in the form of light yellow crystals having a melting point of 51° to 53°C.

The 2,4-dichloro-3-nitro-5,6,7,8-tetrahydroquinoline which was used as the starting material in this example as well as in Example 1 was prepared from the corresponding hydroxy compound (that is, 2,4-dihydroxy-3-nitro-5,6,7,8-tetrahydroquinoline, having a melting point of 224°C with decomposition) by heating with phosphorus oxychloride at a temperature of 135°C. The compound melted at 70° to 71°C after crystallization from petroleum ether.

The dihydroxy compound which was used in the production of the 2,4-dichloro-3-nitro-5,6,7,8-tetrahydroquinoline was prepared in the following manner. 40 g of 2,4-dihydroxy-5,6,7,8-tetrahydroquinoline were stirred for 3 hours with 200 ml of concentrated nitric acid. Upon mixing, the temperature of the reaction mixture rose to about 35°C.

When the temperature of the reaction mixture commenced to fall, the reaction mixture was placed in ice water for 2 hours, and treated with water until turbidity set in. Thereafter, it was filtered with suction and crystallized from aqueous acetic acid. There was obtained 27 grams of the 2,4-dihydroxy-3-nitro-5,6,7,8-tetrahydroquinoline which melted at 244°C, with decomposition.

Example 3: 5.2 grams of 2,4-dichloro-3-nitro-5,6-cyclopentamethylene pyridine were heated at reflux for 1½ hours in 40 milliliters of a 15% solution of potassium hydroxide in methanol. After cooling, the reaction mixture was acidified with alcoholic hydrochloric acid, filtered with suction to remove the potassium chloride present and concentrated. The residue was taken up in ether and washed with water. The 2,4-dimethoxy-3-nitro-5,6-cyclopentamethylene pyridine, which remains behind after evaporation of the ether, was crystallized from 90% methanol. The product was obtained in a yield of 75% of theory in the form of light yellow crystals of melting point 53° to 55°C.

The 2,4-dichloro-3-nitro-5,6-cyclopentamethylene pyridine, which was used as the starting material in this example, was prepared by heating the corresponding dihydroxy compound (that is, 2,4-dihydroxy-3-nitro-5,6-cyclopentamethylene pyridine of melting point 238° to 239°C) at 60°C for 2 hours in phosphorus oxychloride. The compound was obtained in the form of yellowish crystals having a melting point of 68° to 70°C.

Example 4: 20 grams of 2,4-dichloro-3-nitroquinoline were introduced portionwise at 5°C while stirring into a solution prepared from 7.6 grams of sodium and 200 milliliters of absolute methanol.

After stirring for 48 hours at 20° to 25°C, the solution was adjusted to pH 5.8 with glacial acetic while cooling with ice and, subsequently, it was concentrated in a vacuum at 40°C bath temperature. The residue was dissolved in low-boiling petroleum ether, the solution washed with water, dried with sodium sulfate and evaporated. Upon recrystallization from low-boiling petroleum ether, there was obtained 16.0 grams (83% of theory) of 2,4-dimethoxy-

3-nitroquinoline having a melting point of 69° to 70°C.

Example 5: By the procedure described in Example 4, using sodium ethylate in absolute alcohol in place of the methanolic solution of sodium, there was obtained 2,4-diethoxy-3-nitroquinoline, in the form of yellow crystals, having a melting point of 56° to 57°C.

FLORAL FRAGRANCES

JASMINE

Unsaturated Decalactones

L.G. Heeringa, R.J. Fehn, J.D. Grossman and B.D. Mookherjee; U.S. Patent 3,531,501; September 29, 1970; assigned to International Flavors & Frangrances Inc. describe a process for the preparation of unsaturated δ-decalactone. In view of the limited availability of natural jasmine, and its commercial importance in producing high grade fragrances, synthetic substitutes have become desirable. Since certain lactones constitute part of the fragrance impression of jasmine, and 2-(cis-penten-2'-yl-1') pentanolide, the δ-lactone of 5-hydroxy-7-decenoic acid, is known to constitute an important constituent of the essence of Italian jasmine, a commercially feasible synthesis for this lactone has been sought.

A number of routes for the production of such lactones from various starting materials are available, although they are rather complicated. One of the known methods of synthesis for the δ-lactone of 5-hydroxy-7-decenoic acid begins with the reaction of cyclopentanone with pyrrolidine to form pyrrolidylcyclopentene, and subsequent treatment of the unsaturated alicyclic ring with bromopentyne to provide pentynylcyclopentanone.

The prior art suggests that a Baeyer-Villiger reaction could be used to produce the lactone from the pentynylcyclopentanone, but the prior art further demonstrated that treating alkynylcyclopentanone with peracids provided a mixture of materials without the formation of any detectible amounts of the desired lactone. In order to produce the desired intermediate, a multistep method was devised by E. Demole et al and reported in *Helvetica Chimica Acta* 45, 1256 (1962).

In showing a synthesis for the lactone, Demole et al describe that attempts to oxidize the material to the lactone directly utilizing either perbenzoic acid, meta-chloroperbenzoic acid, or trifluoroperacetic acid, all of which were thought to be reagents specific to oxidize the ring and thereby produce the lactone, were unsuccessful. Accordingly, the synthesis finally arrived at utilized a complex process involving reduction of the acetylenic bond in the pentynylcyclopentanone, formation of the cyclic alcohol, bromination and lactone formation, followed by a reduction to obtain the unsaturated lactone ring.

This process comprises treating alkynylcyclopentanone with certain unsubstituted aliphatic percarboxylic acids at temperatures in the range of 10° to 50°C to form the alkynyl δ-lactone. The alkynyl lactone so formed can be further selectively hydrogenated to provide the alkenyl derivatives. Such δ-alkenyl lactones are useful in the preparation of perfumes and fragrance compositions. The alkynylcyclopentanones treated according to the process include 2-(pentyn-2'-yl) cyclopentanone. It is preferred that the starting material be relatively pure to avoid the formation of unwanted by-products and to facilitate purification of the desired lactone. Such alkynylcyclopentanones can readily be prepared by treating cyclopentanone with a secondary amine such as pyrrolidine or piperidine under acidic conditions to form the corresponding enamine such as 1-pyrrolidylcyclopentene-1 and subsequently alkylating the enamine so obtained with 1-bromopentyne-2.

The choice of the percarboxylic acid is most important in obtaining any significant yield of the desired product from the reaction, and accordingly aliphatic percarboxylic acids are used. The lower aliphatic percarboxylic acids having up to about 4 carbon atoms are most desirable, and performic, peracetic, and perpropionic acids are preferred. The best results are generally obtained with peracetic acid.

The yield of alkynyl lactone can be improved or the rate of reaction can be increased by incorporating catalytic amounts of certain strong protonic acids into the reaction system. These protonic acids may be added directly into the system or may first be mixed with the peracid material. When such protonic acids are used, only small amounts are required, that is, up to about 0.5% of the percarboxylic acid. It is especially preferred to utilize as strong protonic materials sulfuric acid and organic sulfonic acids such as methane sulfonic, p-toluene sulfonic, and the like. The following examples illustrate the process. Unless otherwise indicated, all ratios, proportions, parts, and percentages are by weight.

Example 1: A 50 ml Erlenmeyer flask is fitted with a stirrer, a thermometer, and cooling means, and 15 grams (0.1 mol) of pentynylcyclopentanone as prepared above is introduced into the flask. The flask is cooled to maintain a temperature of 20° to 25°C while 21 grams (0.11 mol) of 40% peracetic acid containing about 1% sulfuric acid is added over a 45 minute period. The mass is then maintained under agitation for 3 hours, at which point the GLC monitoring indicates formation of the desired product with a small amount of the original starting material still present. Accordingly, 7 grams (0.037 mol) of 40% peracetic acid is added, and the mixture is stirred for an additional 1 hour.

At the end of the additional 1 hour stirring period, the reaction mixture is transferred to a separatory funnel, and an equal volume of water and 50 ml of benzene are added. After mixing, the upper organic layer is separated from the aqueous layer and washed 3 times with 50 ml of 5% aqueous sodium bicarbonate. The organic layer is further washed twice with 50 ml of aqueous saturated sodium chloride, dried over anhydrous magnesium sulfate and filtered. The benzene is then removed on a rotary evaporator. Instrumental analysis shows the major product formed is the δ-lactone of 5-hydroxy-7-decynoic acid having the structure

$$O=\!\!\!\underset{O}{\bigcirc}\!\!\!-CH_2-C\equiv C-CH_2-CH_3$$

Example 2: Two equal portions of 28.5 grams (0.16 mol) of pentynylcyclopentanone are treated with 35 grams (0.18 mol) of 40% peracetic acid containing about 1% sulfuric acid so that the peracetic acid is in approximately 16% excess over the theoretical amount. In each instance the peracetic acid is added to the cyclopentanone at 20° to 25°C, over a 1 hour interval. The reaction mixtures are stirred for approximately 5 hours, while the course of the reaction is monitored by GLC analysis of the reaction mixture.

After the 5 hour period 50 ml of an aqueous 50% saturated salt solution is added to each reaction mixture together with 25 ml of benzene. The organic layers in each of the two vessels are separated and washed 3 times with 100 ml of aqueous 50% saturated sodium chloride solution and then once with saturated sodium chloride solution. The washed mixtures are dried over anhydrous magnesium sulfate and filtered. The fractions are then distilled on a micro still to obtain pure product. This material is substantially the pure δ-lactone of 5-hydroxy-7-decynoic acid. Similar results are obtained by substitution of propionic acid for peracetic acid.

Selective Hydrogenation — The lactone prepared above in the amount of 27.5 grams is then placed in a Parr reaction vessel with 20 grams of isopropanol and 0.3 gram of a palladium on calcium carbonate catalyst. The mixture is hydrogenated with 0.15 mol of hydrogen at 27° to 55°C with a pressure falling from 49 to 36 psig over the reaction period.

After hydrogenation the material from the Parr apparatus is filtered to remove solids, and the isopropanol is recovered on a rotary separator. The mixture is then distilled on a micro still at a temperature of 108° to 117°C, at 0.5 mm Hg. GLC analysis shows the reaction products to be approximately 60% of the desired cis-isomer and 30% of the trans-isomer of the δ-lactone of 5-hydroxy-7-decenoic acid. The liquid pure cis-isomer has an n_D^{20} of 1.4860. In other hydrogenations conducted according to the foregoing procedure, the product assayed 90% cis-isomer with smaller amounts of the trans-isomer and saturated material.

Example 3: The following perfume composition illustrates the use of compositions made by the process.

Ingredients	Percent by Weight
Phytol	25
Phytyl acetate	10
Hexyl cinnamic aldehyde	6
Benzyl acetate	30
Benzyl alcohol	5
Benzyl benzoate	10
Indole	0.5
Hexenyl pentanone	1.5
Linalool	10
δ-Lactone of 5-hydroxy-7-decenoic acid produced according to the process of Example 2	2

This perfume formulation is an important part of the fragrance of absolute essence of jasmine flower. This perfume composition is incorporated into a soap formulation at the 0.1% level to provide an excellent jasmine scent in the soap.

2-Cyclopenten-1-ones from Acetals

J.L.E. Erickson, F.E. Collins, Jr. and R.T. Dahill, Jr.; U.S. Patent 3,402,181; September 17, 1968; assigned to The Givaudan Corporation describe a process for preparing 2-cyclopenten-1-ones and related intermediates. The process is represented as follows:

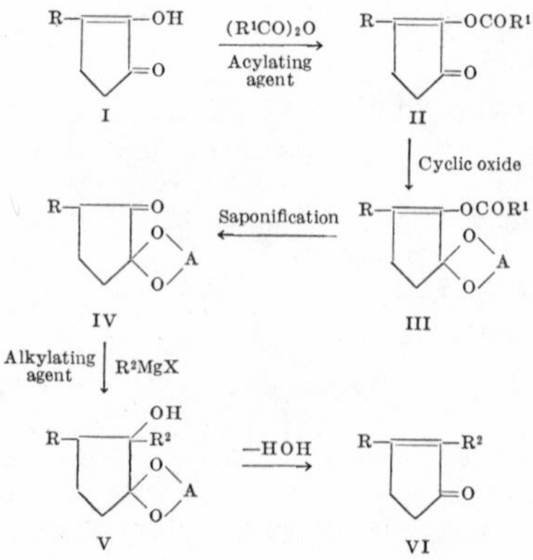

where R is H or alkyl such as methyl, R^1 and R^2 are selected from the group consisting of aryl, alkyl, aralkyl and cycloaliphatic radicals, and A is an alkylene chain having at least 2 carbon atoms, which may have one or more of the hydrogen atoms substituted, e.g., with alkyl radicals, and X is a member selected from the group consisting of chlorine, bromine and iodine. R, R^1, and R^2 may be the same or different. The radicals in R, R^1 and R^2 may be saturated or unsaturated. The intermediates (IV) are useful in perfumery, and as flavors, as well as intermediates for pharmaceuticals.

Cyclopenten-1-one Esters

A process described by *P. Oberhänsli; U.S. Patent 3,754,016; August 21, 1973; assigned to Givaudan Corporation* is concerned with cycloalkenone esters of the general formula

(3)

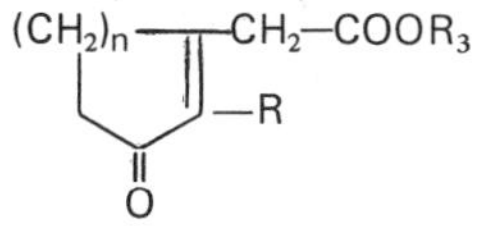

$$(CH_2)_n—CH_2—COOR_3$$
$$—R$$
$$O$$

where R is a hydrogen atom, lower alkyl, lower alkenyl or lower alkynyl, R_3 is lower alkyl and n is 1 or 2. These cycloalkenone esters can be obtained by reacting an enol ether of the general formula

(1)

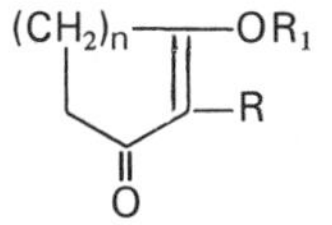

$$(CH_2)_n—OR_1$$
$$—R$$
$$O$$

where R and n signify the same as above and R_1 is lower alkyl, in alkaline, anhydrous reaction medium with a compound of the general formula

(2)

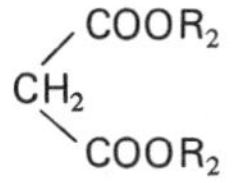

$$CH_2 \begin{array}{c} COOR_2 \\ COOR_2 \end{array}$$

where the radical R_2 signifies lower alkyl.

The esters of general formula (3) can be used as intermediate products for the manufacture of valuable odorants, especially those of the jasmine series, into which they can be converted by hydrogenation or by saponification and decarboxylation. Thus, for example, 2-(2'-pentynyl)-3-keto-1-cyclopentenyl acetic acid metal ester may readily be converted by catalytic hydrogenation (using a Lindlar catalyst) and subsequent hydrogenation of the reaction product (using lithium in ammonia) into the valuable odorant methyl jasmonate, 2-(2'-pentenyl)-3-keto-cyclopentyl acetic acid methyl ester; odoriferous principle of jasmine absolute.

Example 1: (a) Sodium methylate is manufactured from 3.57 grams of sodium and 125 ml of dry methanol. 17.0 grams of malonic acid dimethyl ester and 11.5 grams of 3-methoxy-2-(2'-pentynyl)-2-cyclopenten-1-one are then added and the mixture is boiled at reflux for 16 hours. The solution is cooled and 7.75 grams of glacial acetic acid are added dropwise below 10°C. Most of the methanol is evaporated off, the residue taken up in water and shaken with ether. After drying and evaporation of the ether the crude product still contains malonic acid dimethyl ester. By means of fractional distillation there are obtained 11.15 grams of pure 2-(2'-pentynyl)-3-keto-1-cyclopentenyl acetic acid methyl ester of BP 150°C/0.02 mm. This corresponds to a yield of 79%.

(b) The methyl ester thus obtained can be converted into the valuable odorant methyl jasmonate, 2-(cis-2'-pentyl)-3-ketocyclopentenyl acetic acid methyl ester as follows.

7.65 grams of the 2-(2'-pentynyl)-3-keto-1-cyclopentenyl acetic acid methyl ester in 100 ml of absolute ethanol are hydrogenated in a conventional manner in the presence of 0.76 grams of Lindlar catalyst (palladium catalyst partially deactivated with lead). The calculated amount of hydrogen has been taken up after 2 hours. The catalyst is filtered off and the solution evaporated. After distillation of the residue, there are obtained 6.75 grams of 2-(cis-2'-pentenyl)-3-keto-1-cyclopentenyl acetic acid methyl ester of BP 86° to 88°C under 0.005 mm. Yield: 88%.

1.46 grams of lithium are dissolved in 500 ml of dry, distilled ammonia and cooled to −75°C. 9.0 grams of the 2-(2'-cispentenyl)-3-keto-1-cyclopentenyl acetic acid methyl ester obtained are thereupon added dropwise and the mixture is stirred at −75°C for 10 minutes. 11.7 grams of ammonium chloride are then added, the cooling bath is removed and the ammonia is expelled. Water is thereupon added and the mixture shaken with ether in a conventional manner. After distillation there are obtained 4.65 grams of methyl jasmonate of BP 130°C/0.005 mm; n_D^{20} 1.4780. Yield: 50%.

(c) The 3-methoxy-2-(2'-pentynyl)-2-cyclopenten-1-one used as the starting material can be obtained as follows. 33.2 grams of sodium bicarbonate are dissolved in 300 ml of distilled water. To this solution there are added portionwise 17.6 grams of 1,3-cyclopentanedione and 27.75 grams of 2-pentynyl bromide are subsequently added dropwise. The mixture is stirred at 60°C for 64 hours. After cooling, the reaction mixture is extracted with ether and the aqueous phase acidified with 7% aqueous hydrochloric acid. 2-(2'-pentynyl)cyclo-pentane-1,3-dione of MP 148° to 150°C is thus obtained. Yield: 37%.

A solution of 16.0 grams of 2-(2'-pentynyl)cyclopentane-1,3-dione in 100 ml of tetrahydro-furan is treated with an excess of etheral diazomethane solution. After 10 minutes, the solvents are evaporated in vacuum and the residue is distilled. 13.85 grams of 3-methoxy-2-(2'-pentynyl)-2-cyclopenten-1-one of BP 142° to 150°C under 0.03 mm are thus obtained. Yield: 80%.

Example 2: A sodium methylate solution is manufactured from 2.45 grams of sodium and 60 ml of dry methanol. 138 grams of malonic acid dimethyl ester are then added and subsequently 6.6 grams of 3-methoxy-2-methyl-2-cyclopenten-1-one are added portion-wise as solid substance. After 3 hours boiling at reflux, 6.3 grams of glacial acetic are added dropwise below 10°C to the cooled mixture. Most of the methanol is evaporated off in vacuum and the residue treated with 250 ml of ether. The precipitated sodium ace-tate is filtered off and the filtrate concentrated. By fractional distillation there are re-covered 5.9 grams of pure 2-methyl-3-keto-1-cyclopentenyl acetic acid methyl ester of BP 72° to 78°C under 0.02 mm. This corresponds to a yield of 70%.

3,5,5-Trialkoxycyclopent-2-en-1-ones

M.E. Vandewalle; U.S. Patent 3,803,219; April 9, 1974; assigned to Pfizer Inc. describes 2-substituted 3,5,5-trialkoxycyclopent-2-en-1-ones having the formula:

(1)

$$
\begin{array}{c}
OR^2 \\
R^1 \diagdown \\
O = \boxed{} - OR^2 \\
OR^2
\end{array}
$$

where —R^1 is selected from the group consisting of lower alkyl, alkenyl, alkynyl, 3,3-di-phenyl-allyl, methoxy-lower alkyl, and 6-carboxyhexyl, the lower alkyl, alkenyl, and alkynyl having from 1 to 7 carbon atoms; and where —R^2 is methyl or ethyl. The com-pounds are useful in the preparation of 3-substituted cyclopentan-1,2-diones, and 2,3-sub-stituted cyclopent-2-en-1,4-diones and their 1-ketals. The intermediates of Formula (1) are preferably prepared from 3-substituted cyclopentan-1,2,4-triones of the following formula.

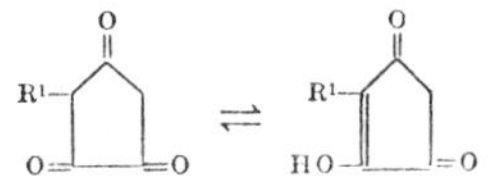

These intermediates are prepared by reaction with an orthoformic acid ester of the formula $HC(OR^2)_3$:

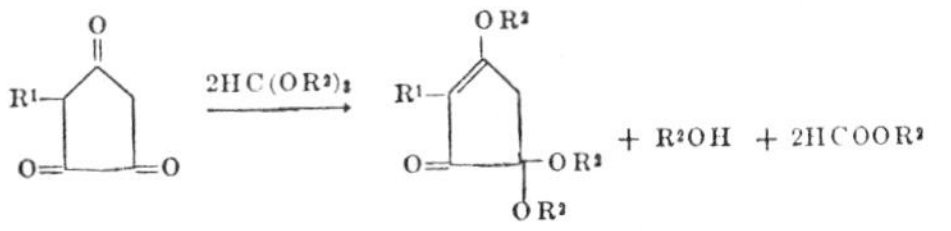

Example: (a) 3-Methyl-cyclopentan-1,2,4-trione — Powdered sodium 161 grams (7 mols) was added to a mixture of tert-butanol (3 liters) and dry toluene (1 liter) in a flask equipped with a stirrer, condenser and dropping funnel, and the mixture was heated under reflux with stirring until the sodium had begun to react. A mixture of butanone 252 grams (3.5 mols) and diethyl oxalate 1,127 grams (7.7 mols) was added during 30 minutes to the refluxing suspension of sodium tert-butoxide, and after maintaining reflux for a further 5 hours, the solution was cooled and treated with concentrated hydrochloric acid, 700 ml.

The precipitated sodium chloride was filtered off, and the filtrate was evaporated to small bulk under reduced pressure. The residue of crude oxalyl ester was hydrolyzed by heating under reflux with hydrochloric acid 2.5 N (2 liters) for 90 minutes. The solution was then cooled, concentrated under reduced pressure, and extracted with ether. The ether extract was evaporated, and water was removed from the residue by addition of benzene followed by azeotropic distillation. A small amount of oxalic acid was filtered off, and the filtrate was purified by crystallization from benzene. It had MP 161°C. Yield: 335 grams (76%).

(b) 2-Methyl-3,5,5-triethoxy-cyclopent-2-en-1-one — 3-Methyl-cyclopentan-1,2,4-trione 56 grams (0.44 mol), triethyl orthoformate 163 grams (1.1 mols) and a catalytic amount 0.2 grams of p-toluenesulfonic acid were dissolved in dry ethanol 1,000 ml and the mixture was heated. The ethyl formate, BP 55°C, generated was allowed to distill through an efficient reflux condenser, and after about 4 hours the temperature of the distillate had risen to the boiling point of ethanol. Ethanol was then removed by distillation under reduced pressure, the residue was extracted wtih ether, and the ether layer was washed with aqueous sodium carbonate solution (5%) and dried (Na_2SO_4).

The ether was then distilled off and the residue was warmed with isooctane (800 ml). After removal by filtration of some undissolved material, the isooctane solution deposited crystals of the desired product, MP 60°C. Yield: 90 grams (78%). Hydrolysis of the mother liquor with dilute aqueous sodium hydroxide yielded an appreciable amount of trione starting material, so that the absolute yield was rather higher. Analysis: found, 63.3% C, 8.80% H; required for $C_{12}H_{20}O_4$, 63.1% C, 8.84% H.

3-Oxocyclopentylacetic Acid Esters

E. Demole; U.S. Patent 3,288,833; November 29, 1966; assigned to Firmenich et Cie, Switzerland describes materials which are racemic compounds of the general formula

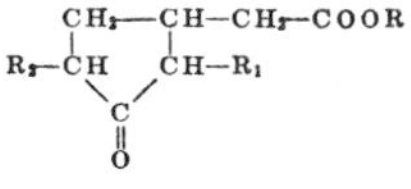

where one of the symbols R_1 and R_2 represents hydrogen and the other an unsubstituted alkenyl group having 5 carbon atoms, and R represents methyl or ethyl. The alkenyl radiical represented by R_1 or R_2 can be, e.g., a cis- or trans-1-penten-1-yl, cis- or trans-2-penten-1-yl, cis- or trans-3-penten-1-yl, 4-penten-1-yl or 3-methyl-2-buten-1-yl radical. A preferred class of the compounds represented by the above formula includes those in which the alkenyl radical is unbranched and has its double bond in the 2,3-, 3,4- or 4,5-position and in which R is methyl or ethyl, preferably methyl.

Those compounds of the above formula in which R_1 or R_2 is a —CH_2—CH=CH—C_2H_5 or —CH_2—CH=C(CH_3)$_2$ group are obtained by condensing a methyl or ethyl 3-oxo-cyclopentyl-acetate with a cyclic secondary amine in order to obtain a mixture of two isomeric enamines, subjecting the mixture to the action of a substituted allyl halide, e.g., the cis- and trans-isomers of 1-bromo-2-pentene or 1-bromo-3-methyl-2-butene, and hydrolyzing the reaction product in order to obtain a mixture of methyl or ethyl 2- and 4-(2-alkenyl)-3-oxo-cyclopentylacetates and, if desired, separating the individual position isomers from their mixture. The following examples illustrate the use of the compounds of this process in perfumery.

Example 1: A composition having a chypre type fragrance was prepared by blending the ingredients listed below in the proportions set forth:

Base Composition	Parts by Weight
Santal oriental	60
Bourbon vetiver	40
Patchouli	20
Bergamot	150
Synthetic neroli	20
Synthetic rose	60
Rose absolute (Grasse)	15
Jasmine absolute (Grasse)	20
Oak moss absolute (50% in ethyl phthalate)	60
Labdanum resinoid (50% in ethyl phthalate)	60
Zenzoin resin (Siam; 50% in ethyl phthalate)	30
Vanillin	5
Ylang	45
Methylionone	60
Coriander	5
Civet (10% in ethyl phthalate)	30
Musk ketone	60
Coumarin	60
Heliotropin	30
Linalyl acetate	90
Cinnamyl acetate	30
Sweet orange oil	40
Additive	
Methyl 2-(cis-2-penten-1-yl)-3-oxo-cyclopentyl acetate	10

The additive imparts to the fragrance of the base composition a more floral note and enhances the effect of the jasmine absolute contained in this composition.

Example 2: A composition having a floral type fragrance was prepared by blending the ingredients listed below in the proportions set forth:

Base Composition	Parts by Weight
Methyl-nonyl-acetaldehyde (1% in ethyl phthalate)	20
Undecanal (1% in ethyl phthalate)	10
Bergamot	60
Ylang	30
Hydroxycitronellal	180
Phenethylol	120
Geraniol	45
(-)-Citronellol	45

(continued)

Base Composition	Parts by Weight
Linalool	30
Heliotropin	30
Methylionone	60
Anisaldehyde	10
Isoeugenol	5
Benzyl acetate	60
Amyl cinnamic aldehyde	30
Purified styrax (50% in ethyl phthalate)	45
Civet (10% in ethyl phthalate)	45
Musk ketone	55
1,1-dimethyl-6-tert-butyl-4-acetyl-indane	5
Orange blossom absolute	5
Jasmine absolute (Grasse)	25
Rose absolute (Grasse)	20
Vetiveryl acetate	40
Santalol	20
Additive	
Methyl 4-(cis-2-penten-1-yl)-3-oxo-cyclopentyl acetate	5

The additive exalts the jasmine note of the base composition.

Aryl-Alkylenones

M.G.J. Beets and W.J. Wiegers; U.S. Patent 3,173,955; March 16, 1965; assigned to International Flavors & Fragrances I.F.F. (Nederland) NV, Netherlands have found that unsaturated aryl aliphatic ketones of the general structure (1) in which Ar is phenyl or methylphenyl and in which R_1 and R_2 are hydrogen or lower alkyl with a total number of carbon atoms not exceeding two, are outstanding perfumes.

(1)
$$Ar-\underset{\underset{CH_3}{|}}{\overset{\overset{CH_3}{|}}{C}}-CH_2-\overset{\overset{O}{\|}}{C}-\underset{\underset{R_1}{|}}{C}=\underset{\underset{R_2}{|}}{CH}$$

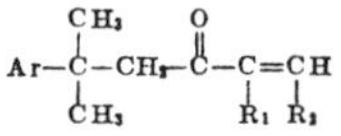

Especially in the case where Ar is phenyl, R_1 is methyl and R_2 is hydrogen, the compound (2) represents material of extraordinary intensive and valuable odor.

(2)

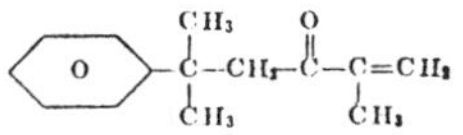

Although 2,5-dimethyl-5-phenyl-hexen-1-one-3 (2) has a strong interesting and definite odor, it is easy to blend into specific and widely varying types of perfumes in relatively large amounts. It shows an excellent tenacity and can be used in perfume compositions as well as in articles in which such compositions are used such as soaps, cosmetics, powders, aerosols, creams and lotions.

2,5-Dimethyl-5-Phenylhexen-1-one-3 — 106 grams (0.40 mol) of 2-acetoxy-2,5-dimethyl-5-phenyl-hexanone-3 were introduced at a pressure of 100 to 110 mm (nitrogen atmosphere) into a reactor consisting of a glass tube packed with glass helices at 350° to 400°C during 4 hours. The crude reaction product was washed to neutral reaction and fractionated through a 16-plate Vigreux column. The yield was 75 to 80%. The product is stabilized with a small amount of one of the usual inhibitors such as hydroquinone. In unstabilized form it shows a tendency to dimerize. Howerver, upon heating (distillation) the dimer dissociates easily and the monomer can always be recovered in nearly quantitative yield. Melting point semicarbazone: 156.4° to 157.0°C.

2,5-Dimethyl-5-(4'-Methylphenyl)Hexen-1-one-3 and 2,5-Dimethyl-5-(3'-Methylphenyl)Hexen-1-one-3 — 2,5-dimethyl-5-(methylphenyl)-hexanol-2-one-3 (mixture of m- and p-isomers) was obtained by condensation of toluene with tetramethyl-tetrahydrofuranone according to Bruson. The corresponding acetate was pyrolyzed as above. A mixture of about 72% para-and 28% meta-isomers of the desired product was obtained in 70% yield. Colorless liquid with strong odor, the rose character of which is shifted somewhat towards the woody note. The two isomers could be separated by gas liquid partition chromatography.

2,5-Dimethyl-5-Phenylhexen-1-one-3 — In a 250 ml distillation flask, fitted for continuous azeotropic water separation were placed 55 grams of xylene, 5.5 grams of toluene-sulfonic acid and 55 grams (0.25 mol) of 2,5-dimethyl-5-phenylhexanol-2-one-3. The solution was refluxed for 30 minutes during which period nearly the theoretical amount of water was separated. The xylene solution was washed and fractionated. The product contained only traces of 1,1,4,4-tetramethyl-tetralone (MP 74.8° to 75.3°C).

2,5-Dimethyl-5-Phenylhexen-1-one-3 — 110 grams (0.5 mol) of 2,5-dimethyl-5-phenyl-hexanol-2-one-3 were introduced into a reactor consisting of a glass tube packed with 17.5 grams of boric anhydride on 45.5 grams of pumice in nitrogen atmosphere at 100 to 110 mm and at 260°C in 2½ hours. Since the conversion was incomplete, the treatment was repeated twice until analysis of the crude product showed the absence of starting material. The crude reaction product was washed and fractionated through a 16-plate Vigreux column. The yield was 65% of theory.

2-Methyl-3-(3',4'-Methylenedioxyphenyl)Propanal

M.G.J. Beets and H. Van Essen; U.S. Patent 3,185,629; May 25, 1965; assigned to International Flavors & Fragrances I.F.F. (Nederland) NV, Netherlands have found that 2-methyl-3-(3',4'-methylenedioxyphenyl)-propanal of the structure below is an outstanding olfactory ingredient in perfume-containing compositions:

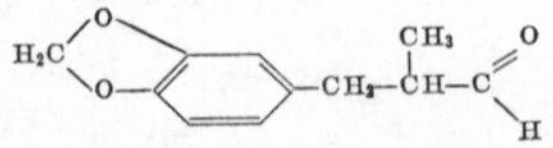

It shows an exceptional tenacity. A strip of filter paper was moistened with 2-methyl-3-(3',4'-methylenedioxyphenyl)-propanal to which 1% of a normal antioxidant, e.g., hydroquinone, had been added and kept for 2 months in contact with air at room temperature. After this period the odor was still strong and undegenerated. The following examples illustrate perfume oils in which 2-methyl-3-(3',4'-methylenedioxyphenol)-propanal is used as an olfactory ingredient, in a mixture with the indicated additional components in the given amounts.

Example 1: A perfume oil having a cyclamen character was made by mixing together the following ingredients:

	Parts by Weight
2-Methyl-3-(3',4'-methylenedioxyphenol)-propanal	50
Hydroxycitronellal	12
Linalool	4
Alpha-ionone	5
Linalyl acetate	4
Geraniol ex Java citronella oil	3
Phenyl ethyl alcohol	5
Musk ketone	2
Amyl cinnamic aldehyde	5
Benzyl acetate	5
Terpineol	5

Example 2: A perfume oil having a jasmine character was mixed from the ingredients shown on the following page.

	Parts by Weight
2-Methyl-3-(3',4'-methylenedioxyphenyl)-propanal	50
Amyl cinnamic aldehyde	13
Benyl acetate	10
Linalool	5
Linalyl acetate	5
Hydroxy citronellal	5
Heliotropin	4
Phenyl ethyl alcohol	8

ROSE

Indeno[1,2-d]-m-Dioxin Derivatives

B.J. Heywood and O. Meresz; U.S. Patent 3,496,193; February 17, 1970; assigned to May & Baker Limited, England describe 2,4-dialkyl-4,4a,5,9b-tetrahydroindeno[1,2-d]-m-dioxin derivatives of the general formula:

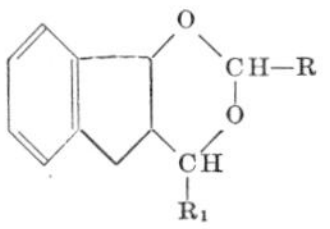

where R and R_1 are the same or different and each represents a methyl, ethyl, propyl, iso-propyl or butyl group. Preferably R and R_1 are the same, the compound wherein they both represent methyl, i.e., 2,4-dimethyl-4,4a,5,9b-tetrahydroindeno[1,2-d]-m-dioxin, being of particular value in perfumery.

The compounds of the above formula are prepared by the reaction of indene with:
(a) when the groups represented by R and R_1 are the same, an aldehyde of the formula RCHO (where R is as defined) or (b) when the groups represented by R and R_1 are different, an equimolecular mixture of aldehydes of the formulas RCHO and R_1CHO, where R and R_1 are as defined.

The reaction is carried out in the presence of formic acid, which serves as a solvent for the reactants and as a catalyst for the reaction. If desired, the reaction mixture may also contain one or more of an inert organic solvent, e.g., petroleum ether, an antioxidant, e.g., hydroquinone, and an acid catalyst, e.g., perchloric acid. The reaction is preferably carried out at ambient temperature.

Example 1: A heterogeneous mixture of 90% formic acid (400 ml), acetaldehyde (280 ml), petroleum ether (BP 60° to 80°C, 650 ml), indene (232 ml) and hydroquinone (0.75 gram) was treated with solid carbon dioxide to flush out air and stirred at room temperature for 3 days. The reaction mixture was then diluted with water (1 liter) and the organic layer separated and washed successively with water, saturated aqueous sodium bicarbonate solution, and water.

After drying over magnesium sulfate and evaporation of the solvent, the product was distilled under high vacuum and the fraction BP 63° to 67°C at 0.05 mm Hg (112.8 grams) collected and redistilled to give 2,4-dimethyl-4,4a,5,9b-tetrahydroindeno[1,2-d]-m-dioxin (79.4 grams), BP 64° to 65°C at 0.05 mm Hg, which possessed a rose odor similar to that of *Rosa damascena*. Gas-liquid chromatography at 150°C showed it to be a mixture of two components corresponding to geometric isomers in the ratio 1.8:1, richer in the more volatile component.

Example 2: Indene (116 ml), propionaldehyde (200 ml), 90% formic acid (160 ml) and petroleum ether (BP 40° to 60°C, 200 ml) were mixed and stirred vigorously at room temperature for 72 hours. The mixture was diluted with water (1 liter). The organic layer was separated and washed successively with water, saturated aqueous sodium bicarbonate solution, and water. After drying over anhydrous sodium sulfate and evaporation of the solvent, the product was distilled under high vacuum to give 2,4-diethyl-4,4a,5,9b-tetrahydroindeno[1,2-d]-m-dioxin (38.5 grams) BP 94° to 98°C at 0.065 mm Hg, which possessed a light, fresh, woody odor with floral overtones. Gas-liquid chromatography at 150°C indicated the presence of two components corresponding to geometric isomers in approximately equal proportions.

Examples of compound perfume bases are as follows. Parts are by weight, and where a solution is mentioned, this is to be understood to mean a solution in an odorless solvent commonly used in the art, e.g., diethyl phthalate, or benzyl alcohol.

Example 3:

	Parts by Weight
2-Phenyl ethyl alcohol	53.50
Rhodinol	30.00
Geraniol	5.00
2-Phenyl ethyl propionate	0.50
Aldehyde C9	0.10
Linalol ex Bois de Rose Oil	0.20
Methyl ionone	3.00
Rose absolute 10% solution	1.00
Eugenol	1.00
Mimosa Concrete	1.50
2,4-Dimethyl-4,4a,5,9b-tetrahydroindeno[1,2-d]-m-dioxin	1.50
Phenyl acetic acid	1.20
2-Phenyl ethyl phenyl acetate	1.50

Example 4:

	Parts by Weight
2-Phenyl ethyl alcohol	53.00
Rhodinol	30.00
Rhodinyl acetate	0.50
Geraniol	5.00
2-Phenyl ethyl propionate	0.50
Aldehyde C9	0.10
Linalol ex Bois de Rose Oil	0.20
Methyl ionone	3.00
Rose absolute 10% solution	1.00
Eugenol	1.00
Mimosa Concrete	1.50
2,4-Dimethyl-4,4a,5,9b-tetrahydroindeno[1,2-d]-m-dioxin	1.50
Phenyl acetic acid	1.20
2-Phenyl ethyl phenyl acetate	1.50

Esters of Cyclododecanoic and Cycloundecanoic Acids

P. Lafont and Y. Bonnet; U.S. Patent 3,227,742; January 4, 1966; assigned to Rhone-Poulenc SA, France describe the preparation of cycloundecanecarboxylic acid, a liquid boiling at 118°C under 0.06 mm Hg, and cyclododecanecarboxylic acid. Cyclododecanecarboxylic acid possesses interesting choleretic activity. It may be esterified by methods of esterification known per se by means of aliphatic or aromatic alcohols free from functional groups to give products of high boiling point which can be used as plasticizers for vinylic and cellulosic polymers. Some of these esters, and in particular the methyl and ethyl esters, have, with a rose characteristic, a very persistent woody and fruity odor, which makes them interesting for the preparation of perfumes. The odoriferous lower alkyl esters of cycloundecanecarboxylic acid and cyclododecanecarboxylic acid may be represented by the structural formula:

$$Q\overset{O}{\underset{\|}{C}}-OR$$

where Q is a radical of the group consisting of cycloundecyl and cyclododecyl, and R is an alkyl group of 1 to 2 carbon atoms. The process for the preparation of cycloundencane-carboxylic acid comprises reacting a 2-halogenocyclododecanone with an alkali hydroxide in a medium selected from the homologous aliphatic alcohols and mixtures of water and a water-miscible solvent for the halogenocyclododecanone, and acidifying the reaction mass.

The halogenocyclododecanone employed as starting material is preferably 2-chloro-cyclo-dodecanone or 2-bromo-cyclododecanone. The starting materials, i.e., the 2-halogenocyclo-dodecanones, are readily obtained in excellent yields by halogenation, at a temperature of 18° to 22°C, of cyclododecanone in solution in an organic solvent such as benzene, ether or chloroform. The halogenation is limited to the monohalogenoketone stage by intro-ducing exactly the theoretical quantity of halogen. The following examples illustrate the process.

Example 1: Into a spherical three-necked 500 cc flask provided with a central stirrer, a condenser and a supply funnel is run a solution of 14 grams of potassium hydroxide in 140 cc of ethanol, and the mixture is boiled. A solution of 13.05 grams (0.05 mol) of 2-bromo-cyclododecanone in 50 cc of ethanol is thereafter added in half an hour with good stirring. An abundant precipitate of potassium bromide forms. After refluxing for a fur-ther hour, the ethanol is distilled off. Water and diethyl ether are then introduced and the neutral fraction is extracted with diethyl ether.

From the ethereal solution thus obtained, there is then extracted 1.7 grams of neutral product consisting of 2-ethoxy-cyclododecanone, BP 83°C under 0.03 mm Hg, giving a 2,4-dinitrophenylhydrazone of MP 121° to 121.5°C. The aqueous fraction, freed from the neutral fraction, is acidified, and then extracted with diethyl ether. The ethereal solution thus obtained is dried over anhydrous sodium sulfate and the ether is driven off by distilla-tion. There are thus obtained 8.2 grams of acid fraction (yield 83%) consisting of cyclo-undecanecarboxylic acid, which boils at 118°C under 0.06 mm Hg and gives an anilide melting at 149°C and an amide melting at 175° to 176°C.

On esterification of this acid with methanol or ethanol by conventional methods, methyl cyclododecanecarboxylate, BP 79° to 80°C under 0.15 mm Hg, and ethyl cycloundecane-carboxylate, BP 85°C under 0.05 mm Hg, are respectively obtained. When in the fore-going process the ethanol solution of potassium hydroxide is replaced by sodium alcohol-ate (1.3 grams of sodium dissolved in 80 cc of anhydrous methanol) there is obtained, from 13.05 grams of 2-bromo-cyclododecanone, 8.6 grams of 2-methoxycyclododecanone MP 56°C and only 330 mg of cycloundecanecarboxylic acid.

The 2-bromo-cyclododecanone employed as starting material is prepared as follows. Into a three-necked 1-liter spherical flask provided with a central stirrer, a condenser and a sup-ply funnel are run 12.8 grams of cyclododecanone (i.e., 0.4 mol) and 500 cc of dry diethyl ether. Bromine (24 cc, i.e., 0.4 mol) is added drop by drop at 20° to 25°C in one and a half hours, and the mixture is then stirred for a further hour.

The ethereal solution thus obtained is then twice washed with 200 cc of water and then dried over anhydrous sodium sulfate, and all the ether is evaporated. The oil obtained is dissolved at 40°C in 200 cc of petroleum ether. On cooling, there separate in the form of crystals 86 grams of 2-bromo-cyclododecanone, MP 53.5°C (yield 85%), giving a 2,4-dinitro-phenylhydrazone, MP 174°C.

Example 2: By proceeding as in Example 1, but dissolving the 14 grams of potassium hy-droxide in 60 cc of water and 60 cc of dioxan (instead of 140 cc of ethanol) and the 13.05 grams of 2-bromo-cyclododecanone in 50 cc of dioxan (instead of ethanol), there are obtained 6.8 grams of cycloundecanecarboxylic acid (i.e., 68%) in addition to 3.2 grams of 2-hydroxycyclododecanone, which compound has already been described by Prelog, *Helv. Chim. Acta* 30, 1741 (1947).

Acetals of p-Menthanediol-3,8

Y.R. Naves and P.A. Ochsner; U.S. Patent 3,461,138; August 12, 1969; assigned to The Givaudan Corporation describe a family of cyclic acetals. These compounds have the formula:

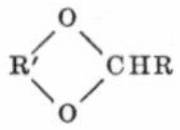

where R' is a bivalent terpenic moiety selected from

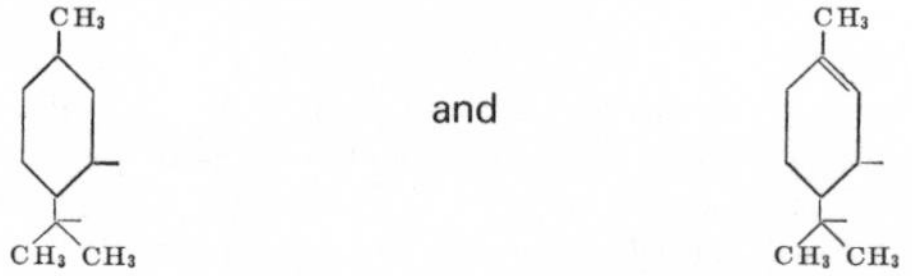

and

the dash lines denoting that the 3 and 8 position carbon atoms have unsatisfied valences, which positions, in the first formula given above, are each linked to an O, and R is a member selected from the group consisting of H, an alkyl radical having from 1 to 7 carbon atoms, and an alkylene radical having from 1 to 7 carbon atoms. Among specific compounds described are the acetals of p-menthanediol-3,8 and acetaldehyde; the formal of p-menthanediol-3,8; an acetal of p-menthene-1-diol-3,8; an acetal of p-menthanediol-3,8 and isovaleric aldehyde; and an acetal of p-menthanediol-3,8 and benzaldehyde.

In general, the acetals may be prepared by reacting a diol with one or more aldehydes having up to 8 carbon atoms, in the presence of an acidic reagent. The diols may be, e.g., menthoglycol, neomenthoglycol, or the corresponding para-menthene-1-diol-3,8 reactants. As aldehydes, aliphatic, cycloaliphatic or aromatic aldehydes may be used which may be saturated or unsaturated. Specific examples of suitable catalysts for use in the process are calcium chloride, ammonium chloride, sulfuric acid and orthophosphoric acid.

Example 1: Acetal of (-)Menthoglycol and Acetaldehyde — To 35 grams of (-)menthoglycol, there was added 14.5 grams of acetaldehyde and 5 grams of powdered calcium chloride. The mixture was permitted to stand for 8 days at room temperature. The contents were then treated with pentane, washed in salt water, dried and distilled. There was obtained 38 grams BP_{15} = 101° to 102°C. Elementary analysis yielded $C_{12}H_{22}O_2$.

Acetal of (+)Neomenthoglycol and Acetaldehyde — The same procedure, beginning with (+)neomenthoglycol, gave the acetal BP_{15} = 100° to 101°C. Elementary analysis gave the composition, $C_{12}H_{22}O_2$. The odor of the acetals is rosy, green and fresh. The acetal of menthoglycol is slightly minty.

Example 2: (a) Into a flask provided with an agitator, a thermometer, a dropping funnel, and a brine refrigerant, 300 grams of a mixture of sulfuric acid and water in equal parts by weight was placed. The contents was chilled at 0°C, and then a cooled mixture of 100 grams of (+)beta-citronellal and 150 grams of acetaldehyde was introduced under agitation over a period of 30 to 40 minutes, without permitting the temperature to go above 5°C. After this addition, agitation was continued for 30 minutes and then the mixture was poured over 500 grams of crushed ice. After extraction with petroleum ether, BP = 60° to 80°C, the contents were washed and neutralized.

Upon distillation and fractionation over a spinning band column, 92 grams of acetals were obtained. These were obtained as the acetal of neomenthoglycol, followed by the acetal of menthoglycol, with all of the characteristics of the preparation mentioned in Example 1. Repetition of the process, starting with (±)beta-citronellal gives acetals having no rotatory power, identified as being the same as the above preparations by the time of retention of vapor chromatography and by the infrared spectra.

(b) Part (a) of this example was repeated, except that the sulfuric acid was replaced by 250 grams of orthophosphoric acid. There was obtained 83 grams of acetals having substantially the same properties as those obtained in part (a) of this example.

β-Phenylethyl Alkylene Glycol Borate Compound

I.S. Bengelsdorf; U.S. Patent 3,239,421; March 8, 1966; assigned to United States Borax & Chemical Corporation describes the preparation of 2-(β-phenylethoxy)-4,4,6-trimethyl-1,3-dioxa-2-borinane having the formula

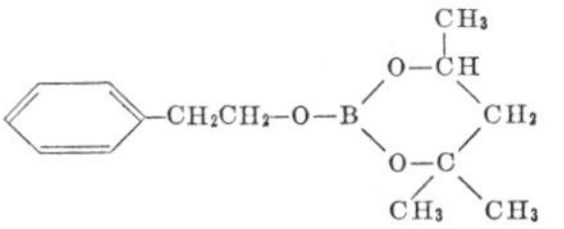

$$C_6H_5-CH_2CH_2-O-B \underset{O-C(CH_3)_2}{\overset{O-CH(CH_3)}{<}} CH_2$$

which is useful as a constituent of perfume formulations. The borate is readily prepared by reaction of β-phenylethanol with the hexylene glycol monoborate (2-hydroxy-4,4,6-trimethyl-1,3-dioxa-2-borinane) or a lower alkoxy derivative of the glycol monoborate, as illustrated by the equation

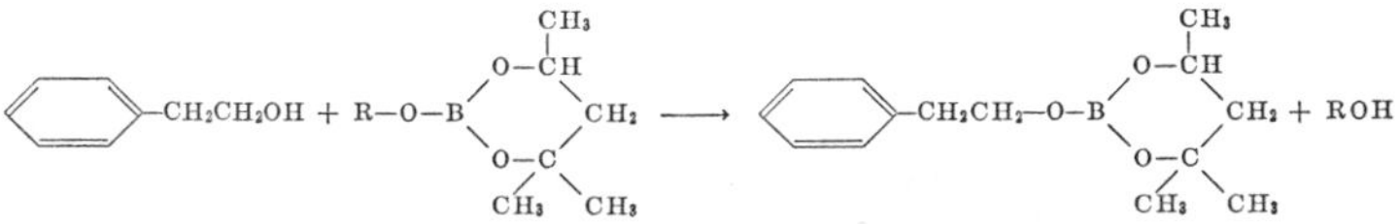

$$C_6H_5-CH_2CH_2OH + R-O-B \underset{O-C(CH_3)_2}{\overset{O-CH(CH_3)}{<}} CH_2 \longrightarrow C_6H_5-CH_2CH_2-O-B \underset{O-C(CH_3)_2}{\overset{O-CH(CH_3)}{<}} CH_2 + ROH$$

where R is hydrogen or a lower alkyl group having, for example 1 to 4 carbon atoms. The following example illustrates the preparation of the compound.

Example: A solution of 61.08 grams (0.5 mol) of β-phenylethanol and 72.0 grams (0.5 mol) of hexylene glycol monoborate in 175 ml of cyclohexane was stirred in a 500 ml flask at reflux temperature. The by-product water was removed as it was formed by means of a Dean-Stark trap. Refluxing was continued until the theoretical amount of water had been taken off (about 4 hours).

The cyclohexane was removed by distillation under reduced pressure to give 123.3 grams of crude product as an oily residue. The crude product was distilled under reduced pressure and 2-(β-phenylethoxy)-4,4,6-trimethyl-1,3-dioxa-2-borinane collected at 99°C/0.2 mm. The compound of this process is an oily liquid having a very pleasant, sweet, rose-like odor, which is useful as a constituent of perfume formulations.

β-Phenylethyl Alcohol

According to *T. Wood; U.S. Patent 3,579,593; May 18, 1971; assigned to Givaudan Corporation* β-phenylethyl alcohol suitable for perfumery use is prepared in excellent yields by the hydrogenation of styrene oxide in the presence of Raney nickel and palladium and fractionally distilling the alcohol. The following examples illustrate the process.

Example 1: *(a)* 240 grams of pure sytrene oxide was charged into the 500 ml stainless steel bomb of an autoclave along with 28 grams of 85% methanol (aqueous), 2 grams of sodium bicarbonate, 10 grams of Raney nickel catalyst and 1 gram of palladium on carbon (1%) catalyst. The autoclave was evacuated and hydrogen was introduced up to a pressure of 50 psi. The temperature was increased to 30°C and agitation was begun. The temperature was allowed to rise to 40°C and hydrogen was continued until absorption stopped (2 hours) and close to the theoretical amount of hydrogen had been absorbed. The temperature was then increased to 100°C and the pressure of hydrogen was raised to 200 psi and agitation was continued for 2 hours longer. The batch was cooled, removed from the autoclave, filtered, and distilled at 1 mm Hg pressure. There was obtained 232 grams of pure β-phenylethyl alcohol, BP 68° to 69°C (1 mm), free of ethylbenzene and suitable for perfumery use. This material was soluble to the extent of 2 ml in 100 ml of water producing a clear solution. The yield was 96.6% based on styrene oxide.

(b) When the above procedure of part (a) was repeated omitting the palladium catalyst, using instead 1 gram of active carbon, and the Raney nickel, the yield was only 212 grams of β-phenylethyl alcohol (88.3% yield) and the product was unacceptable for perfumery use because it contained traces of ethylbenzene and failed to pass both odor and water-solubility requirements. Vapor-phase chromatography showed that the original crude from the autoclave contained about 10% of ethylbenzene.

(c) When the hydrogenation was carried out as in (a) above except that both palladium metal catalyst and active carbon were omitted, only Raney nickel being used, the crude from the autoclave contained 10% of ethylbenzene and the yield of β-phenylethyl alcohol was 209 grams (87.0% yield). The product was unacceptable for perfumery use for the same reasons as in (b) above.

(d) When the hydrogenation was carried out as in (a) above except that 5% palladium on active carbon (1 gram) was substituted for the 1% palladium on active carbon, there was obtained 230 grams of pure β-phenylethyl alcohol (96% yield) suitable for perfumery use without further processing.

(e) When the hydrogenation was carried out as in (a) above except that 5% platinum on active carbon (1 gram) was substituted for the 1% palladium on active carbon, there was obtained a crude which contained 10.6% of ethylbenzene and gave 211 grams of distilled β-phenylethyl alcohol (88% yield). This was not suitable for perfumery use and failed both the odor and water-solubility tests because of the presence of a small amount of ethylbenzene.

(f) When the hydrogenation was carried out as in (a) above except that 50 mg of palladium black (finely divided palladium metal without carrier) was substituted for the 1% palladium on active carbon, there was obtained 219 grams of pure distilled β-phenylethyl alcohol suitable for perfumery use without further processing.

Example 2: *(a)* 120 grams of pure styrene oxide was charged into the 500 ml stainless steel bomb of an autoclave along with 160 grams of methanol, 5 grams of Raney nickel catalyst, and 0.5 gram of palladium on carbon (5%) catalyst. After evacuation of the autoclave hydrogen was introduced up to a pressure of 50 psi. Hydrogenation was conducted at room temperature with agitation until the absorption stopped (2 hours) and close to the theoretical amount of hydrogen had been taken up. The temperature was then increased to 70°C and the batch stirred under hydrogen at 50 psi for 3.5 hours. The batch was cooled, removed from the autoclave, filtered, distilled for removal of methanol, and vacuum-distilled at 1 mm Hg pressure. There was obtained 113 grams of pure β-phenylethyl alcohol (94.3%) free of ethylbenzene and suitable for perfumery use.

(b) When the hydrogenation of styrene oxide was carried out as in (a) above except that the recovered catalyst mixture from (a) was used, there was obtained 116 grams of pure β-phenylethyl alcohol (96.7%), free of ethylbenzene and suitable for perfumery use.

Acetylenic Carbinols

R. Marbet; U.S. Patent 3,379,777; April 23, 1968; assigned to Hoffmann-La Roche Inc. describes acetylenic carbinols having the formula

$$(1) \qquad R-H_2C-Z-CH_2-CH_2-CH-CH_2-CH-C\equiv CH$$
$$\qquad\qquad\qquad\qquad\qquad\qquad \underset{CH_3}{|} \qquad \underset{OH}{|}$$

in which the symbol R represents hydrogen or a lower alkyl group; and in which the symbol Z represents

$$-CH-CH- \quad \text{and} \quad -C{=\!\!=\!\!=}C-$$
$$\underset{CH_3}{|}\ \underset{R}{|} \qquad\qquad \underset{CH_3}{|}\ \underset{R}{|}$$

the symbol R representing hydrogen or a lower alkyl group, are described. The acetylenic carbinols are characterized by their fine fragrance and are used in the production of perfumes and other scented compositions.

The compounds of Formula 1 are readily prepared. In a preferred preparative method, an aldehyde having the formula

$$(2) \qquad R-H_2C-Z-CH_2-CH_2-CH-CH_2-CHO$$
$$\underset{CH_3}{|}$$

in which the symbols R and Z have the same meaning as in Formula 1, is ethynylated. In general, ethynylation of the aldehyde of Formula 2 is carried out, using techniques known per se, by reacting the aldehyde with acetylene or with an acetylide. The condensation of the Formula 2 aldehyde with acetylene or with an acetylide compound is effected, conveniently, in the presence of a solvent. Liquid ammonia has been found to be particularly well suited for use as the solvent for the reaction.

In one particular example, there is used as the starting material, crude citronellal-containing essential oils, such as, citronella oil. These oils have a well-known, somewhat unpleasant penetrating odor with an accompanying rancid fatty side note which, in time, becomes especially unpleasant. Ethynylation thereof produces oils having a fresh rose-like odor which is particularly distinguished by its excellent lasting properties.

3,7,7-Trialkyl-5-Heptenol

H.E. Davis; U.S. Patent 3,394,169; July 23, 1968; assigned to Eastman Kodak Company describes compositions which are 3,7,7-trialkyl-5-heptenols of the formula

$$\overset{R^2}{\underset{|}{}} \qquad\qquad \overset{R^3}{\underset{|}{}}$$
$$R_1{-}CH{-}CH{=}CH{-}CH_2{-}CH{-}CH_2{-}CH_2{-}OH$$

in which each of R^1, R^2 and R^3 is lower alkyl, and esters of such alcohols. These alcohols, esters and pyran derivatives are useful as intermediates in the manufacture of perfumes.

In accordance with the process for preparing a 3,7,7-trialkyl-5-heptenol, a 3,7,7-trialkyl-5-oxoheptanal is reduced. The reduction of the 3,7,7-trialkyl-5-oxoheptanal can be carried out by hydrogenation in the presence of a solid hydrogenation catalyst or chemically with a reducing agent, e.g., an alkali metal borohydride such as sodium borohydride, an alkoxyborohydride, an alkali metal hydride, etc.

The reaction product from the catalytic reduction of the 3,7,7-trialkyl-5-oxoheptanal contains either a 2-(2,2-dialkylethyl)-4-alkyltetrahydropyran or a 3,7,7-trialkyl-5-hydroxyheptanol or a mixture thereof. The 3,7,7-trialkyl-5-hydroxyheptanol is then esterified to form a diester of 3,7,7-trialkyl-5-hydroxyheptanol and the diester is subjected to pyrolysis under carefully controlled conditions to form a 3,7,7-trialkyl-4-heptenol ester and a 3,7,7-trialkyl-5-heptenol ester. The 3,7,7-trialkyl-5-heptenol ester is then saponified to form 3,7,7-trialkyl-5-heptenol. Alternatively, the mixture of 3,7,7-trialkyl-4-heptenol ester and 3,7,7-trialkyl-5-heptenol ester can be saponified to form a mixture of 3,7,7-trialkyl-4-heptenol and 3,7,7-trialkyl-5-heptenol. The following examples illustrate the preparation of a 3,7,7-trialkyl-5-heptanol in accordance with the process.

Example 1: Ethanol (70 ml), 3,7-dimethyl-5-oxooctanal (70 grams, 0.41 mol) and a copper chromite catalyst (Harshaw 1106-P) were heated in an autoclave at 150°C and 2,500 psi hydrogen pressure until no further hydrogen was absorbed. The catalyst was removed and the 3,7-dimethyl-1,5-octanediol (53 grams) distilled, BP 124° to 125°C/1.5 mm.

Example 2: The diacetate of the 3,7-dimethyl-1,5-octanediol (34 grams, 0.13 mol) of Example 1 was diluted with an equal volume of benzene and passed through a Vycor tube 1" x 12" packed with Vycor chips and heated to 370°C with an electric furnace. The addition rate was approximately 1 ml per minute. The effluent, by gas chromatography, was a mixture of acetic acid, benzene, 3,7-dimethyl-4-octenyl acetate and 3,7-dimethyl-5-octenyl acetate.

The 3,7-dimethyl-4-octenyl acetate and the 3,7-dimethyl-5-octenyl acetate were distilled at 58°C under 0.5 mm. NMR and infrared data agreed with the proposed structure. By gas chromatography the product was approximately a 50-50 mixture of the 3,7-dimethyl-4-octenyl acetate and 3,7-dimethyl-5-octenyl acetate. On saponification a mixture of the corresponding unsaturated alcohols was obtained. These alcohols have an odor very similar to that of citronellol, an important article of commerce.

Example 3: The preparation of 2-(2,2-dialkylethyl)-4-alkyltetrahydropyran is as follows. Ethanol (70 ml), 3,7-dimethyl-5-oxooctanal (70 grams, 0.41 mol) and 7 grams of a supported nickel catalyst (Girdler G49A) were heated in an autoclave at 125°C and 2,000 psi hydrogen pressure until no further hydrogen was absorbed. The catalyst was removed and the product distilled. By gas chromatography the product was a mixture of the cis (90 to 95%) and trans (5 to 10%) isomers of the 2-isobutyl-4-methyltetrahydropyran.

The products and by-products of the process are useful in the perfume industry. Thus 2-isobutyl-4-methyltetrahydropyran, a preferred 2-(2,2-dialkylethyl)-4-alkyltetrahydropyran, which is produced as a by-product in the hydrogenation of 3,7-dimethyl-5-oxooctanal, is commonly called dihydro rose oxide and is described in *Bull. Soc. Chim. France, 1961, 645-57.* This compound, which has a pleasant odor, is useful in the formulation of perfumes or in perfumed soaps, and toilet articles. The compound 3,7-dimethyl-5-octen-1-ol, a preferred 3,7,7-trialkyl-5-heptenol, produced in the process, has a pleasant odor somewhat similar to citronellol and is useful in the perfume and flavoring industries as a substitute for citronellol.

Reconstituting Natural Citronella Oil

R.P.T. Young; U.S. Patent 3,579,468; May 18, 1971; assigned to SCM Corporation describes reconstituted citronella oil in which at least a portion of the naturally occurring d-citronellal in the natural oil is replaced by substantially equivalent weight proportion of dl-citronellal.

Natural citronella oil is a commodity originating in Formosa and other remote places. It contains approximately equal weight proportions of geraniol, citronellol and d-citronellal, the latter being optically active. Natural citronella oil is used for its odor value in perfumes, and the d-citronellal fraction is useful in making hydroxy citronellal, also a perfumery chemical.

This process is based on the finding that replacement of part or all of the naturally-occuring d-citronellal in citronella oil by an optically inactive (dl) citronellal does not materially affect the odor value of the natural citronella oil or hydroxy citronellal made therefrom. Thus, the reconstituted natural citronella oil of this process is one in which at least a portion of the naturally-occurring d-citronellal is replaced by a substantially equivalent weight proportion of dl (racemic) citronellal.

The reconstitution of natural citronella oil can be done most simply by fractionally distilling (topping) d-citronellal from the remainder of the citronella oil distillant under reduced pressure, e.g., 10 to 20 mm Hg absolute, and replacing it with a substantially equivalent proportion of dl-citronellal. The latter product can be made by disproportionating and purifying a mixture of geraniol and nerol, which in turn can be synthesized from myrcene.

Example: Natural Formosan citronella oil is charged into a kettle equipped with an efficient fractional distillation column, condenser, reflux return, and other appurtenances to fractionally distill at a pressure of 10 mm Hg absolute. Virtually all the naturally-occurring d-citronellal is topped off by fractional distillation. The distilland is cooled, and a proportion of dl-citronellal (racemic) of the same weight as the d-citronellal distillate is blended into the distilland.

The optically inactive material added does not occur in nature, but is a synthetic product, Samples of the resulting reconstituted natural citronella oil are subjected to organoleptic evaluation for odor value in perfumes and odorants by a panel expert in these arts. They rate the product equivalent to the natural citronella oil which was thus reconstituted. Additionally, when dl-citronellal is fractionated from the reconstituted oil and converted into hydroxy citronellal, the panel detects no appreciable difference between the hydroxy citronellal so made and that made from the d-citronellal fraction of the same natural citronella oil.

Isolation of Rhodinal

E.H. Eschinasi; U.S. Patent 3,244,752; April 5, 1966; assigned to Givaudan Corporation has succeeded in preparing a substantially rich mixture of rhodinal and in isolating substantially pure rhodinal from mixtures containing citronellal, with or without isopulegol. It has been confirmed that rhodinal has the formula: 3,7-dimethyl-7-octenal, in contradistinction with citronellal, which has the formula: 3,7-dimethyl-6-octenal. The two formulas may be represented as follows:

$$CH_2=\underset{\underset{CH_3}{|}}{C}-CH_2-CH_2-CH_2-\underset{\underset{CH_3}{|}}{CH}-CH_2-CHO \quad \text{and} \quad CH_3-\underset{\underset{CH_3}{|}}{C}=CH-CH_2-CH_2-\underset{\underset{CH_3}{|}}{CH}-CH_2-CHO$$

   Rhodinal   Citronellal

The process comprises treating a mixture containing rhodinal and citronellal, with or without isopulegol, with a borating agent at an elevated temperature in the presence of a catalyst which selectively favors the isomerization of citronellal into isopulegol without affecting rhodinal. The pure rhodinal is then isolated from the mixture by distilling it from the resulting isopulegol borate.

The substantially pure rhodinal made in accordance with the process has a distinctly different, more refined and true rose odor than its isomer, citronellal. The presence of just a few percent of citronellal, with its pungent melissa and citronellal odor, subdues and covers the fine rosy, aliphatic smell of the substantially pure rhodinal, i.e., rhodinal of at least 90% purity. In like manner, the delicate, honey-rose odor of substantially pure rhodinal is adversely affected by a few percent of the sharper but less fragrant citronellol.

It has been found that the formyl, acetyl and isopropyl esters of rhodinal possess unusual odor qualities, making them especially suitable for use as practical perfume agents. Rhodinyl acetate has a rich and fragrant honey-rose note with five times the esthetic desirability of citronellyl acetate. Rhodinyl formate has a rich and natural-smelling rose leaf note with five times the esthetic desirability of the corresponding citronellyl formate.

Example 1: 830 grams hydroxycitronellal (Laurine Givaudan) is introduced at a rate of 100 ml per hour at 350°C into a Pyrex column, 100 cm long and 25 mm in diameter, containing 200 grams of ¼" to ⅛" mesh activated alumina. The reaction product (758 grams) is separated from the water (71 ml) and distilled. Crude rhodinal (528 grams) is collected. It shows by gas liquid chromatographic analysis 75% rhodinal, 12% citronellal and 13% isopulegol. The residue of 210 grams consists mainly of unreacted hydroxycitronellal good for reworking. The crude distilled rhodinal (528 grams) containing a total of about 25% citronellal-isopulegol mixture is mixed with 16 grams of boric anhydride; 5 grams of silica gel and 300 ml of toluene and is then refluxed at 130° to 135°C with a Dean Stark trap.

After about 1 hour, no more water (ca 8 ml) is formed and the solvent is evaporated. The pure rhodinal is then distilled from the residual isopulegol borate in a 95% yield. It shows a rhodinal content of over 98 to 99% with only traces of isopulegol present, semicarbazone MP 73°C from ethanol, 2,4-dinitrophenylhydrazone MP 73° to 74°C from ethanol.

Example 2: Rhodinol — Rhodinal (103 grams) in 100 ml dry ether was added to a solution of lithium aluminum hydride (8 grams) in dry ether (250 ml) within 15 minutes. The reaction mixture was refluxed for 1 hour, then decomposed with 5 ml of ethyl acetate followed by 100 ml of water. The slurry was then carefully acidified with diluted sulfuric acid, washed with water, and neutralized. After evaporation of the solvent, the rhodinol was carefully distilled in a 100 cm Connon-packed (Ni) column and the main cut (70 grams) was collected. The infrared spectrum shows strong methylenic ($C=CH_2$) absorption bands at 6.1 and 11.3μ.

ROSE OXIDE

Reaction of Aliphatic Carboxylic Acid and Citronellol

R.L. Markus; U.S. Patent 3,166,576; January 19, 1965; assigned to Stepan Chemical Co. describes a process for the preparation of the compounds cis- and trans-2-(2'-methyl-1'-propenyl)-4-methyltetrahydropyran commonly called Rose Oxide. Rose Oxide is a compound which has found widespread use in the perfume industry because of its pleasant odoriferous nature. It is obtained naturally as an extract from Bulgarian rose oil and Geranium bourbon. The sources of these raw materials are limited, their costs are extremely high, and the necessary extraction and purification procedures which need be followed to obtain the desired end product are elaborate, costly and time consuming.

As a consequence, much time and effort has been spent in attempts to synthesize these compounds. However, these attempts have generally resulted in time consuming, tedious and costly procedures which result in poor yields of the desired end product. According to this process, cis- and trans-2-(3'-methyl-1'-propenyl)-4-methyltetrahydropyran are prepared by a method which comprises reacting a lower aliphatic carboxylic acid with citronellol or citronellyl acetate in the presence of an allylic oxidizing agent thereby causing an allylic rearrangement in an alpha position to the double bond in the citronellol or citronellyl acetate to take place thereby forming an intermediate compound which spontaneously cyclizes, neutralizing the cyclized compound with a soluble alkali to form the methyltetrahydropyran and recovering the methyltetrahydropyran from the reaction medium.

Example 1: Through a warm stirred suspension of 460 grams (0.67 mol) of Pb_3O_4 in 124.8 grams (0.8 mol) of citronellol, air was bubbled at the rate of 400 ml per minute. The temperature of the system was maintained at 65°C and glacial acetic acid 580 grams (9.66 mol) was introduced within about one half hour period of time. Thereupon heating was continued for about another half hour until the red lead dissolved and the test against KI-starch paper turned out to be negative. Upon cooling, dilution with water and neutralization, the oil layer was separated yielding an oil (78.5 grams) consisting of Rose Oxide (26.3%) and recoverable citronellol (71.7%) besides citronellyl acetate (3.61%) as determined by gas chromatography and fractional distillation. The following examples were carried out according to the general procedure set forth in Example 1 above.

Example 2: To a mixture of 31.2 grams of citronellol of 65% purity and 217.5 grams of lead tetroxide was added 225 cc of propionic acid. Upon completion of the reaction and after cooling, dilution with water and neutralization, Rose Oxide was recovered from the reaction medium.

Example 3: To a mixture of 31.2 grams of citronellol of 65% purity and 145 grams of lead tetroxide was added 20 ml of acetic acid and 30 cc of n-propanol. Upon completion of the reaction and after cooling, dilution with water and neutralization, Rose Oxide was recovered from the reaction medium.

Example 4: To a mixture of 31.2 grams of citronellol of 65% purity and 115 grams of lead tetroxide was added 138 cc of acetic acid and 200 cc of benzol. Upon completion of the reaction and after cooling, dilution with water and neutralization, Rose Oxide was recovered from the reaction medium.

Example 5: To a mixture of 31.2 grams of citronellol of 65% purity and 115 grams of lead tetroxide was added 138 cc of acetic acid and 16 cc of methanol. Upon completion of the reaction and after cooling, dilution with water and neutralization, Rose Oxide was recovered from the reaction medium.

Rose Oxide by Pyrolysis of Citronellol Derivative

D. Böse and K. Pfoertner; U.S. Patent 3,657,278; April 18, 1972; assigned to Givaudan Corporation describe a commercially-feasible process for making Rose Oxide, by pyrolyzing 3-chloro-2,6-dimethyl-1-octen-8-ol, which is easily produced from the known, inexpensive and abundant citronellol, 2,6-dimethyl-1-octen-8-ol.

The pyrolysis yields a mixture of cis- and trans-isomers of Rose Oxide in which the cis-isomer, particularly valuable from a fragrance point of view, predominates. The pyrolysates thus obtained can be purified by the usual purification methods (e.g., by vacuum distillation and/or column chromatography on silica gel).

Example 1: 3-Chloro-2,6-dimethyl-1-octen-8-ol — A solution of 2 grams of 2,6-dimethyl-2-octen-8-ol in 250 ml of carbon tetrachloride was treated, dropwise, with a solution of chlorine in carbon tetrachloride while a nitrogen stream, at the rate of 4 liters per minute, was simultaneously led through the reaction solution. The reaction was stopped as soon as no more starting material was detectable by thin layer chromatography. The solvent was then drawn off in water-jet vacuum at 30°C and the residue was chromatographed on silica gel (0.05 to 0.2 mm) with a 95:5 mixture of petroleum ether and acetone, at 40° to 50°C. 3-chloro-2,6-dimethyl-1-octen-2-ol was obtained. IR: 908, 3,083, 1,646, 3,344, 1,060 cm^{-1}. Yield 97%.

Example 2: Rose Oxide (Purification by Chromatography) — 3-Chloro-2,6-dimethyl-1-octen-8-ol, as obtained in accordance with Example 1, was dropped into a flask heated to 260°C (wall temperature). A nitrogen stream of about 1 liter per minute was simultaneously led through the flask. The pyrolysis products leaving the flask with the nitrogen stream were condensed and chromatographed on silica gel (0.05 to 0.2 mm). The silica gel was eluted with 95:5 mixture of petroleum ether and acetone at 40° to 50°C. From 5.57 grams of 3-chloro-2,6-dimethyl-1-octen-8-ol, besides 3.73 grams of unreacted starting material, there was obtained 0.98 grams of cis,trans-2-(2'-methyl-1'-propenyl)-4-methyltetrahydropyran, in the ratio of cis:trans of 2:1.

4-Methyl-2-(2-Methyl-1-Propen-1-yl)Tetrahydropyran

G. Ohloff; U.S. Patent 3,328,426; June 27, 1967; assigned to Firmenich & Cie, Switzerland describes a process for the manufacture of cyclic ethers, in particular of 4-methyl-2-(2-methyl-1-propen-1-yl)-tetrahydropyran (1) and 4-methyl-2-(2-methyl-1-propen-1-yl)-dihydropyran (2) which are known compounds having interesting odoriferous properties.

According to the process, the compounds (1) and (2) are prepared by reacting 2,6-dimethyl-2,3-epoxy-octan-8-ol or 2,6-dimethyl-2,3-epoxy-cis-6-octen-8-ol with a secondary amine in order to open the epoxy nucleus and introduce a secondary amino group into position 3, oxidizing the resulting amino-alcohols in order to form 3-N,N-disubstituted-2,6-dimethyl-3-amino-octan-2,8-diol 3-N-oxide or 3-N,N-disubstituted-2,6-dimethyl-3-amino-6-cis-octen-2,8-diol 3-N-oxide, and subjecting the N-oxides to a cyclizing pyrolysis. It is advisable to treat the product of the pyrolysis by acidic agents in order to remove basic impurities which may be present and to obtain the cyclic ethers in an olfactorily pure form.

Example 1: 172 grams (1 mol) of (+)-2,6-dimethyl-2,3-epoxy-octan-8-ol were heated for

96 hours in an autoclave at 150°C together with 50 grams (1.1 mol) of dimethylamine (100%). The reaction product was then distilled in a high vacuum and at a constant boiling temperature. Practically no residue was left. There were obtained 208 grams (96.3% of the theory) of 2,6-dimethyl-3-dimethylamino-octan-2,8-diol. BP = 124° to 126°C/0.01 mm. Nitrogen content, calculated from $C_{12}H_{27}NO_2$: N, 6.45%; found, 6.46 and 6.27%.

To a solution of 108.5 grams (0.5 mol) of 2,6-dimethyl-3-dimethylamino-octan-2,8-diol in 110 ml of methanol there were added within 40 minutes, while cooling with ice and stirring vigorously, 75 grams (0.75 mol) of a 34% aqueous H_2O_2 solution. The reaction mixture was then slowly heated to room temperature and allowed to stand for 24 hours. The phenolphthalein test for amines was then negative. The excess H_2O_2 was then destroyed by the addition of 0.5 gram of platinum black and stirring for 3 hours. After filtering off the catalyst the solvents were separated in a rotatory evaporator. 115.5 grams of a syrupy residue were obtained. As analyses showed, it consisted of 2,6-dimethyl-3-dimethylamino-octan-2,8-diol 3-N-oxide. The yield was 99% of the theory.

The N-oxide was then directly subjected to pyrolysis without any purification. 100 grams of the syrupy oxidation product were introduced dropwise into a flask heated to 150°C and which was connected with distillation equipment maintained under a vacuum of 10 torr. 64 grams of a mixture of the cis- and trans-isomers of (+)-4-methyl-2-(2-methyl-1-propen-1-yl)-tetrahydropyran were collected in the receiver. Yield: 84% of the theory. In order to remove the last traces of malodorous basic by-products the pyrolysis product was extracted once with 2% aqueous sulfuric acid. The purified product had the following physical constant: BP = 56°C/0.12 mm.

Example 2: 172 grams (1 mol) of (–)-2,6-dimethyl-2,3-epoxy-octan-8-ol were heated for 60 hours at 150°C in an autoclave together with 1,000 ml of an aqueous 25% dimethylamine solution. The excess dimethylamine was removed from the reaction product by distillation in a rotatory evaporator. The residue yielded, after distillation in a high vacuum, 186 grams of pure 2,6-dimethyl-3-N,N-dimethylamino-octan-2,8-diol. BP = 125° to 127°C at 0.01 mm. Nitrogen content calculated from $C_{12}H_{27}NO_2$: N, 6.45%; found, 6.61% Yield: 85.6% of the theory.

108.5 grams (0.5 mol) of the N,N-dimethylamino compound were reacted in the manner described in Example 1 in the same amount of methanol with 75 grams of a 34% aqueous H_2O_2 solution. When the phenolphthalein test was negative, the excess H_2O_2 was destroyed by the addition of 0.5 gram of platinum black, and after the usual treatment there were obtained 115.5 grams of 2,6-dimethyl-3-N,N-dimethylamino-octan-2,8-diol 3-N-oxide. The yield was 99% of the theory.

The pyrolysis of 100 grams of the N-oxide under the conditions set forth in Example 1 yielded 66 grams of (–)-4-methyl-2-(2-methyl-1-propen-1-yl)-tetrahydropyran, corresponding to a yield of 87% of the theory. The traces of basic by-products were removed by extraction with 2% aqueous sulfuric acid. According to the gas-chromatographic analysis the purified product consisted of a mixture of the cis- and trans-isomers in a ratio of 53% of the cis-isomer to 47% of the trans-isomer. The mixture had the following constant: BP 58°C/0.12 mm.

A. Eschenmoser, C.F. Seidel and D. Felix; U.S. Patent 3,161,657; December 15, 1964; assigned to Firmenich & Cie, Switzerland describe the preparation of 2-(2-methyl-1-propen-1-yl)-4-methyl-tetrahydropyran which can be represented by the following structural formula:

The tetrahydropyran derivative represented by the above formula forms two isomers which have the cis- and trans-configuration, respectively, with regard to the substituents in the positions 2 and 4. Each of these isomers exists in optically active forms.

According to this process, the tetrahydropyran derivative is prepared by subjecting to an acid-catalyzed cycling reaction a member selected from the group consisting of 1-hydroxy-3,7-dimethyl-4,6-octadiene, 1-hydroxy-3,7-dimethyl-5,7-octadiene and mixtures. If desired the cis- and trans-isomers of 2-(2-methyl-1-propen-1-yl)-4-methyl-tetrahydropyran can be individually separated from the cyclization product.

Ring Closure Using Dihydroxy Compounds

G. Ohloff, E. Klein and G. Schade; U.S. Patent 3,252,998; May 24, 1966; assigned to Studiengesellschaft Kohle mbH, Germany describe a process for the production of cyclic 5- or 6-membered ethers by intramolecular splitting-off of water from dihydroxy compounds with ring closure, which is characterized in that, 3,4-ethylenically unsaturated acyclic terpenes which have a hydroxyl or perhydroxyl group in the 2-position, a hydroxyl group or an enolizable keto group in the 8- or 7-position and if desired further double bonds, with the basic hydrocarbon structure

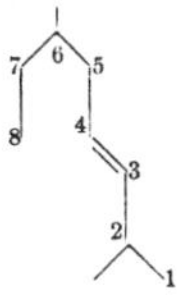

are dehydrated under cyclizing conditions with displacement of the allyl of the double bond from the 3-position into the 2-position. As starting materials for the process, diols of the following general structural formula may be used

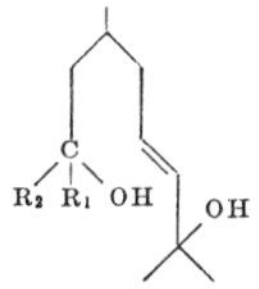

in which a perhydroxyl group may be present at the C_2 instead of the hydroxyl group. A typical reaction scheme according to the process is given below.

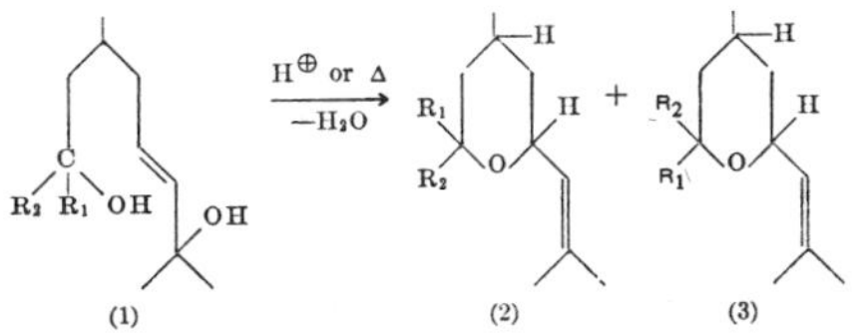

In the case where $R_1 + R_2 = H$, the starting material (1a) would be 2,6-dimethyl-3-octene-2,8-diol and the products (2a or 3a) would be 4-methyl-2-[2'-methylpropene-(1')-yl]- tetrahydropyran. In order that the process may be more fully understood the following examples are given (where appropriate the reactants and products are identified with reference to the above reaction scheme).

Example 1: 200 grams of a crude mixture of hydroxyhydroperoxides, as directly obtained in the photo-sensitized autoxidation of β-citronellol are treated with a brisk current of steam and the oil passing over is collected in a receiver. After half an hour, the steam distillation is complete. Gas chromatography shows that the 48.4 grams of isolated oil consists of 90% of a mixture of the two diastereomeric oxides (2a) and (3a). Yield: 25% of the theory.

Example 2: 200 grams of glycol (1a) are heated in a reaction vessel having a packed column mounted thereon at a bath temperature of 150°C under a vacuum of 1 mm. A continuous splitting-off of water is observed, with distillation of the mixture of oxides (2a) and (3a) at 74°C. After 2 hours, the distillation is complete. 171.8 grams are obtained, which corresponds to a theoretical yield of 96% of (2a) and (3a). Gas chromatography shows that the oxide separated from the water consisted of 99% of substantially equal parts of (2a) and (3a).

Example 3: 250 grams of a glycol mixture obtained by Na_2SO_3 reduction of photo-oxidation products of citronellol were treated with steam in the presence of 100 cc of a saturated aqueous oxalic acid solution. There were thus collected in a receiver 123 grams of a pure mixture of oxides (2a) and (3a). Yield: 92% of the theory. The same result is obtained with a yield of over 90% of oxide mixture when employing glycol mixtures obtained by reduction of the photo-oxidation products of acetoxycitronellol, citronellal and citronellic acid or their esters, for example by $LaAlH_4$.

2-(2-Methyl-1-Propenyl)-2,4,6-Trimethyldihydro-4,5-Pyran

A. Cahn, R.R. Winnegrad and A.H. Gilbert; U.S. Patents 3,455,957; July 15, 1969 and 3,309,276; March 14, 1967; both assigned to Lever Brothers Company have found that a certain dihydropyran imparts an intense top note to rose and enhances the rose note of a perfume blend. The compound has the following structure:

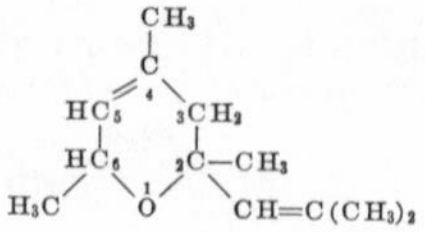

This structure, i.e., 2-(2-methyl-1-propenyl)-2,4,6-trimethyldihydro-4,5-pyran, includes the related isomeric structure. It is necessary to have 2-methyl-1-propenyl in the 2-position. For example, if the 2-position has n-hexyl or i-butyl, the dihydropyran is not a perfume. Dihydropyrans with other substituents in the ring, e.g., 2-i-butyl-4,6-dimethyldihydro-4,5-pyran and 2-(1-propenyl)-4,6-dimethyldihydro-4,5-pyran, also do not have any perfumy properties.

It has been found that this perfume may be provided by reacting 2-methyl-2,4-pentanediol directly with mesityl oxide in a homogeneous aqueous solution. Therefore, a separate step is not required in this in situ process to form 4-methyl-4-pentene-2-ol as an intermediate product. The reaction is generally conducted in the presence of an acid catalyst, e.g., sulfuric acid, with refluxing. After the reaction is complete, e.g., after 24 hours, the solution is cooled, neutralized and distilled to form 2-(2-methyl-1-propenyl)-2,4,6-trimethyldihydro-4,5-pyran, a perfume. The following examples illustrate the process.

Example 1: Mesityl oxide 98 grams (1 mol) and 2-methyl-2,4-pentanediol 130 grams (1.1 mol) were refluxed for 24 hours in 1 ml of concentrated sulfuric acid and 5 ml of water. The solution was cooled, neutralized with alcoholic sodium hydroxide and distilled to yield 45 grams (25%) of an oil (BP 72° to 83°C/11 mm). This oily reaction product, i.e., 2-(2-methyl-1-propenyl)-2,4,6-trimethyldihydro-4,5-pyran, was a light yellow perfume.

Example 2: Perfume compositions were formed from 2-(2-methyl-1-propenyl)-2,4,6-trimethyldihydro-4,5-pyran and other compounds. These compositions are indicated in the table shown on the following page. Both composition (1) and composition (2) indicated in the table add an intense top note to rose.

Ingredients	Compositions, parts by weight	
	(1)	(2)
Citronellol	200	400
Geraniol	100	
Phenyl ethyl alcohol	200	
Ionone	30	
Benzyl acetate	100	
Benzoylphenone		100
Phenyl ethyl acetate		60
Artificial musk		10
2-(2-methyl-1-propenyl)-2,4,6-trimethyldihydro-4,5-pyran	50	200

Photosensitized Oxidation of Acyclic Terpenes

G.O. Schenck, G. Ohloff and E. Klein; U.S. Patent 3,382,276; May 7, 1968; assigned to Studiengesellschaft Kohle mbH, Germany describe a process for the photosensitized oxidation of ethylenically unsaturated compounds with molecular oxygen and with initial introduction of perhydroxyl groups onto one carbon atom of the double bond and simultaneous displacement of the double bond towards the allyl position and, if desired, subsequent reduction of these oxidation products of the first stage, and is characterized in that with selective oxidation on the C—C multiple bond, there are subjected to the process those unsaturated compounds which contain oxygen-containing groups as well as at least one C—C double bond the oxidation products so formed being if required reduced in a manner known per se.

Particularly suitable starting materials for the process are those which contain oxidation-sensitive oxygen-containing functional groups and are at least ethylenically unsaturated in one position. Examples of such starting materials are unsaturated alcohols, aldehydes, ketones, carboxylic acids and their derivatives such as esters or the like. As starting material acyclic terpenes such as

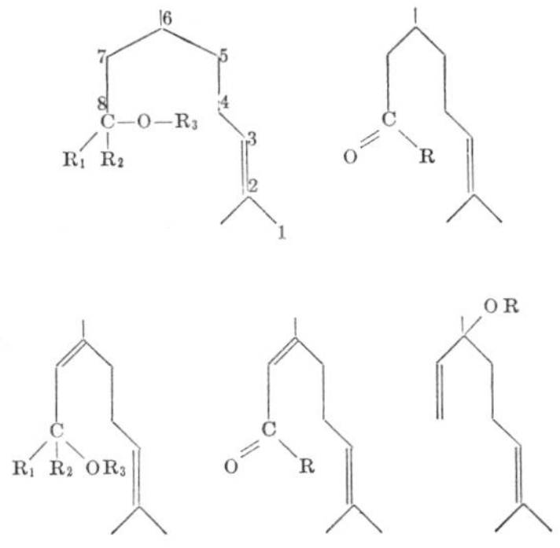

where R is a member selected from the group consisting of hydrogen, acyl, straight and branched chain saturated and unsaturated aliphatic hydrocarbons, hydroxy, and alkoxy, R_1 and R_2 are each a member selected from the group consisting of hydrogen, straight and branched chain saturated and unsaturated aliphatic hydrocarbons, and R_3 is a member selected from the group consisting of hydrogen and acyl.

By the process, that is with oxidation at the double bond and simultaneous displacement of the double bond into the allyl position, an additional oxygen-containing functional group is introduced into the carbon structure without requiring changes by oxidation in the oxygen-containing groups which are already present. The fact that this process produces results which were to a high degree unexpected is immediately apparent if the known sensitivity to oxidation of the aldehyde group is considered. The specific effect of the oxidation process according to the process is emphasized by the fact that an undesired oxidation at the oxygen-containing functional group can be avoided even in the presence of this group which is extremely sensitive to oxygen. The following examples illustrate the process.

Example 1: A solution of 1,000 grams of citronellol in 800 cc of methanol is exposed to light under oxygen in the presence of 4 grams of Bengal pink at room temperature in a lighting apparatus with an oxygen circulation and dipping lamp arrangement (HGH 5000, 900 watt). Oxygen absorption is practically complete after 160 liters have been absorbed in 18 hours. The quantity corresponds to an oxygen absorption of 100% of the theoretical.

The strongly peroxidic reaction solution is poured into an ice-cooled saturated aqueous solution of 2,000 grams of sodium sulfite (20% excess of the theoretical) with vigorous stirring. After stirring for 1 hour in an ice-cold condition, the reaction solution is heated for another hour to 70°C. The organic layer is then separated from the aqueous phase and the reaction mixture is subjected to a vacuum distillation. In this way, a glycol mixture is obtained, having the following physical constant: BP 99° to 101°C/0.01 mm. Yield: 1,080 grams of glycol mixture = 98% of the theoretical.

Example 2: A solution of 196 grams of (+)-citronellyl acetate in 780 cc of methanol takes up 30.5 liters of oxygen over 6 hours in the presence of 1 gram of Bengal pink in the experimental apparatus as described in Example 1. The reaction product is distilled off from the solvent and it is conducted slowly into a solution of 262 grams of triphenyl phosphine in 400 cc of dioxane with ice-cooling and vigorous stirring. By decanting off or filtering with suction, the triphenyl phosphine oxide which has formed is separated from the remaining reaction mixture, and the latter is further purified by removal of the solvent and vacuum distillation. The acetoxy-glycol mixture yielded 185 grams = 88% of the theoretical.

50 grams of monoacetoxy-glycol are heated in 250 cc of a half-normal alcoholic caustic potash solution for 1 hour under reflux. The saponification mixture is then poured into water and the organic layer is distilled in vacuo. The glycol mixture yielded 37 grams = 95% of the theoretical.

VIOLET

α-Irone from 6-Ketodihydrogeraniol

E.H. Eschinasi and M.L. Cotter; U.S. Patent 3,439,042; April 15, 1969; assigned to The Givaudan Corporation describe a process for making 6-substituted ionones. Alpha-irone is a valuable perfume material, as are also the beta- and gamma-irones. They are found as the principal components in violet flowers. Irones may be represented by the following structural formula, in which the encircled 3-carbon atom denotes the fact that double bonds are distributed along the neighboring carbon atoms from the 3-position:

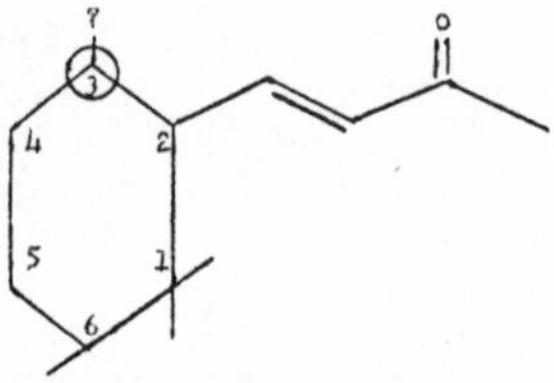

Thus, alpha-irone has the double bond in the 3-4 position, beta-irone has the double bond in the 2-3 position; and gamma-irone has the double bond in the 3-7 position. It is also known that the alpha- and gamma-irones can exist in cis-trans forms. This process involves the discovery that Grignard reaction products containing alpha-hydrogens next to an alkoxy group could be subject to oxidation to carbonyl derivatives by treatment with an excess of carbonyl derivatives such as acetone, or other ketones, or aldehydes and subsequently reacted with the excess carbonyl reagent to give aldol condensation products. The process as applied to making alpha-irone, in essence, may be represented in the following abbreviated form:

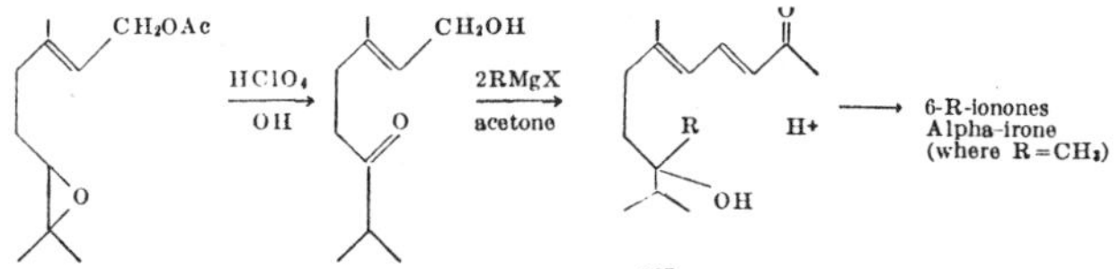

This reaction sequence represents the fact, for example, that when 6-ketodihydrogeraniol, which is obtained in good (60%) yield by the saponification of the perchloric acid-treated epoxydihydrogeranyl acetate, was treated with 2 mols of methyl magnesium halide and then treated with acetone, a hydrated pseudoirone (III) (R = CH_3) is obtained, which upon treatment with mineral acid such as phosphoric acid, was converted to alpha-irone in good yields.

In addition to the 6,9-dimethyl-9-R-9-hydroxy-undeca-3-5-dien-2-one (III), a small amount of 3,7-dimethyl-6-R-2-octen-1-6-diol is also obtained in accordance with the process. The following examples illustrate the process.

Example 1: 6,7-Epoxydihydrogeranyl Acetate — 450 ml of 40% peracetic acid solution containing 17 grams anhydrous sodium acetate is slowly introduced into a mixture of 435 grams geranyl acetate and 450 ml benzene containing 17 grams anhydrous sodium acetate. The addition is made within 30 to 45 minutes under ice water cooling and stirring, the temperature remaining between 10° to 20°C.

After the addition is complete, stirring is continued at room temperature for an additional 2 to 3 hours. The mixture is then washed twice with one volume of saturated sodium chloride solution and then neutralized with 10% soda ash solution and the solvent evaporated. Upon distillation, the main part of the reaction product distills at 113°C at 2 mm pressure; yield 420 to 440 grams. Saponification value 262.5 (theory 264).

Example 2: 6-Ketodihydrogeranyl Acetate — To 150 grams 6,7-epoxydihydrogeranyl acetate and 250 ml dry benzene in a flask provided with good agitation and ice-water cooling, is added dropwise 1.8 grams $HClO_4$ 70% within 10 to 15 minutes and the temperature kept between 10° to 20°C. After stirring for an additional 5 minutes, the mixture is neutralized with 30% NaOH, the solvent evaporated and the reaction product distilled. The main cut BP 109° to 110°C/2 mm, yielded 115 grams containing about 85% of the keto ester (by oximation).

Example 3: 6-Ketodihydrogeraniol — 315 grams 6-ketodihydrogeraniol acetate, 120 grams KOH, 60 ml water and 550 ml ethanol are heated under reflux for one half hour, then 400 ml aqueous ethanol is distilled off. The reaction mixture is then treated with two volumes of saturated sodium chloride solution, extracted with benzene and distilled. The main cut distills at 115° to 118°C/1 mm; carbonyl value 90% (by oximation); yield 225 to 240 grams.

Example 4: 6,7-Ketodihydrogeraniol Directly from Geranyl Acetate — To 1,108 grams geranyl acetate, 1,100 ml benzene, and 42 grams sodium acetate is added under good agitation, within 2 hours, 1,160 grams 40% peracetic acid containing 42 grams anhydrous sodium acetate at a temperature ranging from 25° to 30°C. After completion of the addition, stirring is continued for two more hours at room temperature and the reaction mixture is then washed twice with two volumes of sodium chloride saturated solution and finally neutralized with 10% Na_2CO_3. The benzene is evaporated leaving about 1,215 grams of a crude 6,7-epoxydihydrogeranyl acetate. The crude epoxide is then slowly fed under good agitation into a flask containing 1,000 ml dry benzene containing 3 grams 70% perchloric acid while the temperature is kept at 10° to 150°C with an ice-water cooling bath. After the addition of about half the epoxide within 25 minutes, an additional 1 gram $HClO_4$ was added, followed by another 2 grams $HClO_4$ after the feeding of three quarters of the epoxide. The whole addition of the epoxide took about 1 hour and was followed by the final addition of 2 grams $HClO_4$ and the reaction was completed by stirring for 10 more minutes at 10° to 15°C (a total of 8 grams 70% perchloric acid was used).

The reaction flask was then fitted with a distilling head and 600 grams 50% aqueous sodium hydroxide was fed within 2 to 3 minutes under agitation. The reaction mixture became viscous and warmed up while benzene distilled off. After 15 minutes agitation, 100 ml water was added and the flask heated to distill off the remaining solvent. An additional 100 ml water was added to dissolve the crystalline salts and the reaction mixture heated under reflux for an additional half hour. The top layer was separated, washed with NaCl saturated solution, slightly acidified with acetic acid and distilled. The main 6-ketodihydro-geraniol distilled at about 115° to 120°C at 1 mm pressure; yield, 470 to 520 grams; carbonyl value 90% (by oximation); a higher boiling cut BP 130° to 135°C at 1 mm (75 to 90 grams) consisted of the 3,7-dimethyl-2,7-dien-1,6-diol.

Example 5: 6,9,10-Trimethyl-9-Hydroxyundeca-3,5-Dien-2-one — To a Grignard reagent prepared from 255 grams methyl iodide in 300 ml ether and 45 grams magnesium in 100 ml ether, was added under ice-water cooling and stirring, 127.5 grams 6-ketodihydrogeraniol in 300 ml dry benzene. After the addition was completed, heating was started and the reaction temperature brought to about 60° to 70°C by distilling off the major part of the ether. The heating and stirring was continued for one and a half hours more. The reaction mixture became viscous and was finally cooled to room temperature by means of an ice-water bath. 500 ml of dry acetone (moisture content 0.11%) was slowly added within 15 to 20 minutes under strong agitation and cooling.

The Grignard reaction product which dissolved as a clear amber solution was heated under agitation and refluxed. After about half an hour a rich precipitate of basic magnesium salt formed and after two hours reflux heating was discontinued and the reaction mixture left overnight at room temperature. A solution of 130 ml acetic acid and 260 ml water was then added to dissolve the magnesium salts and the excess acetone distilled until the pot temperature reached 100° to 110°C. 150 ml water was added to the reaction mixture to dissolve the crystalline salts and the top layer separated.

After extraction with 100 ml benzene, the top layers were combined, washed with water and the solvent evaporated. Upon distillation some water of dehydration of the aldolization products was collected followed by acetone condensation products (mesityl oxide, diacetone alcohol, etc.), and a main cut (30%) consisting of 3,6,7-trimethyl-2-octen-1,6-diol, BP 125° to 130°C at 1 mm; followed by a major cut (40 to 45%) of 6,9,10-trimethyl-9-hydroxy-undeca-3,5-dien-2-one, BP 140° to 145°C at 1 mm, 2,4-dinitrophenylhydrazone MP 177° to 178°C.

Example 6: Alpha-Irone — 4 grams of 6,9,10-trimethyl-9-hydroxy-undeca-3,5-dien-2-one (III) was mixed with 18 grams 85% H_3PO_4 at 30°C and the temperature maintained between 30° to 40°C. The reaction mixture was then decomposed with 100 ml water and extracted with 25 ml benzene. After washing with a saturated NaCl solution, the benzene was evaporated and the alpha-irone mixture distilled at 85° to 95°C at 1 mm, yielding 3 grams having the characteristic violet odor of alpha-irone. The gas liquid chromatography on a 20 M Carbowax column showed the product to consist of a mixture of 18.5% neo alpha-irone; 71.5% neo iso alpha-irone; and 10% beta-irone.

The mixture was almost identical with a product obtained, under the same conditions, from an authentic sample of pseudo-irone. A 4-phenylsemicarbazone MP 174°C was isolated from the mixture which gave no melting point depression with an authentic sample prepared from neo iso alpha-irone.

α-Irone from Epoxide Intermediate

According to a process described by *D.H.R. Barton; U.S. Patent 3,117,982; January 14, 1964; assigned to Fritzsche Brothers, Inc.* irone and related compounds are produced from the available compound ψ-ionone by a simplified procedure using as an essential intermediate an epoxide of ψ-ionone. When ψ-ionone, which has the formula

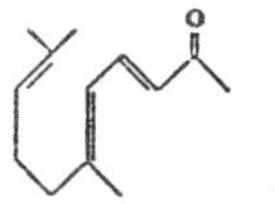

is reacted with reagents which convert a carbon-carbon double bond to an epoxide group, more particularly organic peracids, for example, perbenzoic acid, monoperphthalic acid and peracetic acid, the unconjugated double bond can be selectively epoxidized and the compound having the formula

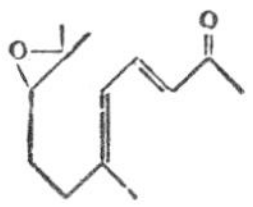

is formed in good yield. The reaction may be carried out by reacting ψ-ionone preferably in solution in an inert solvent, for example, ether or benzene, with an organic peracid, such as peracetic acid, perbenzoic acid or monoperphthalic acid. The reaction is advantageously carried out at reduced temperatures, for example, 0°C.

The epoxide shown above is a particularly useful intermediate in the synthesis of known synthetic perfumes. By reaction of the epoxide, after suitable protection of the ketonic carbonyl, with Grignard reagents, or metal alkyls, it is possible to form ketols which may be cyclized to 6-alkyl ionones. Thus, by using a methylating metal derivative it is possible to prepare the 6-methyl-ionone, irone. The following examples illustrate the process.

Example 1: ψ-Ionone Epoxide — ψ-Ionone (15 grams) in ether (50 ml) was treated at 0°C with stirring with monoperphthalic acid (15 grams) in the same solvent (300 ml) and left for 24 hours. The solution was washed successively with aqueous sodium hydrogen carbonate, with 1 N aqueous sodium hydroxide and then with water. The dried sodium sulfate solution gave on distillation ψ-ionone epoxide (13 grams), BP 118°C/0.7 mm.

Example 2: ψ-Ionol Epoxide — ψ-Ionone epoxide (13 grams) in methanol (200 ml) at 0°C was treated with sodium borohydride (½ mol) until the ketonic function had been reduced [ultra-violet control: disappearance of the band at 291 mμ and appearance of a new band (ϵ = 20,000 approximately) at 240 mμ]. The excess of sodium borohydride was destroyed with acetic acid and then a slight excess of sodium hydrogen carbonate was added. The methanol was removed in vacuo, the residue extracted into ether, dried with sodium sulfate and then distilled to furnish ψ-ionol epoxide (12 grams), BP 105°C/0.2 mm.

Example 3: 2,3,6-Trimethylundeca-6,8-Dien-2,10-Diol — Magnesium (6 grams) was converted to the Grignard reagent using methyl bromide (20 ml) in purified tetrahydrofuran (200 ml). To this solution was added slowly with stirring ψ-ionol epoxide (12 grams) in the same solvent (120 ml) and left for one hour. The reaction mixture was then refluxed for 4 hours, cooled, treated with excess of saturated aqueous ammonium chloride at 0°C. After ether extraction and drying over sodium sulfate the ether and tetrahydrofuran were removed in vacuo at 40°C. The residue could not be distilled due to decomposition but it analyzed correctly for the expected glycol.

Example 4: 2,3,6-Trimethylundeca-6,8-Dien-2-ol-10-one — The glycol of Example 3 (10.3) grams) in dry ether (500 ml) was shaken with active MnO$_2$ (105 grams) at room temperature and the progress of the oxidation followed in the ultra-violet. After 48 hours there was no further increase in the intensity of the band at 291 mμ (ϵ = 18,000). Removal of the MnO_2 by filtration and of the ether in the usual way gave a residue (10 grams) which had λ maximum 291 mμ (ϵ = 18,000) and showed an OH band in the infrared (3,625 cm^{-1}).

Example 5: Synthesis of α-Irone — The ketol, 2,3,3-trimethylundeca-6,8-dien-ol-10-one (10 grams) was added dropwise with good stirring to phosphoric acid (90%; 30 ml) at 30°C and the mixture stirred for 15 minutes. Excess of ice water was added and the cyclized product extracted into ether. The ether was removed and the residue steam distilled to give an oil, BP 73°C/0.3 mm, λ maximum 228 mμ (ϵ = 11,200) and ca 290 mμ (ϵ = 2,000), the latter band indicating the presence of some β-irone.

LILY OF THE VALLEY

1-Hydroxymethyl-1-Methyl-3-Isopropylidenecyclopentane

A process described by *P.J. Teisseire and A.M. Galfre; U.S. Patent 3,743,671; July 3, 1973; assigned to SA des Etablissements Roure-Bertrand Fils & Justin Dupont, France* is concerned with cyclopentane compounds of the Formula 1

(1)

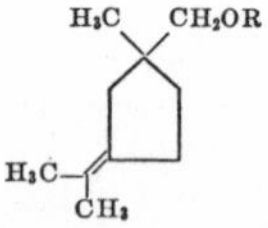

where R represents a hydrogen atom or the acyl residue of a fatty or aliphatic (including cycloaliphatic) or aromatic carboxylic acid containing from 1 to 8 carbon atoms. The process for the manufacture comprises isomerizing a bicyclohexane compound of the Formula 2

(2)

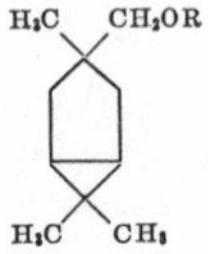

where R has the meaning given above, in the presence of an acid as an isomerizing agent; and, where R in Formula 1 represents hydrogen, saponifying an ester resulting from the isomerization to the corresponding alcohol; and to the utilization of the compounds of Formula 1 for perfumery purposes.

The alcohol of the process, 1-hydroxymethyl-1-methyl-3-isopropylidene-cyclopentane (compound of Formula 1 where R = H), is distinguished by a characteristic odor of lily-of-the-valley and lilac and can accordingly be used as an odorant for perfumery purposes.

Example 1: 20 grams of 3-hydroxymethyl-3,6,6-trimethyl-bicyclo[3.1.0]hexane are dissolved in 600 ml of diisopropyl ether containing 5 ml of concentrated hydrochloric acid. The solution is allowed to stand at room temperature for 24 hours. The solution is worked up by washing with water, then with 5% aqueous sodium bicarbonate and again with water. The diisopropyl ether solvent is then distilled off and the residue is distilled under reduced pressure.

There is thus obtained 19.5 grams of crude product which is shown, by gas-chromatographic analysis, to contain about 30% by weight of 1-hydroxymethyl-1-methyl-3-isopropylidene-cyclopentane. After purification by means of preparative gas chromatography, there is obtained 5.1 grams of pure 1-hydroxymethyl-1-methyl-3-isopropylidene-cyclopentane, smelling of lily-of-the-valley and lilac. The 3-hydroxymethyl-3,6,6-trimethyl-bicyclo[3.1.0]-

hexane used as the starting material may be prepared as follows. 245 grams (1.8 mol) of 3-carene are added over one hour to 4,600 ml of a 0.58 N ethereal solution of monoperphthalic acid at 0°C. The reaction mixture is allowed to stand for 24 hours, during which time the temperature rises to about 20°C. The reaction mixture is worked up by washing with water, then with 5% aqueous sodium bicarbonate and again with water. The product is then dried over anhydrous sodium sulfate and the solvent is evaporated off. There is obtained 180 grams of α-epoxy-carane having a BP of 65°C/5 mm.

20 grams (0.13 mol) of α-epoxy-carane are conducted in the vapor state through a glass tube of 20 mm diameter and 50 mm long filled with Celite (0.2 to 0.3 mm particle size) and heated externally to 180° to 190°C. There is obtained 19 grams of crude product from which, after rectification, 17 grams of 3-formyl-3,6,6-trimethyl-bicyclo[3.1.0]hexane is isolated. BP 55°C/5 mm.

37.5 grams (0.25 mol) of 3-formyl-3,6,6-trimethyl-bicyclo[3.1.0]hexane are dissolved in 400 ml of petroleum ether. This solution is added over 2 hours to a solution of 70 ml (0.38 mol) of diisobutyl aluminum hydride in 800 ml of petroleum ether. The mixture is then refluxed for 2 hours. The reaction product is worked up by pouring it into cold dilute sulfuric acid. The organic layer is then washed with water, then with 5% aqueous sodium bicarbonate and again with water.

The product is then dried over anhydrous sodium sulfate and the solvent evaporated off. 37 grams of crude product are obtained from which ca 30 grams of 3-hydroxymethyl-3,6,6-trimethyl-bicyclo[3.1.0]hexane of BP 56°C/2.5 mm, MP 31° to 32°C, are isolated by rectification. This alcohol may be quantitatively esterified to the corresponding acetate with a mixture of acetic anhydride and pyridine.

Example 2: An odorant composition having a lilac note containing 1-hydroxymethyl-1-methyl-3-isopropylidene-cyclopentane is prepared as follows:

	Parts by Weight
Terpineol extra	90
Cinnamyl alcohol	80
Phenylethyl alcohol	310
Anisaldehyde	30
Linalool	20
Linalyl acetate	10
Benzyl acetate	20
Ylang-ylang oil, 2nd fraction	10
Styrax-oil rectified; 10% solution in ethyl phthalate	30
Phenylpropyl alcohol	30
Cyclamen alcohol	10
Hydroxy-citronellal	100
1-Hydroxymethyl-1-methyl-3-isopropylidene-cyclopentane	260

Cyclopropyl Alkenols

M. Julia; U.S. Patent 3,342,877; September 19, 1967; assigned to Rhone Poulenc SA, France describes organic compounds of the formula:

(1) 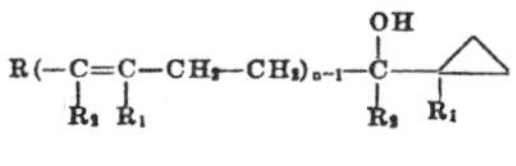 $R(-C=C-CH_2-CH_2)_{n-1}-\overset{OH}{\underset{R_2\ R_1}{C}}-\triangle$
           $\quad R_2\ R_1$

in which R represents an alkyl group, R_1 represents a hydrogen atom or an alkyl or aralkyl group, R_2 represents an alkyl group and n is 2 or 3, the groups shown between parentheses being the same or different. The compounds are useful in the art of perfumery and the preferred compounds from this standpoint are those in which the alkyl groups contain at most 3 carbon atoms and the aralkyl group, if present, is the benzyl group. These products may be prepared by the action of a ketone of the Formula 2

$$(2) \qquad\qquad \underset{\triangledown}{\overset{R_1}{\mid}}\text{-CO-}R_2$$

where R_1 and R_2 have the meanings given above, on an organomagnesium compound of the general Formula 3

$$(3) \qquad\qquad R(-\underset{R_2}{\underset{\mid}{C}}=\underset{R_1}{\underset{\mid}{C}}-CH_2-CH_2)_{n-1}MgX$$

in which X represents a halogen atom such as chlorine or bromine and the other symbols have the meanings given above. The reaction may be effected in any suitable organic solvent, for example, diethyl ether. The resulting complex is then hydrolyzed, for example, by means of a saturated solution of ammonium chloride.

Example 1: 65 grams of 1-bromo-4-methyl-pent-3-ene in solution in 200 cc of ether are added in 3 hours to 10 grams of magnesium covered with 20 cc of diethyl ether. The mixture is heated under reflux for 1 hour and a solution of 33.6 grams of methyl cyclopropyl ketone in 300 cc of diethyl ether is slowly added to the solution, cooled at 5° to 10°C. After standing for one night, the complex mixture is hydrolyzed by a saturated ammonium chloride solution and there is obtained, in a yield of 80%, 6-methyl-2-cyclopropyl-hept-5-en-2-ol, which is a colorless liquid boiling at 115° to 118°C under 20 mm Hg and at 72°C under 1 mm Hg.

Example 2: 67 grams of 6-methyl-2-cyclopropyl-hept-5-en-2-ol are vigorously agitated at room temperature with 160 cc of 48% hydrobromic acid. After extraction with petroleum ether, washing and drying over potassium carbonate, there are obtained 76 grams of 1-bromo-4,8-dimethyl-nona-3,7-diene, which is a colorless liquid boiling at 88° to 92°C under 1 mm Hg.

A solution in 100 cc of ether of 35 grams of 1-bromo-4,8-dimethyl-nona-3,7-diene is added to 3.6 grams of magnesium covered by 25 cc of ether. The reaction is started by heating and is maintained throughout the addition of the bromo derivative, which lasts 3 hours. A solution of 12.6 grams of methyl cyclopropyl ketone in 50 cc of ether is thereafter added in 2 hours with cooling. By treating as in Example 1, there are obtained 17.5 grams of 6,10-dimethyl-2-cyclopropyl-undeca-5,9-dien-2-ol, which is a colorless liquid boiling at 128° to 132°C under 1 mm Hg and at 96° to 98°C under 0.02 mm.

Example 3: 91 grams of 6-methyl-2-cyclopropyl-oct-5-en-2-ol are treated with hydrobromic acid by the procedure of Example 2 and give 106 grams of 1-bromo-4,8-dimethyl-deca-3,7-diene; BP 115° to 117°C/15 mm. 31.6 grams of 1-bromo-4,8-dimethyl-deca-3,7-diene are converted into the magnesium compound, which is thereafter reacted with 8.4 grams of acetylcyclopropane by the procedure of Example 2. There are thus obtained 12.5 grams of 6,10-dimethyl-2-cyclopropyl-dodeca-5,9-dien-2-ol, BP 120° to 122°C/0.08 mm.

The product of Example 1 has an odor of the linalool family, free from the earthy smell which is often found in this product, and having a striking fresh tonality with a highly desirable rustic tinge tending toward the elder stem. The product of Example 2 has a hyacinth note and can be used in hyacinth compositions. It is a heart product. The product of Example 3 has an odor of the linalool family, the fragrance of which is both roseate and more rustic. The product of Example 3 has a waxy odor with a lily-of-the-valley and lilac tone, which diffuses well.

LILAC

2-(1'-Hydroxymethylethyl)-5-Methyl-5-Vinyltetrahydrofuran

S. Wakayama and A. Komatsu; U.S. Patent 3,764,567; October 9, 1973; assigned to Takasago Perfumery Co., Ltd., Japan describes the compound 2-(1'-hydroxymethylethyl)-5-methyl-5-vinyltetrahydrofuran which is an essential oil of a lilac flower. This compound consists of four stereoisomers and is useful as an ingredient to be incorporated in floral perfumes. This compound is obtained by selectively reducing the formyl radical of 2-(1'-formylethyl)-5-methyl-5-vinyltetrahydrofuran

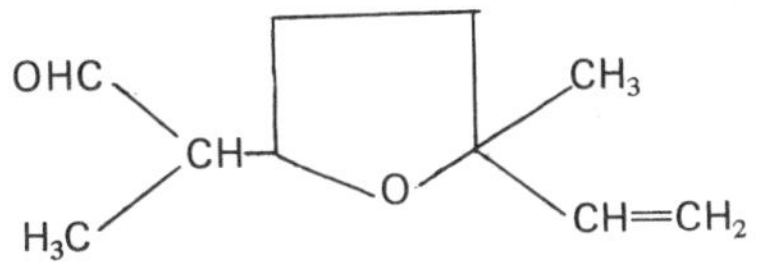

Reducing agents, suitable for selectively reducing the formyl radical of the compound shown in the above formula, include sodium borohydride, lithium aluminum hydride, and lithium borohydride. The Meermein Ponndorf reduction process which employs aluminum alcoholate as the reducing agent may also be used.

The gas chromatographic analysis of the lilac alcohol obtained by the above described processes proves that the lilac alcohol so produced consists of a mixture of four isomers, the same as those found in the essential oil of the natural lilac flower.

LAVENDER

Hexahydro-4,7-Methanoindene

H.C. Saunders; U.S. Patent 3,446,755; May 27, 1969; assigned to Universal Oil Products Company describes a perfume composition containing 3a,4,5,6,7,7a-hexahydro-4,7-methanoindene, substituted in one of the 5 and 6 positions with an oxo group.

Spike lavender oil, also known as Spanish spike oil or aspic, is a natural essential oil derived from the plant, *Lavandula latifolia,* which grows wild in many of the Mediterranean countries, with the principal commercial crop growing chiefly in Spain. This natural oil, consisting of a mixture of a large number of substances such as camphor, borneol, linalool, and cineol, has a fresh and herbaceous odor with a somewhat dry-woody undertone which renders such oil highly useful for perfumery application.

This natural oil, however, like other products derived from plants, and especially wild, uncultivated plants, suffers from the disadvantage of fluctuating supply and quality due to such uncontrollable factors as crop-growing weather. Obviously, therefore, a synthetic replacement for spike lavender oil which is stable in supply and quality would be highly desirable in the perfume industry, which depends upon a constant and stable supply of natural spike lavender oil for a large number of commercial products.

The synthetic lavender oil of this process may be used to replace the natural spike lavender oil constituent of perfumes either in whole or in part and thus create new perfume compositions.

Example 1: A synthetic spike lavender oil comprising 3a,4,5,6,7,7a-hexahydro-4,7-methanoindene substituted in one of the 5 and 6 positions with an oxo group was sampled on a perfume blotter and the odor was compared with the odor of natural spike lavender oil. It was observed that the synthetic spike lavender oil had a fresh and herbaceous odor with a somewhat dry-woody undertone which closely resembled the odor profile of natural spike lavender oil.

Example 2: A bouquet-type soap perfume was prepared using natural spike lavender oil according the the following formula.

Components	Parts by Weight
Spike lavender oil	100
Terpineol	200
Rosewood	200
Diphenyl oxide	30
Cedarwood	100
Citronella, Java	200
Clove	50
Linalyl acetate	50
Red thyme	20
Styrax resin	20
Musk xylene	20

A second bouquet soap perfume was prepared using the same formula as above, except that the natural spike lavender oil constituent was replaced with 100 parts by weight of 3a,4,5,6,7,7a-hexahydro-4,7-methanoindene substituted in one of the 5 and 6 positions with an oxo group.

The odor profiles of the above two bouquet soap perfumes were compared and were found to be substantially similar especially in respect to both having fresh, refreshing notes which characterize perfume compositions containing natural spike lavender oil.

In related work, *H.C. Saunders; U.S. Patent 3,271,259; September 6, 1966; assigned to Universal Oil Products Company* describes a synthetic lavandin oil comprising a mixture of 3a,4,5,6,7,7a-hexahydro-4,7-methanoindene having an oxo substituent in one of the 5 and 6 positions and 5-acetoxy-5-vinyl-2,3,3a,4,5,6,7,7a-octahydro-4,7-methanoindene.

Example: A lavender-type cologne was prepared having the following formula using natural lavandin oil.

Components	Parts by Weight
Natural lavandin oil	19
Oil bergamot	25
5,7-diisopropyl-3,4-dihydrocoumarin	1
7-acetyl-1,1,3,4,4,6-hexamethyl-tetralin, 5% alcohol	1
Linalool	10
Oil Petitgras	5
Allyl phenylpropionate	½
Oil coriander 10%	½
Oil neroli bigarade	½

A second cologne was prepared using the same formula as above, except that the natural lavandin oil constituent was replaced with 19 parts by weight of synthetic lavandin oil comprising a mixture of 18 weight parts of 5-acetoxy-5-vinyl-2,3,3a,4,5,6,7,7a-octahydro-4,7-methanoindene and 1 weight part of 3a,4,5,6,7,7a-hexahydro-4,7-methanoindene substituted in one of the 5 and 6 positions with an oxo group.

The odor profiles of the two cologne compositions were compared and were found to be substantially similar especially in respect to both having fresh, refreshing notes which characterize perfume compositions containing natural lavandin oil.

Demethyl-cis-Sabinene Hydrate

W.I. Fanta and W.F. Erman; U.S. Patent 3,591,643; July 6, 1971; assigned to The Procter

& *Gamble Company* describe a process for the preparation of demethyl-cis-sabinene hydrate comprising the steps of (1) cyclizing 2-methyl-3,6-heptanedione with a base in a suitable solvent to form 3-isopropyl-2-cyclopentenone; (2) reducing the 3-isopropyl-2-cyclopentenone with a suitable reducing agent to obtain 3-isopropyl-2-cyclopentenol; and (3) reacting the 3-isopropyl-2-cyclopentenol with appropriate reagents to form demethyl-cis-sabinene hydrate. Sabina ketone, sabinene and cis- and trans-sabinene hydrates can readily be prepared from the demethyl-cis-sabinene hydrate, if desired.

These are valuable compounds for reconstituting a large number of essential oils, including lavender, lavendin, spearmint, and savin. These and other oils which can be reconstituted utilizing the compounds derived from the process provide highly valuable perfume and flavor bases. The following examples illustrate the process.

Data listed in all of the examples were obtained by means of the following techniques unless otherwise indicated. Infrared spectra were determined on a Perkin-Elmer Model 137 Spectrophotometer; ultraviolet spectra were determined in ethanol on a Perkin-Elmer Model 202 Spectrophotometer. Nuclear magnetic resonance (nmr) spectra were determined in carbon tetrachloride with a Varian Model HA–100 Spectrometer with chemical shifts measured relative to tetramethylsilane (10τ). The nmr data are noted by position, integration, multiplicity, coupling constant (in Hz), and assignment. Gas-liquid chromatography was accomplished with an Aerograph Model 202B using a flow rate of 100 ml/min on 5 feet by 0.25 inch columns packed with 20% FFAP (Carbowax 20M terminated with nitroterephthalic acid) on 60/80 mesh Chromosorb P.

Example 1: A dry, 2 liter flask fitted with an addition funnel and nitrogen inlet was charged with a solution of 51.6 grams of 2-methyl-3,6-heptanedione in 580 ml of 2% aqueous sodium hydroxide and 180 ml of ethanol. A nitrogen atmosphere was introduced and the mixture was heated under reflux with good mechanical stirring for 4.5 hours. The reaction was diluted with a brine solution and the product was isolated with ether. Removal of the magnesium sulfate dried solvent and distillation afforded 32.18 grams of a faint green product which was purified by distillation. Comparison of the physical constants and infrared and nuclear magnetic resonance spectra of this material with published results positively identified it as 3-isopropyl-2-cyclopentenone.

A 1 liter flask fitted with a mechanical stirrer, condenser, and addition funnel was charged with a slurry of 5.0 grams of lithium aluminum hydride in 500 ml of ether. The flask was cooled in an ice bath and a solution of 32.18 grams of 3-isopropyl-2-cyclopentenone in 100 ml of diethyl ether was added with good stirring over 15 minutes. The resulting mixture was stirred 2 hours at room temperature and was decomposed by the cautious addition of 10 ml of water and 8 ml of 10% aqueous sodium hydroxide. After stirring overnight, the reaction was filtered and the solvent was removed to afford 31.8 grams of product. After further purification by distillation, analysis of the product via gas chromatography, and nuclear magnetic resonance and infrared spectra positively identified it as 3-isopropyl-2-cyclopentenol.

A 250 ml flask fitted with a mechanical stirrer, condenser, and septum cap was charged with 7.84 grams of zinc-copper couple. A nitrogen atmosphere was introduced followed by an iodine crystal and 60 ml of ether. Freshly distilled methylene iodine (26.4 grams, 8 ml) was added in one portion and the mixture was heated with good stirring at 40°C for 30 minutes. A solution of 6.42 grams of 3-isopropyl-2-cyclopentenol in 16 ml of diethyl ether was added dropwise over 35 minutes. Heating was discontinued temporarily as the reaction was sufficiently exothermic to maintain reflux. After the addition was complete, the mixture was refluxed for one additional hour and after cooling, the reaction was treated with excess saturated aqueous ammonium chloride and filtered. The solid was washed well with diethyl ether and the resulting filtrate was washed with two portions of 10% aqueous sodium carbonate and brine.

The aqueous layers were back extracted and the combined ether layers were washed with brine and dried over magnesium sulfate. Solvent removal yielded a yellow-green oil which was further purified by distillation. Analyses and spectral data along with a general knowledge of the entire synthetic process positively identified the product as demethyl-cis-sabinene hydrate.

When in the treatment of 2-methyl-3,6-heptanedione with a base and solvent, any of the corresponding bases and solvents listed in H.O. House, *Modern Synthetic Reactions,* page 185, are substituted on an equimolar basis for the sodium hydroxide and water-ethanol in the process of Example 1 substantially equivalent results are obtained in that comparative yields of demethyl-cis-sabinene hydrate are obtained. The only caveat is that the bases and solvents be compatible as shown in *Modern Synthetic Reactions.*

When sodium borohydride, lithium borohydride or a lithium aluminum hydride-aluminum chloride mixture is substituted on an equimolar basis for the lithium aluminum hydride of the process of Example 1 substantially equivalent results are obtained in that comparative yields of demethyl-cis-sabinene hydrate are obtained.

When a dialkyl zinc compound, e.g., diethyl zinc, is substituted on an equimolar basis for the zinc-copper couple of Example 1, substantially equivalent results are obtained in that comparative yields of demethyl-cis-sabinene hydrate are obtained.

Example 2: In a dry, 250 ml flask, a solution of 4.62 grams of demethyl-cis-sabinene hydrate prepared in Example 1 in 75 ml of acetone was oxidized at 0°C with 9 ml of chromium trioxide solution [prepared according to K. Bowden et al, *J. Chem. Soc.,* 39 (1946)] over a 15 minute period. The resulting solution was stirred an additional 10 minutes at 0°C and was then added to brine. Several ether extracts were washed with saturated aqueous sodium bicarbonate, the aqueous layers were back extracted, and the total ether was washed with brine and dried over magnesium sulfate.

Removal of the solvent and distillation afforded 4.05 grams of a faint yellow oil which was further purified by distillation. Comparison of the physical constants, gas chromatographic retention time and infrared and nuclear magnetic resonance spectra of this material with an authentic sample positively identified the product as sabina ketone.

When manganese dioxide or a chromium trioxide-pyridine complex are substituted on an equimolar basis for the chromium trioxide in the process of Example 2, substantially equivalent results are obtained in that comparative yields of sabina ketone are obtained.

Example 3: A dry 250 ml flask fitted with a two-neck adapter, nitrogen inlet and septum was charged with 1.24 grams of a sodium hydride dispersion (61% sodium hydride in mineral oil). A nitrogen atmosphere was introduced and 40 ml of dimethyl sulfoxide (distilled from calcium hydride) was added through the septum. The mixture was then heated at 70°C for one hour, cooled to 0°C and a solution of 11.9 grams of methyltriphenylphosphonium bromide in 40 ml of dry dimethyl sulfoxide was added over 2 minutes at 0°C. The semisolid mixture was allowed to warm to room temperature in order to effect solution. This solution was stirred for 20 minutes at room temperature.

A solution of 1.30 grams of sabina ketone from the process of Example 2 in 20 ml of dry dimethyl sulfoxide was added dropwise over 5 minutes. The resulting dark yellow solution was stirred at room temperature for three hours and was added to water. The mixture was extracted with pentane. Several extracts were combined, washed with water, and brine, and dried over magnesium sulfate. The solvent was removed by distillation. Comparison of the physical constants, gas chromatographic retention time and infrared and nuclear magnetic resonance spectra of this material with an authentic sample positively identified the product as sabinene.

1,5-Dimethylbicyclo[2.1.1] Hexyl-2-Acetic Acid

T.W. Gibson; U.S. Patent 3,468,928; September 23, 1969; assigned to The Procter & Gamble Company describes a photochemical process for the preparation of 1,5-dimethylbicyclo[2.1.1] hexyl-2-acetic acid and esters thereof, utilizing carvone or carvone camphor as a starting material.

The process comprises subjecting a solution of carvone and carvone camphor in a solvent selected from the group consisting of anhydrous alcohol solvents and aqueous solvents to full spectrum ultraviolet radiation to form a 1,5-dimethylbicyclo[2.1.1] hexane compound of the formula

where R is selected from the group consisting of $-CH_2COOH$ and CH_2COOR' and R' is an alkyl radical containing from about 1 to about 10 carbon atoms.

Both carvone or carvone camphor, the starting materials in the above-defined process, are readily obtainable. Carvone, a component of natural occurring spearmint, dill and cara-way oils, is generally purified by rectification and is commercially available. Carvone is also prepared synthetically by the oxidation of limonene.

Carvone camphor is prepared by irradiating carvone with an ultraviolet light source emit-ting radiation of 200 to 280 mμ and/or 320 to 400 mμ but emitting substantially no ra-diation in the 280 mμ to 320 mμ spectrum. Alternatively, special light sources or filters can be used to achieve this result.

The alkyl 1,5-dimethylbicyclo[2.1.1] hexyl-2-acetate compounds have an odor character-ized as dry lavender. This odor is most intense when alkyl is methyl or ethyl and decreases with increasing alkyl chain length. Thus, methyl and ethyl 1,5-dimethylbicyclo[2.1.1]-hexyl-2-acetate are preferred members of this group. These compounds therefore find utility in compositions such as soap bars, room deodorants, personal deodorants, cosmetics, colognes (especially of a floral nature), lavender, spike lavender and lavandin perfumes and the like, where they can be used in amounts of about 0.0001 to about 10% to impart desirable odors to the compositions.

1,5-dimethylbicyclo[2.1.1] hexyl-2-acetic acid has only a very slight odor. However, this compound can be readily converted by conventional esterification to the above-discussed highly useful alkyl 1,5-dimethylbicyclo[2.1.1] hexyl-2-acetate compounds, e.g., treatment of 1,5-dimethylbicyclo[2.1.1] hexyl-2-acetic acid with methanol in the presence of sul-furic acid yields methyl 1,5-dimethylbicyclo[2.1.1] hexyl-2-acetate.

All percentages and ratios in the following examples are by weight unless otherwise indi-cated. The following examples illustrate the process. All carvone used in the following examples was d-carvone, BP 98° to 100°C/10 mm. Use of 1-carvone gives products which are enantiomorphic to those reported herein for d-carvone. Prior to use, the carvone was distilled through a spinning band column, and showed $[\alpha]_D^{25}$ + 51.60°.

Example 1: Irradiation of Carvone to Form Ethyl 1,5-Dimethylbicyclo[2.1.1] Hexyl-2-Acetate — A solution of 1 gram of carvone in 150 ml of absolute ethanol was irradiated with a Hanovia 654 A mercury arc lamp for 20 hours. At this time, vapor phase chromatog-raphy showed only a trace of carvone remaining. The ethanol was removed by vacuum distillation and the residue chromatographed over 30.0 grams of silica gel. Elution with pentane gave about 0.200 gram of a viscous oil which appeared to be dimeric material. Continued elution with 10% ether in pentane gave 0.530 gram of uncontaminated product, ethyl 1,5-dimethylbicyclo[2.1.1] hexyl-2-acetate.

Example 2: Irradiation of Carvone to Form Methyl 1,5-Dimethylbicyclo[2.1.1] Hexyl-2-

Acetate — A solution of 12.14 grams of carvone in 450 ml of methanol was irradiated with a Hanovia 654 A mercury arc lamp for 80 hours. At this time, no carvone remained and the methanol was removed in vacuum. Vacuum distillation of the residue gave 7.07 grams of methyl 1,5-dimethylbicyclo[2.1.1] hexyl-2-acetate (BP$_{5.5}$ 79° to 83°C).

In this example, other aliphatic alcohols can be substituted for methanol to produce the corresponding esters. For example, butyl 1,5-dimethylbicyclo[2.1.1] hexyl-2-acetate is produced when butanol is used as the solvent; hexyl 1,5-dimethylbicyclo[2.1.1] hexyl-2-acetate is produced with hexanol as a solvent; and decyl 1,5-dimethylbicyclo[2.1.1] hexyl-2-acetate is produced with decyl alcohol as the solvent. The compounds of this example have an odor characterized as dry lavender.

Example 3: (a) Formation of Carvone Camphor — A solution of 1.13 grams of carvone dissolved in 100 ml of absolute ethanol in a round quartz flask was irradiated with sixteen 350 mµ Rayonet mercury resonance lamps placed in a circular array. Periodic analysis indicated the formation of carvone camphor with some ethyl 1,5-dimethylbicyclo[2.1.1]-hexyl-2-acetate being formed also. After 108 hours, the mixture was comprised of 34% carvone camphor, 14% ethyl 1,5-dimethylbicyclo[2.1.1] hexyl-2-acetate and 47% carvone. The reaction was then stopped, the solvent removed by distillation, and the carvone camphor purified by gas chromatography.

(b) Irradiation of Carvone Camphor — A solution of 0.0429 gram of carvone camphor dissolved in 5.0 ml of ethanol was irradiated with a Hanovia 608 A mercury arc lamp in a quartz flask for 2 hours and 40 minutes. The ethanol was removed by distillation and the product, ethyl 1,5-dimethylbicyclo[2.1.1] hexyl-2-acetate, was purified by gas chromatography. Analysis of this product was identical to the same product obtained in Example 1.

In this example, other alcoholic solvents can be substituted for the ethanol to produce the corresponding ester. For example, when methanol is substituted for ethanol, methyl 1,5-dimethylbicyclo[2.1.1] hexyl-2-acetate is the product; similarly, decyl alcohol can be used as the solvent to produce decyl 1,5-dimethylbicyclo[2.1.1] hexyl-2-acetate.

Also in this example, an aqueous solvent such as aqueous alcohol, aqueous dioxane, or aqueous ether can be substituted for the ethanol solvent whereby the product is 1,5-dimethylbicyclo[2.1.1] hexyl-2-acetic acid, e.g., use of a solvent comprised of 70% dioxane and 30% water in this example results in the formation of 1,5-dimethyl[2.1.1] hexyl-2-acetic acid as the product.

Linalool by Pyrolysis of Pinan-2-ol

G. Ohloff, E. Klein and G. Schade; U.S. Patent 3,240,821; March 15, 1966; assigned to Studiengesellschaft Kohle mbH, Germany have found that optically active linalool is obtained if the enantiomeric forms of pinan-2-ol or its disastereomers are pyrolyzed. Advantageously optically active cis- or trans-pinan-2-ol is conducted at temperatures between 500° and 650°C, advantageously under reduced pressure, through a suitable pyrolysis oven. By operating discontinuously, there are formed from 50 to 90% of linalool, 5 to 40% of other pyroalcohols, 5 to 15% of hydrocarbons as well as varying amounts of unmodified starting material, depending upon the precise conditions used.

Starting from (+)-cis-pinan-2-ol, the (−)-linalool is obtained, while the (+)-linalool is formed from the (−)-cis-pinan-2-ol or (+)-trans-pinan-2-ol. Mixtures of equal parts of (−)-trans- and (−)-cis-pinan-2-ol give inactive linalool. The racemates of the diastereomeric pinan-2-ols produce exclusively racemic linalool. The optical purity of the diastereomeric bicyclic terpene alcohol which is used as starting material is of major importance in determining the optical activity of the final product.

For the further understanding of the process valency isomerization of the enantiomeric forms of diastereomeric pinan-2-ols is shown in the reaction scheme on the following page.

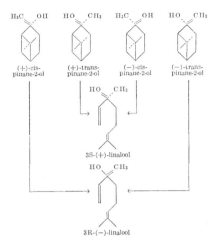

Example 1: 100 grams of (-)-cis-pinan-2-ol (MP 78°C) were introduced through a heated dropping funnel (80°C) into a two-necked flask with a capacity of 250 cc and preheated to 200°C, the flask being provided with a capillary tube for the introduction of inert gas (nitrogen or argon). The spontaneously evaporating alcohol was conducted into a quartz tube with a length of 80 cm and a diameter of 25 cm, this tube being half-filled with sintered filler bodies consisting of quartz and being heated to 570°C by an electrical heating jacket having a length of 1 meter. The entire pyrolysis apparatus was under a vacuum of 2 mm Hg. The pyrolyzate was conducted through a distillation bridge, condensed in a condenser and collected in a receiver.

In this way, 95 grams of a reaction mixture were obtained, and when analyzed by gas chromatography, the mixture consisted of 50% of linalool, 25% of hydrocarbons and 25% of other pyroalochols, in addition to starting material.

Example 2: 100 grams of (+)-cis-pinan-2-ol (MP 77° to 78°C) were pyrolyzed at a temperature of 600°C in the manner described in Example 1. Instead of using a quartz tube as the reaction tube, there was merely employed a smoothly polished tube of stainless steel, which was partially filled with filler bodies of the same material. In this way, 97.5 grams of pyrolyzate could be obtained with a content of 82% of linalool.

Example 3: (-)-cis-pinan-2-ol was reacted, as described in Example 1 or 2, in the presence of 10% of pyridine at a reaction temperature of 600°C. According to analysis by gas chromatography, the pyrolyzate consisted of 93% of dextrorotatory linalool. The hydrocarbon formation could in this case be reduced to 3%.

Alcohols from Diolefin-Magnesium Addition Compounds

According to a process described by *H.E. Ramsden; U.S. Patent 3,711,560; January 16, 1973; assigned to Esso Research and Engineering Company* hydrocarbon polyolefins and oxygenated organic compounds, such as alcohols, glycols, ketones, diketones, and diacids, which compounds contain at least two olefinic sites of unsaturation per molecule are obtained by contacting a diolefin-magnesium addition compound with various reagent systems. The organomagnesium compound has the generic formula $(R')_n Mg$ where R' is a C_4 to C_{40} conjugated diolefin and mixtures and n is an integer varying from 2 to 8.

The organomagnesium compounds employed in the reaction as well as the method used in their preparation are described in U.S. Patent 3,388,179. Typical examples of useful conjugated diolefins include: butadiene, 2,3-dimethyl butadiene, 2-phenyl-butadiene, isoprene 1,4-diphenylbutadiene and myrcene.

The alcohols prepared using the process are useful as odor chemicals for the perfume industry. C_{10} alcohols, prepared from diisoprene-magnesium compositions are particularly important because they are believed to be isomers of linalool (a tertiary $C_{10}H_{18}O$ alcohol) and geraniol (a primary $C_{10}H_{18}O$ alcohol), both naturally occurring substances that are widely used in perfumes.

The following examples illustrate the process. All of the reactions were carried out under an inert nitrogen atmosphere, except where otherwise specified, which atmosphere was controlled under static conditions of a few cm of hydrocarbon pressure by the use of an immersion bubbler. The diolefins employed in the manufacture of the diolefin magnesium adducts were not freed of polymerization inhibitors prior to use and all starting materials were used without prior purification. Time of flight measurements were made on a Bendix spectrometer coupled with a temperature program F&M 500 gas chromatograph. Capillary gas chromatography was obtained with a 300 foot R-column operated at 100°C, the injection block temperature being 150°C, and the detector block being maintained at 160°C.

Preparative gas chromatographic separations were performed in an Aeroprep unit using a 20 foot x ⅜ inch 20% squalane column. Column temperature was maintained at 100°C and the injector and detector blocks were maintained at 200°C. Nuclear magnetic resonance spectra were obtained at 60 mc on a Varian A 60 spectrometer.

Example 1: A 175 ml sample of diisoprene-magnesium was rapidly added to a glass reaction vessel containing a chilled dilute ammonium chloride water solution. The aqueous phase was separated from the organic phase and the organic phase extracted with n-pentane. The resulting pentane solution was washed three times with small quantities of water and then dried over sodium sulfate. This solution was then filtered and introduced into a short path distillation apparatus. Two distillate fractions were obtained.

The first fraction having a boiling point between 165° and 180°C at 760 mm of mercury pressure weighed 16 grams and the second fraction which exhibited a boiling point varying between 138° and 144°C at 26 mm of mercury pressure weighed 2 grams. Both fractions were fragrant terpene-like unsaturated hydrocarbons. Infrared and gas chromatograph analysis showed both fractions to be practically identical. The calculated composition of the hydrocarbon, $C_{10}H_{18}$ contains 86.95 weight percent carbon and 13.05 weight percent hydrogen. The composition obtained from the reaction contained 86.80 weight percent carbon and 13.51 weight percent hydrogen. The calculated bromine number for the composition was 230. The bromine number of the materials secured from the reaction was 208.

Example 2: In a 5 liter, four-neck flask, equipped with an anchor stirrer, thermometer, reflux condenser, and dropping funnel was placed 8 gram atoms (194.4 grams) of magnesium turnings. The magnesium turnings were initiated by contacting the same with 5 ml of ethylene dibromide and 5 ml of tetrahydrofuran. To this mixture was added a solution of 8 mols of isoprene contained in 1,400 ml of tetrahydrofuran. The isoprene and tetrahydrofuran were added with stirring at the reflux temperature of the mixture. The total mixture was added over a period of 7 hours and 56 minutes. At the completion of the addition, the reflux temperature of the mixture was 53°C. At the end of this time the reaction was stopped and restarted the following day where a further 8 mols of isoprene and 700 ml of tetrahydrofuran were added over a period of 8 hours.

Refluxing of this mixture was continued for 48 hours and then a liter of tetrahydrofuran was added and refluxing continued for another 32 hour period. After cooling, the reaction mixture was sampled and the sample was found to contain a 0.21 meq of diisoprene-magnesium/ml of solution.

This solution, after standing under nitrogen atmosphere for a protracted period was then hydrolyzed by contacting the same with 600 ml of methanol, one liter of water and 16 mols of hydrochloric acid as concentrated (12 N) acid. Following contacting, the organic and aqueous layers were separated and the organic layer concentrated in a rotary film evaporator to yield 1,021 grams of terpenes boiling above 80°C at 40 mm of mercury pressure. Theoretical yield would be 1,088 grams of diolefinic material.

Example 3: One mol of diisoprene-magnesium [$(C_{10}H_{16})$Mg] solution is introduced into a flask equipped with a gas inlet tube and air (or oxygen) is bubbled into the mixture until the equivalent of one-half mol of oxygen has been emitted. The solution is then hydrolyzed with 100 ml of water to remove the unreacted tertiary carbon-magnesium linkage. Sufficient dilute hydrochloric·acid (about 2 mols) is added to solublize the $Mg(OH)_2$ and the organic and aqueous layers separated. After removal of solvent, the residual alcohols from the organic layer are subjected to vacuum fractionation. In several repeats of this procedure, mixtures of terpene alcohols having very pleasant odors are obtained.

Example 4: One mol of a diisoprene-magnesium compound is placed in a reaction flask similar to that employed in Example 3. One mol of acetic acid is added very slowly with cooling and vigorous agitation. As soon as this reaction is complete (the partial hydrolysis to remove one-half of the carbon to magnesium bonds, the more reactive one) air or oxygen is bubbled into the mixture. The mixture may be diluted, if necessary, with more tetrahydrofuran or other unreactive solvent. The mixture is then treated with water-hydrochloric acid solution, the resulting organic and aqueous layers separated, the organic layers stripped of solvent and the resulting organic residue fractionated under vacuum conditions.

In this example, those most reactive centers which react readily with oxygen as is shown in Example 3 are removed and the less reactive centers then react with oxygen to give alcohols similar to but different from those obtained in Example 3. Both series were terpene alcohols having delicate and delightful fragrances. This product is quite similar to or contains linalool.

3,4-Alkyl-Substituted Linalools

W.C. Meuly and P.S. Gradeff; U.S. Patent 3,296,080; January 3, 1967; assigned to Rhodia Inc. describe unsaturated alcohols which are tertiary carbinols, corresponding to the general formula

where R_1 is a lower alkyl group other than methyl and containing from 2 to 6 carbon atoms and R_2 is H or a lower alkyl group containing one to five carbon atoms. R_1 and R_2 may form together a trimethylene or tetramethylene group. If R_2 is greater than methyl, R_1 may be methyl. The 4 position of the carbinol may be substituted by two methyl groups in place of H and R_2. These tertiary carbinols can be prepared conveniently from a group of ketones by reacting the ketones with acetylene to form ethynyl carbinols, followed by selective hydrogenation to vinyl carbinols or by reacting the ketones with vinyl magnesium halide to directly yield the vinyl carbinols.

The ketones are formed in a very economical manner which makes the products of the application available at a low cost which further enhances their value as perfumery chemicals. The ketones described in U.S. Patent 3,668,255, are obtained as a mixture of two isomers, if derived from an unsymmetrical starting ketone with a hydrogen atom in each of the two alpha positions. While it is usually possible to separate the isomers by fractional distillation it has been found that the mixed ketones lead to a mixture of two isomeric vinyl carbinols which possess excellent odor characteristics, richer and closer to natural products (which are normally mixtures of related chemicals). The following examples illustrate the process.

Example 1: 154 grams (1.0 mol) 4,7-dimethyl-6-octen-3-one were added with agitation during a 5 hour period into a solution of 1.2 mol vinyl magnesium halide in tetrahydrofuran. The reaction mixture was kept at 15° to 20°C during the addition and held at least another hour after the end of the addition. Then the reaction mixture was poured simultaneously with a 15% ice cold aqueous solution of 70 grams acetic acid, into a large cooled flask under efficient stirring. The resulting solution separated in 2 layers. The top layer containing all the product and most of the tetrahydrofuran was distilled at atmospheric pressure or slight vacuum, in order to remove the solvent.

On fractionation the crude material yielded 155 grams pure 4,7-dimethyl-3-ethyl-1,6-octadien-3-ol in the form of a colorless liquid BP 69°C/1.0 mm. This is a yield of 85% of theory. The product has a very lasting odor related to linalool but with a more flowery character and a definite lily of the valley note. It is much more useful in the perfuming of toilet soap than is linalool.

Example 2: 2-(3-methyl-2-butenyl)-cyclohexanone (166 grams) was treated with vinyl magnesium halide and worked up as described in Example 1. On fractionation 165 grams of 1-vinyl-2-(3-methyl-2-buten-1-yl)-cyclohexanol (cis and trans isomers) was obtained. BP 85° to 89°C/1.0 mm, yield is 85% of theory. The odor is fresh, leafy with a very natural linden type note.

Example 3: 7-methyl-6-octen-3-one is obtained by careful fractionation of the mixture of 3,6-dimethyl-5-hepten-2-one and 7-methyl-6-octen-3-one. The latter boils about 4°C higher than the former, is found in the later cuts of the fractionation and has the following constant: BP 63°C/8 mm. The lower boiling 3,6-dimethyl-5-hepten-2-one has the constant BP 59°C/8 mm. 140 grams (1.0 mol) 7-methyl-6-octen-3-one were reacted with vinyl magnesium halide as in Example 1 and the reaction mass was worked up in the same manner. There were obtained after fractionation 140 grams 7-methyl-3-ethyl-1,6-octadien-3-ol or 83% of theory. The product is a colorless mobile liquid, BP 65°C/1.2 mm. The odor is a powerful and fragrant linalool type, more floral and richer than linalool and with a note of muguet. It is much more lasting than linalool and lends smoothness and coherence to perfume compositions. It is much richer and natural than the known homolog, corresponding to $R_1 = C_2H_5$, $R_2 = CH_3$ in the formula above.

Lavandulol and Lavandulyl Acetate

H. Kappeler and J. Wild; U.S. Patent 3,700,717; October 24, 1972; assigned to Givaudan Corporation describe a synthetic process for producing lavandulol (III) and lavandulyl acetate (V) economically and in pure form.

In the past, lavandulol (III) and lavandulyl acetate (V), which are important constituents of essential oils utilized in perfumes and colognes to provide a lavender fragrance, have been produced commercially from their natural plant source, *Lavandula hybrida.* Various synthetic processes have been provided for synthesizing lavandulol and lavandulyl acetate. However, none of these syntheses has proven commercially or economically feasible.

In this process, the olfactorily-useful lavandulol (III) and lavandulyl acetate (V) are formed synthetically, in pure form and in high yield, from lavandulic acid (II) which is made in a manner by the rearrangement of 2-methyl-3-buten-2-yl β,β-dimethylacrylate (I).

Also, if desired, the lavandulic acid (II) obtained in accordance with this process, may be reduced to lavandulal (IV), converted into a lower alkyl ester (V) or into lavandulic acid nitrile (VI). Lavandulol (III) thus obtained can, if desired, be transformed into an ester (VII). The lower alkyl ester (V) obtained may, like the acid (II), be reduced to lavandulal (IV).

The reactions are shown schematically in the following reaction scheme:

Reaction Scheme

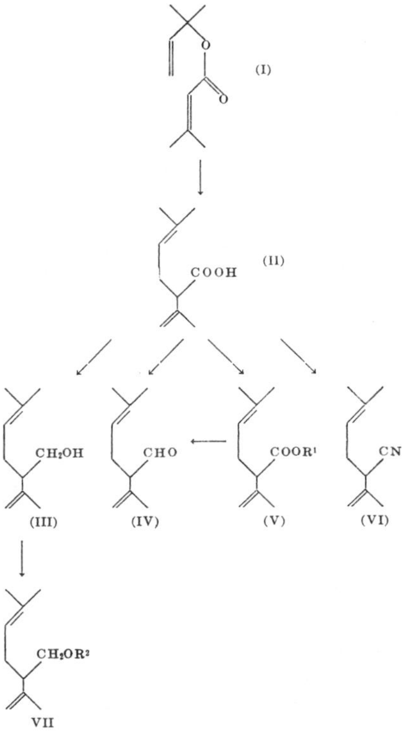

In the above formulas V and VII, R^1 and R^2 respectively have the following significance: R^1 signifies a lower alkyl group, preferably one with 1 to 6 C atoms such as methyl, ethyl, propyl, isopropyl, butyl etc. R^2 signifies the acyl residue of a carboxylic acid, especially a lower alkane carboxylic acid with 1 to 6 C atoms. Examples of such acyl residues are: formyl, acetyl, propionyl, butyryl, isobutyryl, caproyl etc.

The acrylic acid ester of formula I used as the starting material can be obtained readily and in high yields by esterification of β,β-dimethylacrylic acid or of a functional derivative thereof (e.g., the acid chloride) with 3-methyl-1-buten-3-ol (e.g., in the form of the corresponding sodium alcoholate).

The rearrangement of the acrylic acid ester I into lavandulic acid (II) brought about by strong bases proceeds practically quantitatively. The lavandulic acid obtained is completely isomer-free.

Particularly suitable strong bases are strong bases which are capable of splitting off a γ-hydrogen atom in an α,β-unsaturated ester, i.e., alkali hydrides such as sodium hydride: however, there also can be taken in consideration, for example, potassium tert–butylate or butyl lithium.

The rearrangement is conveniently carried out in an inert solvent such as, for example, benzene or toluene at elevated temperature, for example at temperatures between about

50° and 150°C, suitably at reflux temperature, preferably at about 100°C. After completion of the rearrangement reaction, the reaction mixture is conveniently rapidly cooled,
for example by pouring onto ice-water. The lavandulic acid can then be isolated according to methods which are known per se, for example by means of ether-extraction.

The transformation of the lavandulic acid (II) obtained into the corresponding primary
alcohol (lavandulol, formula III), the corresponding aldehyde (lavandulal, formula IV), into
lower alkyl esters V, into the corresponding nitrile (lavandulic acid nitrile, formula VI), as
well as the esterification of the lavandulol thus obtained (for the purpose of producing
esters of formula VII) and the reduction of esters of formula V to lavandulal (IV) can be
carried out in a manner known per se.

The reduction of the lavandulic acid (II) obtained to lavandulol (III) can, for example, be
carried out in ether at lower temperatures, preferably at about 10°C. Lithium aluminum
hydride, for example, is suitable as the reducing agent. Diisobutyl aluminum hydride, for
example, can also be used instead.

The reduction of the lavandulic acid (II) to lavandulal (IV) can, for example, be accomplished with a reducing agent such as diisobutyl aluminum hydride in the presence of a
solvent such as hexane at low temperatures (e.g., at about -70° to -80°C).

In order to produce esters of formula V from lavandulic acid (II), known mild esterification methods can be used. Thus, for example, lavandulic acid methyl ester is obtained
in high yields when lavandulic acid is reacted with 1.1 equivalents of diazomethane at
room temperature. However, one also may secure the same result with methanol and dry
hydrochloric acid as catalyst or when using trimethyl orthoformate in the presence of
acidic catalysts such as ion exchangers, Lewis acids or mineral acids.

The transformation of lavandulic acid (II) into the nitrile of formula VI can, for example,
be brought about by first converting the acid into the amide in a manner known per se
and dehydrating the latter to the nitrile.

The reduction of an ester of formula V to lavandulal (IV) proceeds, for example, with
diisobutyl aluminum hydride as the reducing agent under conditions already stated above
in connection with the reduction of lavandulic acid to lavandulal.

The esterification of lavandulol for the purpose of producing esters of general formula
VII can, for example, be done by reaction of lavandulol (optionally in the form of the
sodium alcoholate) with an acylating agent (e.g., an acid halide such as acetyl chloride).
For the production of, for example, lavandulyl acetate, isopropenyl acetate can also be
used as the esterification agent. The lavandulic acid and its transformation products of
formulas III–VII obtainable in accordance with the process are useful as odorants or as
intermediates.

Monoalkyl-3-Chlororesorcylates

*J.D. Grossman and K.K. Light; U.S. Patent 3,729,430; April 24, 1973; assigned to Inter-
national Flavors and Fragrances Inc.* describe perfume compositions containing certain
monoalkyl-3-chloro ring-substituted resorcylic acid esters which impart to these perfume
compositions and perfumed articles a natural and distinctly oakmoss note without causing discoloration.

Natural oakmoss is commercially important in producing high-grade fragrance compositions. Oakmoss constitutes an important and basic part of the fragrance impression of
chypre and lavender. In view of the limited availability of natural oakmoss synthetic substitutes are desirable and have been long sought.

It has been found that certain alkyl ring-substituted resorcylic acid esters simulate and
resemble the fragrance impression of oakmoss. While a number of routes for the pro-

duction of such resorcylic acid esters are available, they are rather tedious, complicated, generally uneconomical and none have been shown to produce alkyl-3-chloro ring-substituted resorcylic acid esters. For instance, one of these methods, as reported by Sonn in *Berichte,* 62BB, 3012-6 (1929), involves utilization of the rather expensive, and difficultly recoverable, palladium catalyst for the aromatization of mono- or dialkyl ring-substituted hydro alkyl resorcylates. Another method shown by Robertson et al in *J. Am. Chem. Soc.,* pages 313-20 (1930) involves a multistep sequence difficult to perform and tedious to carry out.

Still another method described by Neelakantan et al, *Indian J. Chem.,* 2(12), 478-84 shows the chlorination of methyl 6-methylresorcylate to yield methyl 6-methyl-3,5-dichloro-resorcylate. However, Neelakantan et al did not show production of the alkyl 3-chloro ring-substituted resorcylic acid esters with only one chlorine atom substituted at the (3) position on the benzene ring.

In Canadian Patent 837,131 mono- and dialkyl ring-substituted resorcylic acid esters are shown to be produced by reacting the corresponding dihydroresorcylic acid esters with an oxidative chlorine material. The dihydroresorcylic acid esters are prepared by treating β-ketoalkanoic acid esters with α,β-unsaturated alkyl alkenoates in the presence of an alkali metal alcoholate. The synthesis as set forth is not shown to yield alkyl monochloro ring-substituted resorcylic acid esters.

A process for producing nonaromatized materials having a halogen moiety substituted on the ring is shown by Teitel in German Patent Application 2,002,815 (July 30, 1970) and involves the production of a hydroresorcylic acid ester having the structure:

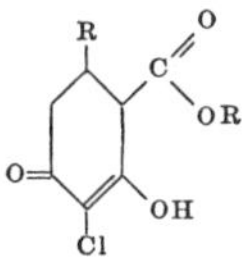

where the R groups respresent alkyl.

The 3-chloro ring-substituted resorcylic acid esters of this process may be represented by the following formula:

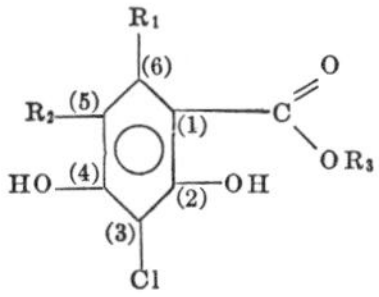

where R_3 and either R_1 or R_2 is a lower alkyl radical containing from 1 to 5 carbon atoms, the other of R_1 or R_2 being hydrogen. Representative of the compounds included within the formula are: methyl 6-methyl-3-chlororesorcylate, methyl 6-ethyl-3-chlororesorcylate, methyl 6-n-propyl-3-chlororesorcylate, ethyl 6-methyl-3-chlororesorcylate, ethyl 6-ethyl-3-chlororesorcylate, ethyl 6-n-propyl-3-chlororesorcylate, ethyl 6-isobutyl-3-chlororesorcylate, n-propyl 6-methyl-3-chlororesorcylate, n-propyl 6-ethyl-3-chlororesorcylate and n-propyl 6-n-propyl-3-chlororesorcylate. The C–1 and C–2 lower alkyl resorcylic esters are preferred as fragrance materials and the methyl esters are most suitable. Particularly preferred is methyl 6-methyl-3-chlororesorcylate by reason of its pronounced and long lasting moss-like odor.

It has been found that monoalkyl-3-chloro ring-substituted resorcylic acid ester, as represented by the formula on the following page where R_3 and either R_1 or R_2 is a lower alkyl radical containing from 1 to 5 carbon atoms (and the other of R_1 or R_2 is hydrogen) can be conveniently and more economically prepared by reacting a mono-ring-substituted dihydroresorcylate ester with an oxidative chlorine material. This process has been found to result in high yields of the products desired and suppresses undesirable side reactions. The following examples illustrate the process.

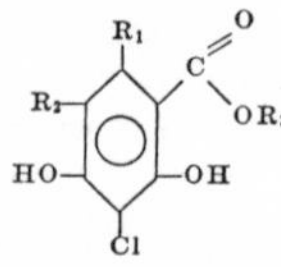

Example 1: Methyl 6-Methyl-3-Chlororesorcylate — Into a slurry of 184 grams (1 mol) of methyl dihydro-6-methylresorcylate in 500 cc of glacial acetic acid is bubbled 140 grams (2 mols) of chlorine gas at a temperature of 15°C. When the addition is complete, the mixture is stirred for ½ hour and then heated to 50°C until evolution of the HCl gas ceases. The solution is cooled and poured into water. The precipitate is filtered, washed with water, 5% aqueous sodium bicarbonate solution, and finally with water. The solid is dried in vacuum yielding 146.4 grams (68%) of methyl 6-methyl-3-chlororesorcylate, MP 139°–40°C. The product is a white crystalline material having a moss-like odor which can be imparted to soap at a level of 0.25%.

Example 2: Perfume Composition — The following mixture is prepared:

Ingredient	Grams
Jasmine liquid, A	15
Rose liquid	5
Solution orris	6
Santal oil El	6
Bergamot	120
Patchouli oil	6
Musk ketone, ⅕ in BB	60
Vetivert oil	5
Methyl 6-methyl-3-chlororesorcylate (tincture ⅕)	200
Coumarin	2
Vanillin	1.5
Heliotropin	2
Rose synthetic	25
Rose otto, Bulgarian	10
Pimento oil	5
Olibanum resinoid	10
Bitter orange oil	4
Ambrette seed oil	2
Musk tincture, 3%	250
Alcohol	4,000
	4,734.5

The foregoing perfume formulation is an important part of chypre essence. The methyl 6-methyl-3-chlororesorcylate is used as a replacement for oakmoss. This perfume is incorporated into a handkerchief perfume at the 0.1% by weight level. The methyl 6-methyl-3-chlororesorcylate gives to this fragrance a natural and distinctly oakmoss note.

Example 3: Methyl 6-Methyl-3-Chlororesorcylate — Into a 5 liter flask equipped with stirrer, thermometer, condenser, gas inlet tube and bubbler are placed the following materials: 3.5 liters of chloroform and 421 grams of methyl 6-methyldihydroresorcylate. Chlorine gas is added while stirring the reaction mass over a period of one hour until the chlorine is no longer taken up and the reaction mass becomes clear. During the bubbling the reaction mass temperature increases from 22° to 37°C. At the end of the reaction, the hydrogen chloride gas ceases to evolve. The solid material is recovered by filtration and weighs 507.1 grams. It is dissolved in 2 liters diethyl ether. The diethyl ether solution is washed using sodium bicarbonate washes until CO_2 no longer evolves in the wash solution. The bicarbonate solutions are extracted with ether and the ether layers combined and washed with 10 volumes of sodium hydroxide at 5°C. The methyl 6-methyl-chlororesorcylate product is recovered by crystallization from the ether layers. 111 grams of dried product is obtained. The structure of the product is shown to be methyl 6-methyl-3-chlororesorcylate by IR, NMR and mass spectral analysis. The product is a white crystalline material having a melting point of 135.8° to 137.8°C. This material has a moss-like odor which can be imparted to soap at a level of ¼%.

In related work *J.D. Grossman, R.S. De Simone, and L.G. Heeringa; U.S. Patent 3,634,491; January 11, 1972; assigned to International Flavors & Fragrances, Inc.* describe a process for the preparation of dialkyl ring-substituted resorcylic acids and esters which comprises reacting a dialkyl ring-substituted dihydroresorcylic acid or ester with an oxidative chlorine source. Certain dialkyl ring-substituted resorcylic acids and esters which are useful in perfumery are obtained.

The dialkyl ring-substituted resorcylic acids and esters of this process may be represented by the following formula:

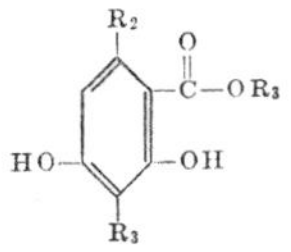

where each of R_1 and R_2 is a lower alkyl radical containing from about 1 to 5 carbon atoms and at least one of R_1 or R_2 contains two or more carbon atoms and where R_3 is hydrogen or a lower alkyl radical preferably containing about 1 to 3 carbon atoms. Representative of the compounds included within the formual are: methyl 3-methyl-6-isopropyl-resorcylate, methyl 3,6-diethyl-resorcylate, methyl 3,6-di-n-propyl-resorcylate, methyl 3,6-di-n-butyl-resorcylate, ethyl 3-n-propyl-6-methyl-resorcylate, methyl 3-methyl-6-ethyl-resorcylate and methyl 3-ethyl-6-methyl-resorcylate.

The resorcylic acids and esters of this process effectively simulate and resemble oakmoss fragrance and are suitable as fragrance materials or in a perfume composition such as a chypre or lavender perfume. The resorcylic esters are preferred as fragrance materials and the methyl esters are most suitable. Particularly preferred is methyl 3-ethyl-6-methyl-resorcylate by reason of its pronounced and long lasting moss-like odor.

GERANIUM

Citronellyl Senecioate

M. Dunkel; U.S. Patent 3,493,650; February 3, 1970; assigned to Universal Oil Products Company describes perfume and deodorizing compositions containing citronellyl senecioate and the use of such compositions to deodorize and eliminate malodors. Citronellyl senecioate is characterized by a geranium odor profile.

Citronellyl senecioate, having the following structural formula on the next page may be prepared by several different methods including for example esterification where citronellol is reacted with senecioic acid in the presence of a catalyst and, if desired, a solvent; transesterification where a lower alkyl ester of senecioate acid, for example, methyl senecioate, is reacted with citronellol in the presence of a transesterification catalyst such as sodium methylate and while continuously removing the lower alkyl alcohol from the reaction mixture as it forms; or by reacting a senecioyl halide, for example senecioyl chloride, with citronellol.

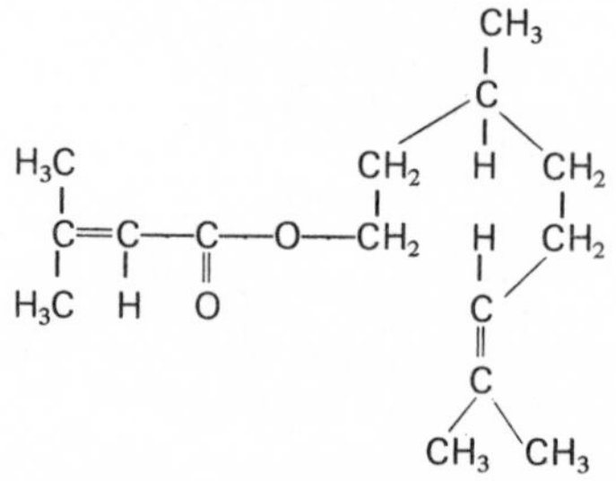

$$
\begin{array}{c}
\text{CH}_3 \\
| \\
\text{C} \\
\diagup \quad | \quad \diagdown \\
\text{CH}_2 \quad \text{H} \quad \text{CH}_2 \\
| \qquad \quad | \\
\text{CH}_2 \quad \text{H} \quad \text{CH}_2 \\
\diagdown \quad \diagup \\
\text{C} \\
\|\\
\text{C} \\
\diagup \diagdown \\
\text{CH}_3 \quad \text{CH}_3
\end{array}
$$

$$
\begin{array}{c}
\text{H}_3\text{C} \qquad\qquad \text{CH}_2 \\
| \qquad\qquad\qquad | \\
\text{C}{=}\text{C}{-}\text{C}{-}\text{O}{-}\text{CH}_2 \\
| \quad | \quad \| \\
\text{H}_3\text{C} \quad \text{H} \quad \text{O}
\end{array}
$$

Example 1: Citronellyl senecioate was prepared by charging about 75 grams (0.75 mol) of senecioic acid, 117 grams (0.75 mol) of citronellol, 100 ml of toluene and 2 grams of methyl sulfonic acid to a reaction flask equipped with an overhead condenser with a water trap. The mixture was heated to reflux (a well temperature ranging from 122° to 135°C) and maintained thereat for about five hours during which time about 12.5 ml of water were collected. The reaction mixture was cooled, washed with an aqueous sodium carbonate solution, then with water, and finally with a saturated sodium chloride solution.

After the toluene was flashed from the washed mixture, the mixture was fractionally distilled to recover about 89 grams of citronellyl senecioate boiling at 165°C at 6 mm Hg and having a refractive index n_D^{20} 1.4670. Analysis by gas-liquid chromatography indicated that the product was 90.5% pure.

Example 2: A geranium-type perfume is prepared using a standard formula having the following composition:

Perfume A

Component	Parts by Weight
Geranium oil	250
Bergamot oil	150
Sandalwood oil	100
Bois de rose oil	100
Patchouli oil	20
Ylang-ylang oil	30
Phenylethyl alcohol	200
Rose otto	10
Isobutyl phenylacetate	40
Cinnamic alcohol	50
Terpeneol	40
Coumarin	10

The perfume is sampled on a perfume blotter and found to have a pleasant geranium top note and odor profile. Two more perfumes, B and C, are prepared except that in perfume B the geranium oil component is replaced with a mixture of 125 parts of natural geranium oil and 125 parts of citronellyl senecioate, and in perfume C the entire natural geranium oil component is replaced by 250 parts of citronellyl senecioate. The perfumes B and C are sampled on perfume blotters and are found to closely resemble perfume A in having similar geranium top notes and odor profiles. In addition it is noted that both perfumes B and C have an improved dryout note, that is, the odor is very persistent particularly the geranium notes.

GENERAL FLORAL

Methyl Pentenyl Dihydropyran

W.T. Somerville; U.S. Patent 3,140,311; July 7, 1964; assigned to International Flavors & Fragrances Inc. has found that one can produce from myrcene, formaldehyde and a mild acid one or more compounds having the formula on the next page where one of the symbols R and R' is oxygen and the other is CH_2. In other words, the formula given is for two isomers in which the —O— is at different positions on the ring at the right, as follows:

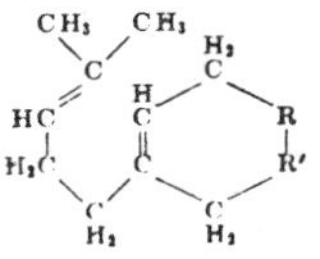

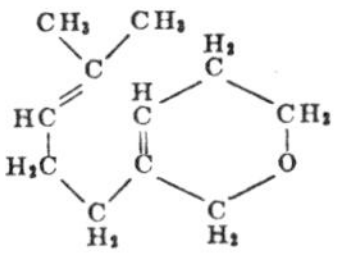

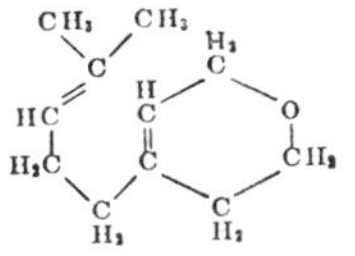

3-(4-methyl-3-pentenyl)-5,6-dihydro-2H-pyran   and   4-(4-methyl-3-pentenyl)-5,6-dihydro-2H-pyran

The mixture of myrcene, formaldehyde and acid is heated and refluxed for several hours. The product is then washed with water and a mild alkali, and the resulting oil is separated and distilled to recover unreacted myrcene, and from the remainder is distilled and recovered the unpolymerized reaction products above mentioned. There is also distilled and recovered a mixture of C_{11} acyclic primary alcohols and mild acid esters thereof, which are subsequently separated from each other. The reaction occurring is as follows:

$$C_{10}H_{16} + (CH_2O)_x \xrightarrow[\text{Heat}]{\text{Acetic acid}} C_{11}H_{18}O \ +$$

Myrcene   Methyl
formaldehyde   pentenyl
              dihydropyran

$$C_{10}H_{15}CH_2OH + C_{10}H_{15}CH_2OCCH_3$$

Primary acyclic   Primary acyclic
C_{11} alcohol   acetate

The methyl pentenyl dihydropyran is a perfume material having a strong refreshing floral odor with rose, muguet, violet and limey character. It is useful in a wide range of perfumes from floral to herb-cologne blends. The C_{11} alcohols are perfume materials having a very rich rose-violet note of distinctive character. The mixture of C_{11} alcohols and their esters is a perfume material having an odor somewhat reminiscent of the above mentioned alcohols, but drier and more herbaceous. The C_{11} alcohol designated as 2-isopropenyl-5-methylene-6-heptene-1-ol is a perfume. It has a powerful, persistent unique and pleasant odor of pronounced violet character. The acetate of the last mentioned alcohol has a natural and individualistic odor. It is also a perfume. It has a pleasant green, plant-like, chrysanthemum- and cologne-like odor. It is useful as part of the perfumes geranium, neroli and bergamot.

Substituted Dimethyl Dihydropyrans

L.M. van der Linde and H. Boelens; U.S. Patent 3,681,263; August 1, 1972; assigned to NV Chemische Fabriek Naarden, Netherlands describe perfume compositions containing as an essential ingredient at least one compound selected from the group consisting of 2,4-dimethyl-6-n-butyl-2,3-dihydro-6H-pyran, 2,4-dimethyl-6-n-butyl-5,6-dihydro-2H-pyran, and 2-methyl-4-methylene-6-n-butytetrahydropyran. The following examples illustrate the process.

Example 1: 354 grams (3 mols) of hexylene glycol together with 0.1 gram of copper sulfate was heated under reflux in a distilling flask during 7 hours. After removal of the water formed by azeotropic distillation, the contents of the flask is fractionated. There is thus obtained 94 grams of 2-methyl-1-pentene-4-ol, boiling point 130° to 132°C. 100 grams (1 mol) of this substance was shaken together with 86 grams (1 mol) of n-pentanal and 1 gram of p-toluenesulfonic acid until the acid has been dissolved. The mixture is then allowed to stand for about 64 hours at room temperature. After 200 grams of benzene has been added, the reaction mixture is washed with a 10% soda solution and then with water until the litmus reaction is neutral.

Benzene and first runnings are distilled under reduced pressure until the temperature of the liquid is about 80°C at 27 mm. 5 grams of potassium bisulfate is then added after which the distillation is continued and a fraction is retained boiling at 76° to 85°C at 12 mm. This fraction is again washed neutral with a 10% soda solution and fractionated. The desired product (78 grams) boils at 65° to 68°C at 6 mm.

Example 2: Geranium Oil Composition

	Grams
The product obtained by the process of Example 1	100
Dimethyl sulfide, 1% in geraniol	40
Isomenthone	30
Geraniol	450
Nerol	50
Citronellol	250
Linalool	10
Eugenol, 10% in geraniol	30
Citral, 10% in geraniol	20
Isopulegol, 10% in geraniol	20
	1,000

Example 3: Rose Geranium Composition

	Grams
Benzyl-isoeugenol	15
Musk ketone	15
11-oxahexadecanolide	10
Dimethyl-benzyl-carbinyl acetate	10
Rhodinol	50
Sandalwood oil OI	50
Patchouli oil	40
Methyljonon	100
Ylang-ylang oil	30
Linalyl acetate	150
Citronellol	150
Phenyl-ethanol	200
The product obtained by the process of Example 1	30
	850

Dialkenyl-Substituted Tetrahydropyran

P. Haynes; U.S. Patent 3,576,011; April 20, 1971; assigned to Shell Oil Company has found that dialkenyl-substituted tetrahydropyran compounds are produced by contacting a conjugated olefinic compound and formaldehyde in the presence of an organophosphine-containing palladium (0) compound as catalyst. By way of illustration, the reaction of butadiene and formaldehyde in the presence of catalytic amounts of tetrakis(triphenyl-phosphine)palladium (0) produces a mixture comprising 2,5-divinyltetrahydropyran and 3,5-divinyltetrahydropyran. The following examples illustrate the process.

Example 1: A mixture of 3 grams of butadiene, 3 grams of a 30% weight aqueous formaldehyde solution, 0.25 grams of tetrakis(triphenylphosphine)palladium (0) and 10 ml of benzene was charged to a 80 ml stainless-steel autoclave. The autoclave was maintained at a temperature of 80°C for about 17 hours. The autoclave was then cooled, and the reaction mixture, composed of a benzene phase and a water phase, was recovered. The benzene phase was separated, dried over magnesium sulfate and distilled to give 2.6 grams of a product mixture (BP 51°C at 3 mm) consisting of 64% 2,5-divinyltetrahydropyran and 36% 3,5-divinyltetrahydropyran. The conversion of butadiene was 67% and the selectivity to divinyltetrahydropyrans was 95%.

A sample of the divinyltetrahydropyran product mixture was separated into the 2,5-divinyltetrahydropyran isomer and the 3,5-divinyltetrahydropyran isomer by gas-liquid chromatography. Examination of the 2,5-divinyltetrahydropyran by infrared spectroscopy indicated bands at 6.09μ, 5.43μ, 3.25μ, 7.03μ, and 9μ. The infrared spectrum of 3,5-divinyltetrahydropyran was extremely similar with minor differences only in the fingerprint region. Mass spectroscopic and nuclear magnetic resonance spectroscopic analysis were consistent with the divinyltetrahydropyranyl structure.

Example 2: By a procedure similar to that of Example 1, a mixture of 3 grams isoprene, 6 grams of 30% weight aqueous formaldehyde, 0.25 gram of tetrakis(triphenylphosphine)-palladium and 10 ml of benzene was contacted at a temperature of 80°C for 17 hours. A good yield of vinyl-substituted and isopropenyl-substituted tetrahydropyrans was obtained. Infrared analysis of the tetrahydropyran product mixture showed a band of 9.05μ (ether linkage) and a band at 6.10μ (olefinic linkage).

Example 3: A fancy perfume composition of a floral type is prepared by mixing the ingredients set forth below.

Ingredients	Parts by Weight
Mixture of divinyltetrahydropyrans prepared as described in Example 1	35
Rhodinol	180
Phenylethyl alcohol	120
Linalool	40
Dimethylacetal of phenylacetaldehyde	30
Amyl cinnamic aldehyde	30
Benzyl acetate	90
Hydroxycitronellal	150
Methylionone	60
Heliotropine	30
Musk ambrette	10
Musk ketone	40
Vanillin	15
Eugenol	15
Benzyl salicylate	25
Bergamot oil	50
Ylang oil	30
Neroli bigarde oil	10
Santalol	20
	1,000

Tetrahydropyran and Furan Ketones

A process described by *H.D. Lamparsky and R. Marbet; U.S. Patent 3,470,209; Sept. 30, 1969; assigned to Givaudan Corporation* relates to ketones and to a process which is characterized in that a γ,δ-unsaturated aldehyde of the general formula

(1)

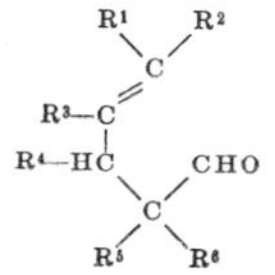

where R^1 represents a lower alkyl group which may be substituted by a free, esterified or etherified hydroxy group; a lower alkenyl, an aralkyl or aryl group, or together with R^2, a lower alkylene group; R^2 is a lower alkyl group, R^3, R^4 and R^5 represent hydrogen atoms or lower alkyl groups; and R^6 represents a hydrogen atom or a lower alkyl or alkenyl group, is reacted with a ketone of the general formula:

(2) 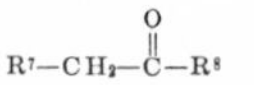
$$R^7-CH_2-\overset{\overset{\text{O}}{\|}}{C}-R^8$$

where R^7 represents a hydrogen atom or a lower alkyl group which may be substituted by a free, esterified or etherified hydroxy group; and R^8 represents a lower alkyl group which may be substituted by a free, esterified or etherified hydroxy group; a lower alkenyl or an aryl group in the presence of an alkaline condensation agent, and the resulting hydroxy-ketone of the general formula:

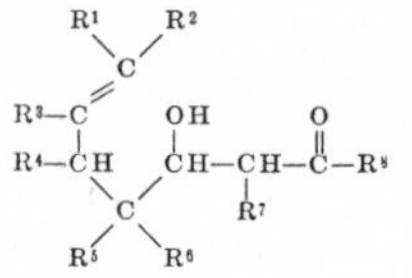

(3)
$$\begin{array}{c}
R^1 \quad R^2 \\
\diagdown \text{C} \diagup \\
R^3-\text{C} \quad\quad \text{OH} \quad\quad \text{O} \\
\| \quad\quad\quad | \quad\quad\quad \| \\
R^4-\text{CH} \quad \text{CH}-\text{CH}-\text{C}-R^8 \\
\diagdown \text{C} \diagup \quad\quad | \\
\quad\quad R^7 \\
R^5 \quad R^6
\end{array}$$

where R^1 through R^8 have the above meaning is cyclized in the presence of an acid cyclization agent.

Depending on the nature of the starting materials used, various diastereomeric tetrahydropyran compounds of the formula:

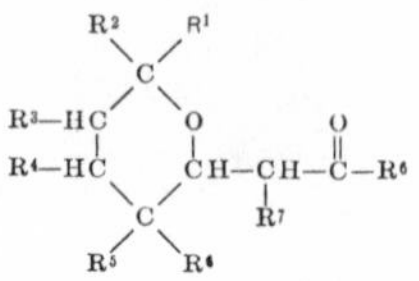

(4)
$$\begin{array}{c}
R^2 \quad R^1 \\
\diagdown \text{C} \diagup \\
R^3-\text{HC} \quad\quad \text{O} \quad\quad \text{O} \\
| \quad\quad\quad\quad\quad \| \\
R^4-\text{HC} \quad \text{CH}-\text{CH}-R^6 \\
\diagdown \text{C} \diagup \quad | \\
\quad\quad R^7 \\
R^5 \quad R^6
\end{array}$$

or the isomeric tetrahydrofuran compounds of the formula:

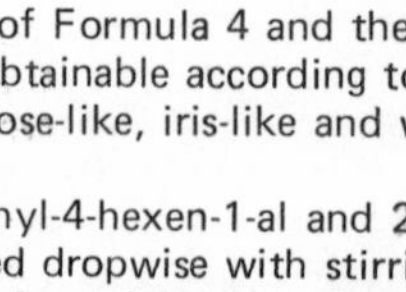

(5)
$$\begin{array}{c}
R^1-\text{CH}-R^2 \\
R^3-\text{C} \longrightarrow \text{O} \quad\quad \text{O} \\
| \quad\quad\quad\quad\quad \| \\
R^4\text{HC} \quad \text{CH}-\text{CH}-R^8 \\
\diagdown \text{C} \diagup \quad | \\
\quad\quad R^7 \\
R^5 \quad R^6
\end{array}$$

or mixtures of compounds of Formulas 4 and 5 result from the ring closure.

The tetrahydropyran compounds of Formula 4 and the isomeric tetrahydrofuran compounds of Formula 5 which are obtainable according to the process are characterized by particular odor notes. As a rule, rose-like, iris-like and wood-notes are prevalent.

Example 1: 56.0 grams of 5-methyl-4-hexen-1-al and 290 grams of acetone are mixed and the resulting mixture is treated dropwise with stirring at 15° to 20°C with a sodium ethylate solution freshly prepared from 0.6 gram of sodium and 10 ml of absolute ethanol. After complete addition, the reaction mixture is stirred for a further 2 hours at 15°C, then neutralized with glacial acetic acid, whereupon the excess of acetone is distilled off on the water-bath. The residue is taken up in 200 ml of ether, the ethereal solution is washed with water and dried. The residue (90 grams) after evaporation of the solvent is distilled in vacuum, the fractions which pass over at 87° to 90°C being collected. Yield: 34.2 grams of 4-hydroxy-8-methyl-7-nonen-2-one, BP 56° to 58°C/0.01 mm.

57.0 grams of distilled 4-hydroxy-8-methyl-7-nonen-2-one are boiled at reflux with stirring for 4 hours with 5.7 grams of concentrated phosphoric acid in 150 ml of benzene. After cooling, the reaction solution is poured on ice, the organic phase is decanted, the aqueous phase is extracted with toluene, the combined organic solution is washed neutral with water, dried and freed from solvent in vacuum. The residue (53 grams) is subjected to fractional distillation. There are obtained 37 grams of 2-acetonyl-6,6-dimethyl-tetrahydropyran, purification of which yields a uniform product of BP 43° to 44°C/1 mm, fruit-like fragrance with camphor-like note.

Example 2: 126 grams of 2,5-dimethyl-4-hexen-1-al are dissolved in 580 grams of acetone. A total of 2.7 grams of sodium methylate is added in small portions with stirring at 10° to 15°C to this solution. Stirring is continued for 2½ hours at 15° to 18°C. The solution is subsequently neutralized with glacial acetic acid and worked up as in Example 1. Yield: 102.5 grams of 4-hydroxy-5,8-dimethyl-7-nonen-2-one of BP 70° to 72°C/0.03 mm.

132 grams of this ketol are boiled at reflux for 4 hours with 13.2 grams of crystallized phosphoric acid in 400 ml of benzene. After working up as in Example 1 there are obtained 87 grams of 2-acetonyl-3,6,6-trimethyl-tetrahydropyran in the form of an isomer mixture. Careful fractionation on the spinning-band column results in concentration (up to 94% purity) of the diastereomer of BP 53° to 54°C/1 mm which had been formed as the main product. The product has a green note which is reminiscent of roses.

Cyclopentenylfuran Derivatives

According to a process described by *G.H. Büchi, C.P. Giannotti, E. Lederer, and H. Wüst; U.S. Patent 3,584,013; June 8, 1971; assigned to Firmenich & Cie, Switzerland* 2-(methyl-methylhydroxymethyl-substituted cyclopentenyl)-3-isopropylfurans are prepared by reduction of corresponding intermediate carbonyl analogs, 2-(methyl-acetyl-substituted cyclopentenyl)-3-isopropylfurans. The ultimate and intermediate furans both having utility as fragrances in perfume compositions. The intermediate is prepared by cyclization of 2-(1,6-dioxo-2-methylheptyl)-3-isopropylfuran which, in turn, is prepared by a 7 step synthesis beginning with condensation of isobutyryl-acetaldehyde dimethylacetal with methyl chloroacetate and ending with cleavage of the 5 membered carbon ring of 1,2-dimethyl-2-(3-isopropyl-2-furoyl)cyclopentanol.

The substituted hydroxyl cyclopentenylfuran derivatives and their carbonyl precursors are particularly useful for enhancing and reinforcing the top note of perfume compositions. They are particularly useful when added to floral-type and chypre-type perfume compositions or synthetic essential oils and are advantageously used in proportions of 0.1 to 5% based on the total weight of a perfume composition, 1 to 3% being a preferred range.

3,6,10-Trimethyl-5,9-Undecadiene-2-one

According to a process described by *W.C. Meuly and P.S. Gradeff; U.S. Patent 3,668,255; June 6, 1972; assigned to Rhodia Inc.* alkylation of aliphatic monoketones is conveniently conducted with sodium or potassium hydroxide in solid form in the presence of an organic amine or ammonia, where the amino nitrogen or ammonia is not a part of nor attached to an aromatic system. Thus, organic amine bases, in their free state or in the form of derivatives such as their salts, organic hydroxy amines, or amino acids; and amine-forming and ammonia-forming compounds which in the presence of alkali form amines or ammonia, can be used. Aromatic amines, such as aniline, dimethylaniline, or heterocyclic nitrogen compounds having an aromatic character, such as pyridine and collidine, are not effective in this process.

The alkylation proceeds in accordance with the following reaction:

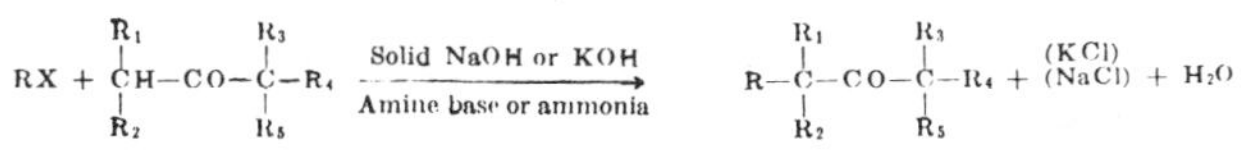

$$RX + \underset{\overset{|}{R_2}}{\overset{\overset{R_1}{|}}{C}}H - CO - \underset{\overset{|}{R_5}}{\overset{\overset{R_3}{|}}{C}} - R_4 \xrightarrow[\text{Amine base or ammonia}]{\text{Solid NaOH or KOH}} R - \underset{\overset{|}{R_2}}{\overset{\overset{R_1}{|}}{C}} - CO - \underset{\overset{|}{R_5}}{\overset{\overset{R_3}{|}}{C}} - R_4 + \overset{(KCl)}{(NaCl)} + H_2O$$

where R is hydrogen, alkyl having from one to about 12 carbon atoms, or alkenyl having from two to about 12 carbon atoms, allyl, propargyl, or cyclohexyl or a benzylaklyl or -alkenyl having from one to about 18 carbon atoms, preferably one to about eight carbon atoms; and R_1 and R_3 or R_2 and R_4 can be taken together to form a ring including the CO group to yield the corresponding cyclopentanone or cyclohexanone derivatives.

The ketones provided by this process that have not previously been known are defined by the formula:

$$R_1 \quad R_3$$
$$CH-C-C-CH_2-CH=C-CH_2-R$$
$$R_2 \quad O \quad R_4 \qquad CH_3$$

In this formula, (1) R is selected from the group consisting of hydrogen, alkyl and alkenyl groups (both straight and branched chain) having from two to about five carbon atoms, and (2) R_1, R_2, R_3 and R_4 are selected from the group consisting of hydrogen and alkyl groups (both straight and branched chain) having from one to about five carbon atoms, and alkylene groups having from two to three carbon atoms where two of R_1 and R_3 or R_2 and R_4 are taken together to form a ring including the

$$\begin{array}{c} C \\ \parallel \\ O \end{array}$$

group, the total number of carbon atoms in R_1, R_2, R_3 and R_4 being from two to about six, and if R_1, R_2 and R_3 are hydrogen, R_4 has at least three carbon atoms. These ketones have a pleasant odor, unlike their lower homologues, and are useful in perfumes and in perfume manufacture.

Example: Into a reaction flask provided with a stirrer were charged 174 grams (3.0 mols) acetone, 76 grams (1.0 mol) allyl chloride, 2 grams (0.025 mol) dimethylamine hydrochloride and 63 grams (1.5 mols) caustic 96% soda flakes. After stirring at 25° to 35°C for 24 hours, the inorganic precipitate was filtered off, and the cake washed with acetone. The organic layer was distilled to separate it into acetone, crude allyl acetone and high boiling residue. VPC analysis and comparison with an authentic sample of allyl acetone indicated a yield of 29% pure allyl acetone. Similar results were obtained when the reaction was carried out at reflux temperature (54°C) for 6 hours.

Halide	Ketone	Alkali metal hydroxide (flake)	Catalyst	Conditions	Yield of theory based on halide
1.0 allyl chloride..	3.0 acetone....	1.5 NaOH	0.025 dimethylamine-HCl...	25-30° C., 1 day...	29% allyl acetone.
do............	.......do........	1.5 NaOH	None.......	....do..........	6% allyl acetone.
1.0 allyl bromide..	4.0 MEK......	1.5 NaOH...	0.04 dimethylamine-HCl...	28° C., 1 day......	22% 1-methyl-1-allyl acetone, and some 1-heptene-5-one.
1.0 1,3-dichloro-2-butene.	3.0 MEK......	1.5 NaOH	0.03 dimethylamine-HCl..........	...do............	22% 3-methyl-6-chloro-5-heptene-2-one.
1.0 1-chloro-5,5,7,7-tetramethyl-2-octene.	3.0 acetone....	1.5 NaOH...	0.04 dimethylamine-HCl....	30° C., 6 hours....	50% 8,8,10,10-tetramethyl-5-undecene-2-one b./ 3.0 mm.; 115° C.; N_D^{20}: 1.4600.
1.0 geranyl bromide.	6.0 MEK......	1.5 NaOH...	0.05 dimethylamine-HCl....	25° C., 2 days.....	34% 3,6,10-trimethyl-5,9-undecadiene-2-one 3 mm.; 110° C.; N_D^{20}: 1.4684.
1.0 benzyl chloride.	3.0 acetone....	1.5 NaOH	0.015 dimethylamine-HCl...	35° C., 5 hours....	30% benzyl acetone.
do............	...do.......	1.5 NaOH	None.......	....do..........	0.5% benzyl acetone.
do............	...do.......	1.5 KOH	0.015 dimethylamine-HCl...	30° C., 5 hours....	22% benzyl acetone.
do............	...do.......	1.5 KOH	None.......	....do..........	4% benzyl acetone.
do............	4.0 MEK......	1.5 NaOH	0.06 dimethylamine-HCl....	25° C., 1 day...	42% 3-methyl-4-phenyl butane-2-one; b./12 mm.; 112° C.; N_D^{20}: 1.5094.
1.0 propargyl bromide.	6.0 acetone	1.5 NaOH	0.03 dimethylamine-HCl...	30° C., 1 day......	24% propargyl acetone.

The 3,6,10-trimethyl-5,9-undecadiene-2-one prepared is a new compound. The substance exhibits outstanding value, as compared with geranyl acetone and ethyl geranyl acetone, the former being the trade name of 6,10-dimethyl-5,9-hendecadien-2-one, and the latter being 6,10-dimethyl-5,9-dodecadien-2-one. The latter two substances are marketed in the perfume industry. 3,6,10-trimethyl-5,9-undecadiene-2-one has a much richer floral-type odor than geranyl acetone and ethyl geranyl acetone, so that it has greater ability to impart a fresh note in many florals, such as rose, lily of the valley, lavender and gardenia. It is better suited than geranyl acetone and ethyl geranyl acetone for reinforcing odor and for blending with a variety of floral compositions. One of its main advantages is that it does not have the sharp and pungent characteristics of geranyl acetone and thus may be used in larger amounts in perfuming compositions to impart roundness, lasting power and stability. Another advantage is that the compound has a more stable odor than geranyl acetone, that is, the odor lasts longer and is not affected by aging.

Dimethyl Acetals of α,β-Acetylenic Aldehydes

P. Bedoukian; U.S. Patent 3,268,594; August 23, 1966 has found that the dimethyl acetals of the α,β-acetylenic aldehydes, $CH_3(CH_2)_nC{\equiv}CCH(OCH_3)_2$ where n is 3 to 7, have strong and pleasant odors.

The diethyl acetals of the α,β-acetylenic aldehydes have been reported. It was significant to find that although the diethyl acetals have faint odors which give them no utility in the perfume or cosmetic products the dimethyl acetals of the process have such odor properties that they are very effective in such products.

The following is one practical procedure for the preparation of four α,β-acetylenic aldehydes listed below. In a suitable apparatus, consisting of a three-neck flask with a stirrer and reflux condenser, are placed 1.25 mols (about 30 grams) of magnesium turnings and 250 ml of anhydrous ether. To this is added gradually, from a separatory funnel, a mixture of 1.3 mols (about 140 grams) of ethyl bromide at a rate to cause gentle refluxing of the ether. At the end of the reaction, the mixture is heated for fifteen minutes under reflux to insure the completion of the reaction. To the reaction mixture is added 1.25 mols (about 110 grams) of 1-octyne mixed with 50 ml of anhydrous ether. This reacts with the ethyl magnesium Grignard liberating ethane and giving 1-octyne magnesium Grignard $CH_3(CH_2)_5C{\equiv}CMgBr$.

Again, the rate of addition is controlled so that a gentle refluxing of the ether takes place. At the end of the reaction the mixture is heated to reflux for a period of half an hour to insure the completion of the reaction. The third step of the reaction consists of the addition of trimethyl orthoformate to the octyne Grignard reagent. In order to obtain higher yields, 1.25 mols (about 130 grams) of trimethyl orthoformate is mixed with 150 ml of toluene and added to the reaction mixture. The mixture refluxes gently on addition of the orthoformate at a proper rate. At the end of the reaction, another 150 ml of toluene is added and the ether is slowly distilled off from the reaction mixture. After the removal of the ether, the mixture is refluxed gently for a period of five hours to insure increased yields.

The thick reaction product containing much precipitated matter is hydrolyzed with excess ammonium chloride solution, washed with water, then with sodium carbonate solution, and subjected to careful fractional distillation. The fraction, 98 grams (about 53% of theory), distilling at 86° to 88°C at 4 mm Hg pressure and having a refractive index of 1.438 and a specific gravity of 0.897 at 20°C is relatively pure dimethyl acetal of 2-nonynal.

Three other homologs of the dimethyl acetals of 2-nonynal prepared by the above operation were found to have the following constant: 2-octynal dimethyl acetal, BP 109°C/22 mm, 2-decynal dimethyl acetal, BP 94°C/2 mm and 2-undecynal dimethyl acetal, BP 106°C/2 mm.

Because of their strong fragrance, and particularly the floral green odors, these compounds may be used very effectively in perfume fragrance formulations. The following are representative perfume fragrance formulations of the process.

Jasmine Fragrance

Benzyl acetate	16
Benzyl alcohol	5
Linalool	8
Linalyl acetate	3
Terpineol	1
Amyl cinnamic aldehyde	6
Cyclamen aldehyde	2
Ylang ylang oil	3
Benzyl salicylate	8
2-nonynal dimethyl acetal	1.25

Rose Fragrance

Geraniol	10
Citronellol	4
Geranyl acetate	3
Phenyl ethyl alcohol	8
Decyl aldehyde	0.1
Phenyl acetaldehyde	0.1
Methyl ionone	4
Clove oil	1
Iso-cyclo citral	0.5
2-nonynal dimethyl acetal	0.5

2-Hexoxyacetaldehyde Dimethyl Acetal

K. Kulka; U.S. Patent 3,764,712; October 9, 1973; assigned to Fritzsche Dodge & Olcott Inc. describes compounds which are hexoxyacetaldehydes, dialkyl acetals of such aldehydes, cyclic acetals of such aldehydes, hemiacetals of such aldehydes and polymeric forms of such aldehydes, such as aldols. The hexoxyacetaldehydes have the formula: R—O—CH$_2$CHO in which R is a monovalent hydrocarbon radical having six carbon atoms.

The monovalent hydrocarbon radical may be a saturated straight or branched chain radical, such as n-hexyl or 2-methyl-n-pentyl or an unsaturated hydrocarbon radical containing one or two double bonds, such as $CH_3CH_2CH_2CH{=}CHCH_2{-}$, $(CH_3)_2C{=}CHCH_2CH_2{-}$ or $(CH_3)_2C{=}CHCH{=}CH{-}$, a straight or branched chain hydrocarbon radical containing a triple bond, such as $CH{\equiv}CCH_2CH_2CH_2CH_2{-}$ and $(CH_3)_2CHC{\equiv}CCH_2{-}$. The alkyl groups in the dialkyl acetals or hemiacetals of this process are lower alkyl containing not more than five carbon atoms and preferably not more than two carbon atoms. Desirably the acetals do not have more than sixteen carbon atoms.

The hexoxyacetaldehydes may be produced by reacting an alkali metal alcoholate of the required alcohol with a chloroacetaldehyde dialkyl acetal. The required alkali metal alcoholate, such as sodium alcoholate, may be produced by reacting the required alcohol with an alkali metal hydride, such as sodium hydride in a nitrogen atmosphere. The reaction which takes place when chloroacetaldehyde dimethyl acetal and the required sodium alcoholate are employed is as follows:

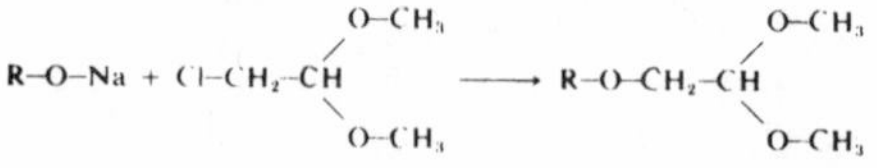

$$R{-}O{-}Na + Cl{-}CH_2{-}\underset{\overset{|}{O{-}CH_3}}{\overset{O{-}CH_3}{CH}} \longrightarrow R{-}O{-}CH_2{-}\underset{\overset{|}{O{-}CH_3}}{\overset{O{-}CH_3}{CH}}$$

Example 1: 2-Hexoxyacetaldehyde Dimethyl Acetal — The reaction was conducted in a nitrogen atmosphere by leading a stream of nitrogen below the surface of the reaction mixture. There were placed in a two liter 3-necked reaction flask 255 grams of n-hexanol. 53.3 grams of sodium hydride as a 54% oil emulsion were added to the n-hexanol contained in the reaction flask under agitation and cooling with an ice water bath over a period of 20 minutes. The reaction was exothermic and the temperature range was maintained at 17° to 30°C. After the addition, the cooling bath was removed. Agitation was continued with nitrogen ebullition over a period of about 4½ hours. At that time, the hydrogen test was negative. The mixture was permitted to stand overnight with agitation. The reaction product was a creamy, slightly yellow suspension. 100 grams of n-hexanol were added to facilitate agitation and the mixture became clear and thin. The mixture was then heated to 117°C. There were added over a period of about 4½ hours below the surface with agitation and nitrogen ebullition 124.5 grams of chloroacetaldehyde dimethyl acetal. The temperature of the reaction mixture was maintained at 120° to 135°C. The mixture refluxed with agitation of 1 hour. It was permitted to stand over a weekend and then refluxed for an additional 7 hours.

The progress of the reaction was followed by infrared (IR) determination and the reaction was terminated upon the substantial disappearance of the IR peak indicative of chlorine. To the cooled reaction mixture was added 1,000 ml of warm water. The solids dissolved and two layers were formed. The layers were separated and the organic part was filtered to liberate it from some muck. The aqueous portion was extracted twice with 200 ml of benzene. The benzene extracts were added to the main organic part. The resulting solution was washed successively with 500 ml of warm water, 500 ml of saturated aqueous sodium bicarbonate solution and twice with 500 ml of water. The benzene was distilled off in vacuum. The residue was fractionated through a 1½ foot Vigreaux column. The results of the fractionation are shown in the following table:

Fraction	Temperature of Vapor, °C	Temperature of Flask, °C	Vacuum in mm	Volume in ml	Weight in Grams	
1	38–66	82–83	33	2	1.8	
2	66–83	83–128	31	280	230.6	Recovered n-hexanol
3	72–88	101	7	7	6.6	Intermediate
4	88–90	101–153	7	100	89.7	Main
5	76	166	7	4	3.4	High fraction
Residue					71.8	

The main fraction had a refractive index (RI) at 20°C of 1.4170. The IR confirmed the presence of 2-hexoxyacetaldehyde dimethyl acetal. The wet analysis indicated an approximate 100% purity.

Example 2: 2-Hexenoxyacetaldehyde Dimethyl Acetal — The same procedure is followed as in Example 1 except that about 255 grams of 2-hexen-1-ol is employed instead of the 255 grams of n-hexanol. The boiling point of the resulting 2-hexenoxyacetaldehyde dimethyl acetal is 110° to 111°C at 15 mm. The refractive index at 20°C is 1.4331.

Example 3: 1,3-Dimethylbutanoxyacetaldehyde Dimethyl Acetal — The procedure described in Example 1 is followed except that 255 grams of 1,3-dimethylbutanol is employed instead of the 255 grams of n-hexanol. The boiling point of the resulting 1,3-dimethylbutanoxyacetaldehyde dimethyl acetal is 86° to 89°C at 15 mm. The refractive index at 20°C is 1.4139.

Example 4: Hyacinth Perfume Composition — A hyacinth perfume composition is prepared by mixing the following:

Components	Parts by Weight
Phenyl acetaldehyde 10%	15
Oil tolu balsam extra	5
Phenylethyl alcohol coeur	15
Cinnamic alcohol	20
Hydroxy citronellal extra	8
Heliotropin	5
Terpineol pure	3
Oil petitgrain Paraguay	4
Benzyl acetate	1
Phenylethyl acetate	2

(continued)

Components	Parts by Weight
α-Ionone white coeur	2
Isoeugenol 10%	5
Oil ylang extra	3
Linalool synth	5
Dimethyl benzyl carbinyl acetate	2
Oil galbanum	1
2-Hexoxyacetaldehyde dimethyl acetal	45
Diethyl phthalate	9
	150

6,7-Epoxycitronellal

G.O. Chase and A.A. Pilarz; U.S. Patent 3,590,053; June 29, 1971; assigned to Givaudan Corporation describe a method for producing 3,7-methyl-6,7-epoxy-octan-1-al from a dialkanoyl derivative of 3,7-dimethyl-2,6-octadien-1-al or from a monoalkanoyl derivative of 3,7-dimethyl-1,2,6-octatrien-1-ol.

3,7-dimethyl-6,7-epoxy-octan-1-al (6,7-epoxy-citronellal) which has the formula:

(1)

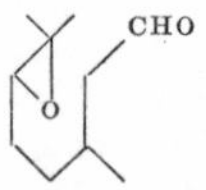

is a known compound, which because of its soft floral odor with a green nuance, is extremely useful as an odorant in the preparation of perfumes and other scented compositions.

In the process, 6,7-epoxy-citronellal of the above formula can be prepared by first epoxidizing either of the following two compounds:

(2a)   (2b)

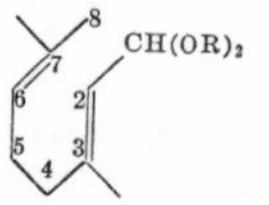

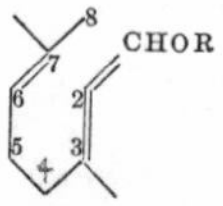

where R is lower alkanoyl, with an organic per-acid to form the corresponding 6,7-epoxy compounds without affecting the double bonds in any of the other positions in the compounds of Formula (2a) or Formula (2b). The 6,7-epoxy compounds are then reacted with an alkali metal bicarbonate and thereafter, catalytically reduced to form the compound of Formula (1).

It has been found that this three-step process produces 6,7-epoxy-citronellal from the compounds of Formula (2a) or (2b) in higher yields than that obtainable by the prior art process. Furthermore, the epoxidation with per-acids of compounds of Formula (2a) or (2b) can be carried out with yields as high as 90% since epoxidation only takes place at the double bond at the 6-position without affecting the double bond in the 1 or 2-positions.

The compounds of Formulas (2a) and (2b) are formed as a mixture from dehydrolinalool by esterification and rearrangement. The mixture containing the compounds of Formulas (2a) and (2b) can be converted to a compound of Formula (1) above. Therefore, the process provides a means for converting the mixture resulting from the esterification and rearrangement of dehydrolinalool into the compound of Formula (1) above so as to provide the compound of Formula (1) above in high yields and with a high degree of purity. The following examples illustrate the process.

Example 1: Preparation of 1,1-Diacetoxy-3,7-Dimethyl-6,7-Epoxy-2-Octene — 152.6 grams of (98% pure) 1,1-diacetoxy-3,7-dimethyl-2,6-octadiene was dissolved in 900 ml of methylene chloride. The solution was stirred and cooled to 10°C. To this was slowly added a solution of 10 grams of sodium acetate trihydrate in 130 ml of aqueous acid solution containing about 40% by weight of acetic acid, about 13% by weight of water and about 41% by weight of per-acetic acid, over a period of 30 minutes. The reaction mixture was cooled to maintain the reaction temperature at a maximum of 20°C during addition. After the addition, the reaction mixture was stirred at room temperature for two hours and allowed to stand at room temperature overnight. The reaction mixture then was added with stirring to one liter of cold tap water.

After separation of the two phases formed, the aqueous acetic acid phase was separated, discarded, and the methylene chloride phase washed to neutrality with saturated sodium bicarbonate solution. The solvent was removed from the neutral, washed extract by distillation. The residue was distilled under reduced pressure. The product, 1,1-diacetoxy-3,7-dimethyl-6,7-epoxy-2-octene, so obtained boiled at 103° to 104°C, under a vacuum of 0.03 mm of Hg. 139 grams of this product was obtained in a purity of 98% as determined by gas chromatography. This represented a yield of 86% based upon the octadiene.

Example 2: Preparation of 3,7-Dimethyl-6,7-Epoxyoctan-1-al from 1,1-Diacetoxy-3,7-Dimethyl-6,7-Epoxy-2-Octene — 270.3 grams of pure 1,1-diacetoxy-3,7-dimethyl-6,7-epoxy-2-octene prepared in Example 1 was mixed with 500 ml of methanol, 146 grams of sodium bicarbonate and 83.4 ml of water under constant stirring. The mixture was heated and refluxed for two hours. The reaction mixture was then cooled to room temperature and 5.4 grams of 5% palladium on charcoal was added. Then hydrogen gas was passed into the reaction mixture at about a pressure of 15 inches of water while the temperature was maintained at 20° to 25°C. After no further hydrogen was absorbed by the reaction mixture, the catalyst was removed by filtration.

The resulting filtrate was concentrated to an oil by distillation under slightly reduced pressures (about 300 to 400 mm Hg). The residual oil was dissolved in about 500 ml toluene and the toluene solution was washed with water to neutrality. The toluene was removed by distillation and the residue was fractionated under reduced pressure. The product obtained from fractionation was 3,7-dimethyl-6,7-epoxyoctan-1-al which boils at 65° to 66°C under a vacuum of 0.1 mm of Hg.

α-Methylene Aldehydes

J.H. Blumenthal; U.S. Patent 3,463,818; August 26, 1969; assigned to International Flavors & Fragrances Inc. describes a process for producing α-methylene- and α-methyl-aldehydes and -alcohols.

Typical compounds include 3,7-dimethyl-2-methylene-6-octenal, having the formula:

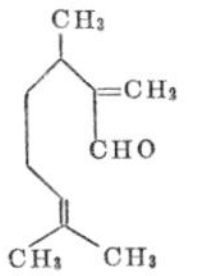

2,3,7-trimethyl-6-octenal, having the formula:

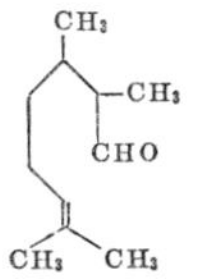

3,7-dimethyl-2-methylene-6-octenol, having the formula:

$$
\begin{array}{c}
\text{CH}_3 \\
| \\
\text{=CH}_2 \\
\text{CH}_2\text{OH} \\
\\
\text{CH}_3 \quad \text{CH}_3
\end{array}
$$

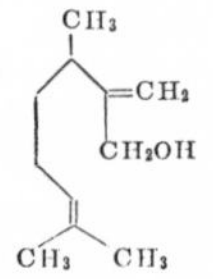

2,3,7-trimethyl-6-octenol, having the formula:

$$
\begin{array}{c}
\text{CH}_3 \\
| \\
\text{—CH}_3 \\
\text{CH}_2\text{OH} \\
\\
\text{CH}_3 \quad \text{CH}_3
\end{array}
$$

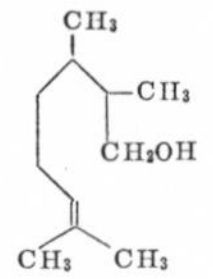

2,3,7-trimethyloctanol, having the formula:

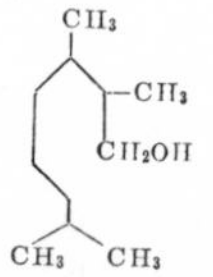

$$
\begin{array}{c}
\text{CH}_3 \\
| \\
\text{—CH}_3 \\
\text{CH}_2\text{OH} \\
\\
\text{CH}_3 \quad \text{CH}_3
\end{array}
$$

and 2,3,7-trimethyloctanal, having the formula:

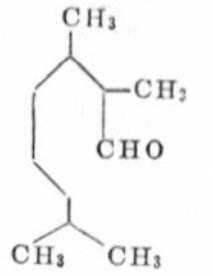

$$
\begin{array}{c}
\text{CH}_3 \\
| \\
\text{—CH}_2 \\
\text{CHO} \\
\\
\text{CH}_3 \quad \text{CH}_3
\end{array}
$$

In carrying out a process for manufacturing compounds of this type, one may employ the reaction using either catalytic or greater quantities of an amine. In carrying out this process, one reacts an aldehyde having the formula RCH_2CHO, where R is an alkyl group having 5 to 10 carbon atoms, e.g., citronellal, with a secondary amine, e.g., diethylamine, and formaldehyde in an aqueous medium to produce α-methylene citronellal.

In Example 1 below a one-step reaction is exemplified, using molar quantities of the reactants. Example 2 shows the same reactants, but using a catalytic quantity of diethylamine, namely a molar ratio of aldehyde to secondary amine of 10:1. Other examples also use catalytic quantities.

Example 1: A mixture of 18 mols of n-decanal, 20 mols of dimethylamine, 20 mols of 37% formaldehyde, 10 mols of sulfuric acid, 2 liters of water and 10 grams of Ionol was adjusted to pH 3.7 and refluxed for 2.5 hours. At this point, only a trace of the starting aldehyde was present by GLC (gas liquid chromatography). After cooling, the oil layer was separated and the aqueous layer extracted with benzene. The combined organic layer was washed neutral with water and the solvent stripped off. The crude oil was rushed-over to yield 2,532 grams of 2-methylene decanal testing 91.2%, by oximation (76% yield of theory based on n-decanal).

Example 2: A mixture of 1 mol of n-decanal, 1 mol of 37% formaldehyde, 0.1 mol of diethylamine, 1 gram of Ionol and 17 cc of water was adjusted to pH 6 with sulfuric acid and then heated in a stirred autoclave for 3 hours at 120°C. The oil layer was separated and washed neutral with water. The crude reaction mixture weighed 190 grams and contained 58% of 2-methylene decanal (by oximation). GLC indicated one major peak with only a trace of the starting aldehyde (65% of theory based on n-decanal). The course of the reaction in the above example is as follows:

$$CH_3 \cdot (CH_2)_7 \cdot CH_2 \cdot CHO + CH_2O + \xrightarrow{(C_2H_5)_2NH} CH_3 \cdot (CH_2)_7 \cdot \overset{\overset{\displaystyle CH_2}{\|}}{C} - CHO$$

(Here the diethylamine is present in catalytic proportions).

Example 3: To a solution of 4,265 grams of water and 1,220 grams of concentrated H_2SO_4 was added 1,750 grams diethylamine, 1,200 grams 37% formaldehyde, 2,266 grams of citronellal (81%) and 24 grams of Ionol. The pH was adjusted to 5.1 and the mixture was heated in a stirred autoclave for 4 hours at 120°C. The oil layer was separated and washed with water to yield 1,820 grams of product containing 8.8 mols of 3,7-dimethyl-2-methylene-6-octenal (by oximation). Fractionation gave the pure product 3,7-dimethyl-2-methylene-6-octenal, BP 84°C/7 mm. It is a perfume having an odor characterized as a powerful citrus fruit aroma very reminiscent of bergamot, and much less coarse than citronellal.

Example 4: A solution of 957 grams of 3,7-dimethyl-2-methylene-6-octenal (prepared as in Example 3) in 957 cc of isopropanol was hydrogenated at 20°C and 115 lb of hydrogen pressure to an uptake of 1 mol of hydrogen, using 45 grams Raney nickel as catalyst. After filtration and removal of the solvent, the crude product was fractionated to give 2,3-7-trimethyl-6-octenal, BP 80°C/5 mm. This product has a fresh, citral-bergamot odor.

Example 5: To 505 grams methanol, 190 grams water, 34.7 grams $NaBH_4$ and 2 grams of a 25% NaOH solution was added with cooling and stirring at 20°C over a period of 1 hour, 247 grams of 3,7-dimethyl-2-methylene-6-octenal (87% aldehyde) prepared as in Example 3. The reaction mixture was stirred for another 20 minutes. An equal volume of water was added and the oil layer separated. The aqueous layer was extracted with benzene and a combined organic layer washed with water and the solvent stripped off. The crude product was fractionated to yield pure 3,7-dimethyl-2-methylene-6-octenol, BP 102°C/4.7 mm. This product is a perfume having an odor characterized as a floral, rose-muguet odor.

Hydroxymethyl-2-Methylocta-2,7-dienes

S. Lemberg; U.S. Patent 3,258,497; June 28, 1966; assigned to International Flavors & Fragrances Inc. describes acyclic primary alcohols and processes for making them from cis- and trans-myrtanol.

The cis- and trans-myrtanol may be prepared from β-pinene by hydroboration followed by oxidation, in accordance with J.C. Braun and G.S. Fisher, *Tetrahedron Letters,* Number 21, pages 9–11, 1960. An alternate synthesis via aluminum alkyl exchange with β-pinene also provides a convenient method of preparation, following the general procedure in the following authors: K. Ziegler, F. Krupp and K. Zosel in *Annalen der Chemie,* volume 629, pages 241–250, of 1960.

It has been found that myrtanol, either as the cis- or trans-isomer, when heated to pyrolysis temperatures in the vapor-phase yields a mixture of the following: (1) 6-methyl-2-vinyl-5-heptene-1-ol and (2) 2-(2-methyl-propenyl)-5-hexene-1-ol , and (3) unreacted myrtanol, formed in accordance with the following reactions:

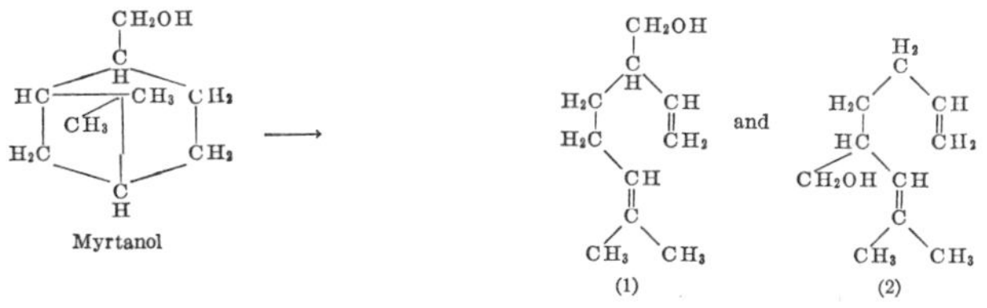

The alcohols formed, (1) and (2), possess a degree of optical activity which is dependent upon the optical activity of the myrtanol used. In general, it is important to conduct the isomerization in the vapor-phase, the temperature ranging from at least 450° to 825°C, under reduced pressure, preferably 20 mm Hg.

The mixture of components has a sweet, soft floral odor like the linalool family, but more earthy green. It is useful in hyacinth and violet-narcisse perfume compositions.

Alicyclic Hydroxyaldehydes

According to a process described by *T. Moroe, A. Komatsu, T. Matsui and K. Ueda; U.S. Patent 3,433,839; March 18, 1969; assigned to Takasago Perfumery Co., Ltd., Japan* myrcene obtained by pyrolysis of β-pinene is used as a starting material. This myrcene is first photo-oxidized to produce a mixture of its hydroperoxides and the resulting mixture is then reduced to produce a mixture of unsaturated alcohols, and the mixture thus obtained is subsequently condensed with a dienophile to obtain a desired mixture of two kinds of alicyclic hydroxyaldehydes respectively represented by the following general formulas:

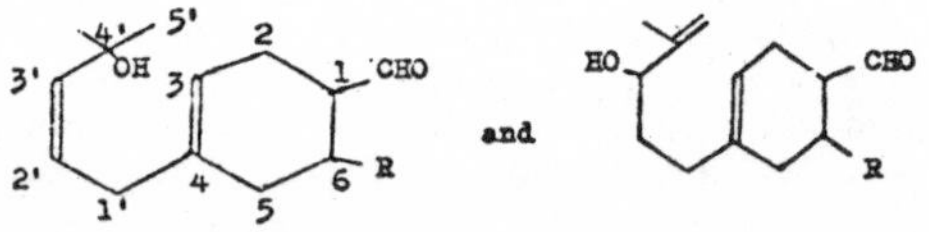

where R is a member selected from the group consisting of hydrogen and a methyl group. This mixture is a valuable perfume material. The following examples illustrate the process.

Example 1: Oxygen was introduced into a solution of 54 grams of myrcene (90% purity) and 5 grams of Rose Bengal in 550 ml of methanol with an oxygen bubbling velocity of 300 ml/min and the system was thereafter irradiated for 8 hours with a high pressure arc lamp using a Pyrex filter during which time the temperature of the reaction solution was kept at 15° to 20°C. The methanol solution of hydroperoxides thus obtained was dropped onto a solution of 100 grams Na_2SO_3 in 600 ml water and stirring was continued at 45° to 50°C for 3 hours and the system was extracted with benzene. After washing, the extract was distilled under reduced pressure and thus there was obtained a mixture of 2-methyl-6-methylene-3,7-octadiene-2-ol (A) and 2-methyl-6-methylene-1,7-octadiene-3-ol (B) where the proportion of A to B was 45:55 according to chromatographic analysis. The yield was 60.0 grams and the product obtained had a floral note, BP 58° to 60°C/0.35 mm Hg.

Further, 200 grams of such mixture of A and B and 110 grams of acrolein were charged into an autoclave and the headspace in the charged autoclave was filled with nitrogen and the reaction was carried out at 130° to 140°C for 4 hours. The reaction product was steam-distilled once to distill off the excess acrolein and after being extracted with benzene, the extract was washed with water and then distilled. Thus, a mixture of 4-(4'-methyl-4'-hydroxy-2'-pentenyl)-3-cyclohexene-1-carboxaldehyde and 4-(4'-methyl-3'-hydroxy-4'-pentenyl)-3-cyclohexene-1-carboxaldehyde was obtained, BP 124° to 133°C 0.6 mm Hg.

Example 2: 100 grams of a mixture of unsaturated alcohols obtained by the process described in Example 1; 70 grams of crotonaldehyde and 2 grams of hydroquinone were charged in an autoclave and the headspace in the charged autoclave was filled with nitrogen. These substances were reacted at 140° to 150°C for 5 hours, and the reaction product was steam-distilled once and then the excess crotonaldehyde was distilled off, after which the residue was extracted with benzene. The extract thus obtained was distilled under reduced pressure to produce a mixture of 4-(4'-methyl-4'-hydroxy-2'-pentenyl)-6-methyl-3-cyclohexene-1-carboxaldehyde and 4-(4'-methyl-3'-hydroxy-4'-pentenyl)-6-methyl-

3-cyclohexene-1-carboxaldehyde. The yield was 80.5 grams, BP 131° to 136°C/0.25 mm Hg.

2-Arylmethylpyromeconic Acids

B.E. Tate and R.P. Allingham; U.S. Patent 3,365,469; January 23, 1968; assigned to Chas. Pfizer & Co., Inc. describe compounds which are of the formula:

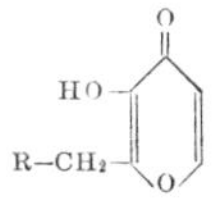

where R is phenyl, naphthyl, substituted phenyl or substituted naphthyl and each of the substituents is alkyl having from 1 to 6 carbon atoms, hydroxy, chlorine, bromine, iodine or alkoxy having from 1 to 6 carbon atoms.

The 2-arylmethylpyromeconic acids of this process are prepared by a modification of the process described in U.S. Patent 3,130,204. The compounds are prepared by reacting pyromeconic acid with an aryl aldehyde and thereafter reducing the intermediate 2-(1-hydroxy-1-arylmethyl)pyromeconic acid, obtained. This process is carried out according to the following sequence:

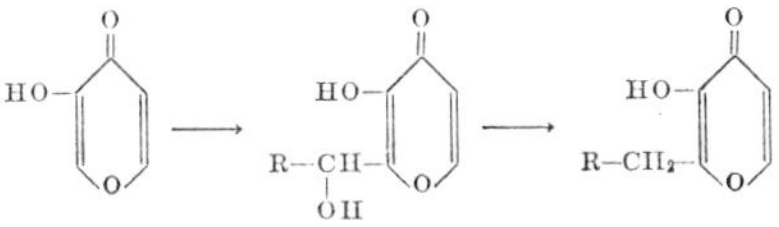

where R is as above. The conversion of pyromeconic acid to 2-(1-hydroxy-1-arylmethyl)-pyromeconic acid is accomplished in excellent yield, by carrying out the reaction at a pH of above about 5, and preferably above about 8. The following examples illustrate the process.

Example 1: 2-Benzylpyromeconic Acid — In an 8 liter stainless steel vessel fitted with a stirrer and an air sparger is placed a suspension of 350 grams of kojic acid in 3,500 ml of water. The pH is adjusted to 11.1 by addition of 256 ml of 50% aqueous sodium hydroxide and then 142 grams (7.1 grams as metal) of a 5% palladium on charcoal catalyst is added. Air is passed into the suspension at a rate of about 2,100 ml/min. The reaction, which is slightly exothermic, is maintained at a temperature of about 20° to 22°C by occasional application of external cooling. After 11 hours the reaction mixture is filtered to remove the catalyst and is treated with 600 ml of concentrated hydrochloric acid. The crystals of comenic acid which precipitate from the pH 0.5 mixture are removed by filtration, washed with a small amount of cold water and are air-dried.

There is obtained 328 grams of product. This is 85.3% of the theoretical yield. Titration data indicate the product to be 99.2% pure; therefore, there is obtained an 84.6% yield of comenic acid as corrected for purity.

In a 150 ml Pyrex flask fitted with a mechanical stirrer and a thermometer and connected through a distillation head to a receiver are placed 10.0 grams of comenic acid, prepared as described, and 30 ml of diphenyl ether. The reaction mixture is stirred and heated by application of a heating mantle. After about 20 minutes, the temperature reaches 225°C and gas is observed to pass into the receiver. When the temperature reaches 245° to 250°C, a vigorous evolution of carbon dioxide is observed. After an additional 40 minutes at 245° to 250°C, the pyromeconic acid is distilled therefrom until no more passes over at an internal temperature of 255°C and a vapor temperature of 230°C. 30 ml of additional diphenyl ether is added to the reaction flask and a second fraction is obtained after distillation at 255°C internal temperature for an additional 1 hour and 10 minutes. The product is suspended in about 5 volumes of hexane, then is removed by filtration, and is recrystallized in 4 volumes of toluene. There is obtained 5.71 grams of pyromeconic acid, MP 113° to 115.5°C. Concentration of the toluene mother-liquors to about $\frac{1}{20}$ volume affords an additional 0.7 gram of somewhat less pure pyromeconic acid. The combined weight of pyromeconic acid obtained represents an 80% conversion.

A solution of benzaldehyde, 53 grams, 0.5 mol, in 175 cc of dioxane is added to a stirred mixture of 56 grams, 0.5 mol pyromeconic acid in 175 cc of water, and sufficient 50% sodium hydroxide to give a final pH of 10.5. The temperature is maintained at 60°C during the addition and for an additional 16 hours. The mixture is acidified (pH 2.5) with HCl and is extracted with chloroform and with ether. Evaporation of the solvents and recrystallization from ethyl acetate affords 45.5 grams, 42% yield of 2-(1-hydroxy-1-phenylmethyl)pyromeconic acid, MP 142° to 143°C. Analysis—Calculated for $C_{12}H_{10}O_4$: C, 66.05; H, 4.62. Found: C, 66.06; H, 4.81.

Concentrated HCl, 35 cc, is added dropwise over 25 minutes to a stirred mixture of 0.1 mol, 21.8 grams, 2-(1-hydroxy-1-phenylmethyl)pyromeconic acid, 13.1 grams, 0.2 mol zinc and 125 cc of 25% aqueous ethanol. The temperature is maintained at 60° to 65°C during addition and for an additional hour of stirring. After filtration and extraction of filtrates and filter cakes and recrystallization of crude fractions from ethyl acetate there is isolated 9.5 grams, 47.5% yield, of product, MP 113° to 115°C. One additional recrystallization from ethyl acetate affords analytically pure 2-benzylpyromeconic acid. Analysis—Calculated for $C_{12}H_{10}O_3$: C, 71.28; H, 4.99. Found: C, 71.16; H, 5.18.

Example 2: 2-benzylpyromeconic acid alone is added to a perfume base solvent at 10 ppm. When the mixture is sprayed into an area it provides a pleasant floral aroma.

Example 3: 2-benzylpyromeconic acid is dissolved in a floral base cologne to provide 1, 50, 100, 250 and 500 ppm, respectively. The odors of the resulting perfume compositions are determined and compared with that of the untreated perfume as a control. The aromas of the 2-benzylpyromeconic acid-containing perfumes are significantly enhanced.

3-Methyldecenoic Acids, Esters and Alcohols

E.P. Demole; U.S. Patent 3,579,550; May 18, 1971; assigned to Firmenich & Cie, Switzerland describes compounds which correspond to the general formula

(1)
$$\underset{\text{CH}_3}{\text{CH}_3-(\text{CH}_2)_4-\text{CH}_n \ldots \text{CH} \ldots \overset{|}{\text{CH}}_{2-n}-\text{CH}_2-\text{R}}$$

where a double bond is located in one of the positions indicated by the dotted lines and where R represents a —COOH or —CH$_2$OH group and n stands for the integer 1 or 2. The compounds of Formula 1 exist both in the cis and trans configurations.

The acids and alcohols represented by Formula 1 have been found to possess interesting odors of a high intensity exceeding substantially the average odoriferous power of many of the common known fragrances. When added to mixtures of other odoriferous ingredients, the compounds also exert a fixing action on these mixtures.

The process for the preparation of compounds 1 with trans configuration comprises (a) saponifying and partially hydrogenating esters of formula

(2)
$$\underset{\text{CH}_3}{\text{CH}_3-(\text{CH}_2)_3-\text{CH}_n \ldots \text{CH} \ldots \text{CH} \ldots \overset{|}{\text{C}} \ldots \text{CH}_{3-n}-\text{COOR}'}$$

containing two conjugated double bonds in two of the positions indicated by the dotted lines and where R' represents an aliphatic radical comprising from 1 to 4 carbon atoms and n stands for the integer 1 or 2, in order to obtain the compounds 1 where R is —COOH, then (b) subsequently reducing the carboxylic groups of the partially hydrogenated products to obtain the compounds 1 where R is a methylol group. The process is illustrated by the following examples where the temperatures are given in degrees centigrade.

Example 1: A perfume composition having a Cassia-like odor was prepared by mixing the following ingredients:

Ingredients	Parts by Weight
Isobutyl salicylate	20
Ethyl salicylate	4
Benzyl acetate	1
Geranyl acetate	1
Eugenol at 10%*	0.5
Ethyl phthalate	49
Geranyl isobutyrate	0.5
Anisaldehyde	1.5
Decanal at 10%*	0.5
Methyl 2-nonynoate at 1%*	1.5
β-Ionone	1
Iris resinoid at 10%*	5
Anisyl acetate	0.5
Benzyl alcohol	5.5
Geraniol	2
Violet leaves abs at 1%*	1.5
Mimosa abs	3

*In diethyl phthalate

By adding to 98 grams of this mixture, 0.5 grams of 3-methyl-4-decenoic acid, 1 gram of 3-methyl-3-decenol and 3-methyl-4-decenol (ratio by weight about 8:2), a very tenacious natural powdery and somewhat fatty odoriferous note was imparted to the perfume composition.

Example 2: A perfume composition of the floral type was prepared by mixing the following ingredients:

Ingredients	Parts by Weight
Ylang extra	7.5
Bergamot	4.5
Synthetic lily-of-the-valley	18
Synthetic jasmine	12
Synthetic rose	9
γ-Methylionone	6
Synthetic carnation	6
Benzyl salicylate	3
Methylnonyl acetaldehyde at 10%*	1
Dodecanal at 10%*	0.5
Undecylenic aldehyde at 10%*	1.5
Isojasmone at 10%*	1.5
Cardamom at 1%*	3
Santalol	1.5
Vetyveryl acetate	4.5
Exaltolide at 10%* (pentadecanolide)	1.5
Natural degreased civet at 10%*	3
4-tert-Butyl-3,5-dinitro-2,6-dimethylaceto-phenone	6
Orange blossom abs at 10%*	2
Rose absolute	1
Bulgarian rose oil	1
Jasmine absolute	2
Vanillin at 1%*	3

*In diethyl phthalate

By adding 1 gram of a 10% solution of 3-methyl-3-decenol in diethyl phthalate to 99 grams of this mixture, the tenacity of the perfume composition was substantially improved.

Example 3: (a) Preparation of a mixture of methyl 3-methyl-2,4-decadien-1-oate and methyl 3-methyl-3,5-decadien-1-oate is as follows. A laboratory vessel was equipped with a reflux condenser and a dropping funnel containing a mixture of 81 grams of methyl 3-methyl-4-bromocrotonate and 52 grams of trimethyl phosphite. A fraction of 20 ml of this mixture was poured into the vessel and heated to 90°C, at which temperature the reaction started. The heat source was removed, and the remainder of the liquid was introduced at such a rate that the reaction proceeded at 90° to 110°C. A temperature of 120°C was maintained for an additional 1½ hours, then distillation yielded 56.4 grams (60.5%) of dimethyl 2-methyl-3-methoxycarbonyl-allyl-phosphonate.

14 grams of sodium amide (in the form of a 50% dispersion in toluene) were suspended in 150 ml of anhydrous tetrahydrofuran at 15° to 20°C under nitrogen. A mixture of 17.5 grams of n-hexanal and 39 grams of the phosphonate as prepared above was added dropwise. Stirring was continued for 1 hour at 25°C and for 1 hour at 50°C, whereupon the whole was allowed to stand overnight at room temperature. 50 ml of a saturated NaCl solution were introduced between 0° and 10°C, and then three extractions with hexane were carried out. The extract was washed twice with a saturated NaCl solution, dried and distilled.

There were obtained 20.47 grams (60%), BP 64 to 66°C/0.001 torr, of a mixture of diene esters which was analyzed by gas chromatography (235°C, 15% silicone oil, column 7.5 m) and comprised the following fractions: (1) 35% of methyl 3-methyl-2,4-decadienoate, cis structure of the double bond at C-2. (2) 15% of methyl 3,5-decadienoate. (3) 50% of methyl 3-methyl-2,4-decadienoate, trans structure of the double bond at C-2. The above mixture was thus composed of a total of 85% of methyl 3-methyl-2,4-decadienoate (mixture of cis and trans) and of 15% of 3,5-diene ester.

(b) The preparation of 3-methyl-3-decenoic acid and 3-methyl-4-decenoic acid 1(R=—COOH) is as follows. 30 grams of the mixture of esters prepared according to (a) of this example, 75 ml of ethanol and 300 ml of N caustic soda were heated to the boil until a clear solution was obtained (about 1½ hours). The solution was cooled to 0°C, and 689 grams of 2% sodium amalgam were introduced portionwise over a period of 4 hours. The solution was stirred for 3 hours at 0°C, then the mercury was separated and the mixture was acidified by means of 10% sulfuric acid. It was extracted three times with ether, the extracts were washed three times with water and then, after the usual treatment, they were distilled to give 22.2 grams (78.5%) of a mixture of acids which could be separated by gas chromatography (200°C, 5% Carbowax, column 2.5 m) and which was composed of the following fractions: (1) 20% of 3-methyl-4-decenoic acid, of trans configuration. (2) 80% of 3-methyl-3-decenoic acid of trans configuration.

Cinnamate Esters of Thujols

V. Hach and H.G. Higson; U.S. Patent 3,708,521; January 2, 1973; assigned to MacMillan Bloedel Limited, Canada describe cinnamate esters of the four isomeric thujanols represented by the following structural formula:

where R^1 and R^2 are different and represent hydrogen or methyl and R^3 and R^4 are different and represent hydrogen or

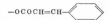

In accordance with the nomenclature proposed by H.C. Brown et al, *J. Organic Chemistry* 34, 3015 (1969), the above products can be named as follows:

R^1	R^2	R^3		R^4	Product name
CH_3	H	$-OCOCH=CH-$ ⬡		H	3-neoisothujyl cinnamate.
CH_3	H	H		$-OCOCH=CH-$ ⬡	3-isothujyl cinnamate.
H	CH_3	$-OCOCH=CH-$ ⬡		H	3-thujyl cinnamate.
H	CH_3	H		$-OCOCH=CH-$ ⬡	3-neothujyl cinnamate.

The odor quality and characteristics of the compounds not only resemble the quality and characteristics of natural styrax, but in odor intensity and persistence they surpass natural styrax. The longer lasting and characteristically styrax note of these esters makes them useful not only for their odor properties but also as effective perfume fixatives in many preparations.

The esters can be prepared by techniques by esterification of the isomeric thujanols with cinnamic acid or suitable derivatives thereof. A particularly useful method of preparing these esters is by the esterification of thujanols using a cinnamoyl halide in a nonaqueous medium. The esters obtained are viscous, colorless liquids having a boiling point in the range of 160° to 165°C at 0.7 mm. The following example illustrates the process.

Example: (—)-3-neoisothujanol (15.2 grams) is dissolved in 24 grams of pyridine and slowly added to a solution of 21.6 grams of cinnamic acid chloride in 200 ml of benzene. During this addition stirring is applied. Subsequently the reaction mixture is heated to reflux for 5 hours. After cooling to room temperature the reaction mixture is filtered through an Al_2O_3 column containing 500 grams of alumina to remove unreacted acid chloride, cinnamic acid and pyridine-HCl. The column is washed with benzene (200 ml) and the benzene eluates are combined, washed with dilute HCl, aqueous $NaHCO_3$ and water. Benzene is evaporated and the crude (—)-3-neoisothujyl cinnamate is distilled in vacuo at 169° to 172°C/1.5 mm Hg. The yield of ester is 22.6 grams (80%). After some hours of cooling the ester crystallizes and has a MP of 28°C.

Elemental analysis—Calculated for $C_{19}H_{24}O_2$ (percent): 80.29 C, 8.45 H, 11.26 O. Found (percent): 80.31 C, 8.44 H, 11.11 O. Purity of the ester was determined by IR spectroscopy (absence of —OH bands, one C=O peak) and by GLC. The latter method showed a single compound. The product has a styrax note and exhibits a stable odor note after several days.

Isobutylhydrocinnamaldehydes

I. Scriabine; U.S. Patent 3,548,006; December 15, 1970; assigned to Rhone-Poulenc SA, France describes certain substituted hydrocinnamaldehydes of superior stability which are useful in perfumery.

It has been found that very desirable properties for use as perfume materials, namely very valuable fragrances and high stability to air oxidation, to acid and alkali, are found in substituted hydrocinnamaldehydes having a molecular weight between 190 and 232, additionally containing an alkyl or alkenyl substituent with at least 4 carbon atoms attached to the benzene ring. The substituent may be an open chain or cyclic, or it may be a closed ring fused with the aromatic benzene ring. For instance, the aromatic ring may be the tetrahydronaphthalene nucleus, in which case the substituent may be viewed as a 4 carbon tetramethylene ring structure, fused to the benzene ring. The substituent may be in the para or in the ortho position, with respect to the aliphatic aldehyde chain, or the product may be a mixture of the two isomers. Substitution on the aromatic ring with groups containing more than 6 carbon atoms, is not advantageous, because the products have insufficient odor strength.

It has also been found that stability is generally favorably affected by a $-CH_2R$ group (primary alkyl) attached to the aromatic ring, rather than $-CH(R)_2$ or $-C(R)_3$ group. Thus, the preferred substances, within the scope of the process have the general formula

$$CH_2CH(R)CHO$$

in which R is either $-CH_3$ or H, and CH_nR^1 is an alkyl or alkenyl group, straight chain or branched, containing between 4 and 6 carbon atoms or a cycloalkyl or fused ring, the latter containing 4 carbon atoms. When CH_nR^1 is an open chain or a fused ring, n is equal to 2, and when CH_nR^1 is a cycloalkyl ring, for instance the cyclohexyl, n is equal to 1.

The substances, within the scope of this process, exhibit the strong floral character of the cyclamen type, but offer infinitely greater possibilities of application than p-isopropyl-alpha-methyl hydrocinnamaldehyde. Being free of the heavy sweetness of this substance, they are far more suitable for general use, and for incorporation into almost unlimited blends, particularly jasmine, rose, honeysuckle, flower of orange, mimosa, lilac, hyacinth, lily and magnolia.

One process as described in U.S. Patent 1,844,013, for preparing these substances consists of reacting the substituted benzaldehyde with acetaldehyde or propionaldehyde, to obtain a substituted cinnamaldehyde, which is then hydrogenated to the substituted hydrocinnamaldehyde. Another process is described by Poizat in French Patent 833,644, and consists of reacting a substituted benzyl chloride with malonic ester or methyl malonic ester, followed by hydrolysis and monodecarboxylation to give the substituted hydrocinnamic acid which is then reduced to the corresponding aldehyde. Very convenient is the process described in U.S. Patent 3,023,247, which comprises reacting an aromatic compound with an unsaturated aldehyde, CH_2=CACHO, or an alken-2-ylidene diacylate, CHB=CACH(OCOR)$_2$, in which A and B are hydrogen atoms or alkyl groups and which may be the same or different.

The reaction is conducted in the presence of a Friedel-Crafts type catalyst, for instance titanium tetrachloride, and a promotor, for instance, boron trifluoride. Hydrolysis of the alken-2-ylidene diacylate to the aldehyde, is required if the diacylate derivative of the aldehyde has been used. This process gives primarily the para isomer, in mixture with varying amounts of the ortho isomer. The content of the para isomer, varies between 70 and 100%, with the ortho isomer in amount between 0 and 30%. When the substituent is the fused tetramethylene ring from tetrahydronaphthalene, the 3,4-tetramethylene isomer is obtained exclusively.

Separation of the para and ortho isomers for all practical purposes, generally, is not necessary, because the mixture is stronger and richer than the pure para isomer alone. The ortho isomer is usually characterized by a very powdery and warm nuance and its presence intensifies the natural character and perfume value of the mixture. The following example illustrates the process.

Example: Preparation of Isobutylhydrocinnamaldehyde — Into a flask, equipped with a mechanical stirrer, dropping funnel and a column, provided with a calcium chloride tube, were placed 9 mols (1,206 grams) of isobutyl benzene, 1.9 mol (369 grams) of titanium tetrachloride and 5.6 grams boron trifluoride diethyl etherate complex. The mixture was cooled under stirring to $-10°C$. A mixture of 1.9 mol (285 grams) of acrolein diacetate and 2 mols (270 grams) of isobutyl benzene was added, from the dropping funnel, which was kept at $-10°C$, by circulation of brine. The addition required 2 hours, while maintaining the inside temperature at $-10°$ to $-14°C$.

After stirring for an additional 1.5 hours, the reaction mixture was poured into 1.5 kg of ice and 300 ml of hydrochloric acid (density 1.18). After separation of the organic layer and extraction of the aqueous layer with 150 ml of benzene, the combined organic layer was washed with 180 ml of water, then with three 200 ml portion of 5% aqueous sodium tartrate solution, and dried over anhydrous magnesium sulfate. The residue (392 grams) after removal of benzene and excess isobutyl benzene by distillation, was the crude enolic acetate.

The crude product from above, 357 grams, was refluxed under nitrogen, 9 hours, with 300 ml 6 N sulfuric acid, 1,500 ml of 95% alcohol, and 0.2 gram hydroquinone. After cooling to 60°C, 750 ml of water were added. The reflux condenser was replaced by a Vigreux column, the alcohol and ethyl acetate formed during the hydrolysis, were distilled off, the residue cooled to 25°C, the organic layer separated and the aqueous layer extracted with three portions 200 ml, 150 ml, and 150 ml, respectively, of ether. The combined ether layer was washed with water until free of sulfate ion and dried over magnesium sulfate. After removal of the ether, vacuum distillation gave 184.5 grams of isobutylhydrocinnamaldehyde, BP 104°C/1.5 mm; yield = 59% of theoretical, based on acrolein diacetate.

Vapor phase chromatography showed that the product was a mixture of the para and ortho isomer, in the proportion of 75:25. The mixture of para and ortho isomers, possesses not only the cyclamen fragrance, but also a fresh, flowery, pollen-like fragrance, and a broad, full odor, reminiscent of sandalwood, iris, lime tree, lilac, labdanum, and especially the mimosa, acacia, cassia and a variety of floral perfumes. The sandalwood and labdanum notes are valuable in compounding amber and oriental type perfumes, in which the latter two natural substances are almost indispensable.

Myrcene-Methacrylonitrile Adducts

R.T. Dahill, Jr.; U.S. Patent 3,714,220; January 30, 1973; assigned to Givaudan Corp. describes an adduct of myrcene and methacrylonitrile which possesses a soft, floral odor which has not been observed in any nitrile previously. The adduct is a mixture of isomers of the following structural formulas

The adduct possesses remarkable stability to light air air, and this stability combined with its lack of color makes it useful as a base for perfumes. The adduct is produced by reacting the components at elevated temperatures in an autoclave. The following example illustrates the process.

Example: A mixture of 426 grams of myrcene, 178 grams of methacrylonitrile and a trace of hydroquinone is charged into a 1 liter stainless steel autoclave equipped with an agitator and a gauge reading to 300 lb. Nitrogen pressure is applied and released 3 times. The mixture is heated with good agitation to a temperature of 150°C for 8 hours. The progress of the reaction is monitored by gas liquid chromatography on an SE 30 column at 225°C. The autoclave is cooled and the reaction mixture removed. This mixture is distilled under water-pump vacuum to remove the unreacted starting materials. The residue is then distilled under a 6 inch fractionating column packed with glass helices to yield the desired adduct consisting of 3-cyano-3-methyl- and 4-cyano-4-methyl-1-(4-methyl-3-pentyl)cyclohexene. BP 103°C/0.5 mm of Hg, yield 249 grams, (64% based on uncovered myrcene).

Gas liquid chromatographic analysis indicates that the product contains two components in the ratio 35 to 65 approximately.

Octahydro-Exo-4,7-Methanoinden-5-Ethyl Glycidate

A process described by S. Chodroff, J. Linsk and A. Zale; U.S. Patent 3,270,061; Aug. 30, 1966; assigned to Norda Essential Oil & Chemical Co., Inc. relates to fragrant compounds which contain an octahydro-4,7-methanoindene structure to which is attached a glycidate group or an aldehyde or a ketone group.

It has been discovered that cyclodiene derivatives, e.g., octahydro-exo-4,7-methanoinden-5-one can be conveniently converted into a variety of fragrant compounds which are valuable in the formulation of perfume oils, for example those used for floral perfumes, soaps, cosmetic creams, baby lotions, etc.

The principal reactant used is a keto derivative of dicyclopentadiene corresponding to the formula

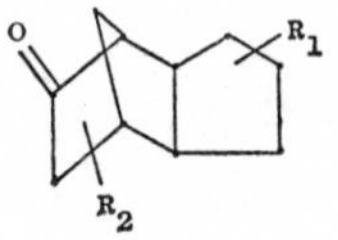

where R_1 and R_2 are identical or different members selected from the group consisting of hydrogen and methyl radicals. While these compounds usually and predominantly consist of the pertinent exo-isomers their corresponding endo-isomers can also be used.

One such particularly suitable and convenient reactant is octahydro-exo-4,7-methanoinden-5-one, i.e., the compound corresponding the above formula where both R_1 and R_2 represent hydrogen atoms. This compound is a liquid which has a MW of 150 and a BP of 129° to 132°C/29 mm. It is readily obtained from dicyclopentadiene via the corresponding monoolefinic alcohol, hexahydro-exo-4,7-methanoinden-exo-5-ol, which is then hydrogenated to give the corresponding saturated alcohol and the latter is finally oxidized to give the desired ketone. See for instance, the description of such a preparation by Bruson et al, JACS, 67, 726 (1945).

The keto compound, e.g., octahydro-exo-4,7-methanoinden-5-one, can be converted to a glycidate, e.g., octahydro-exo-4,7-methanoinden-5-ethyl glycidate. This can be done by reacting it in the presence of an alkali metal hydride such as sodium or lithium hydride or a corresponding alkoxide such as sodium ethoxide with a C_1–C_4 alkyl alpha-chloroacetate ester such as $ClCH_2COOC_2H_5$. The corresponding alpha-chloropropionate and alpha-chlorobutyrate esters may be used similarly but these will eventually yield a ketone product where the use of the chloroacetate leads to an aldehyde product. The resulting glycidate ester then can be converted to the corresponding glycidic acid, e.g., by saponification of the ester followed by acidulation of the resulting salt.

The glycidic acid can be readily decarboxylated to give the corresponding aldehyde, e.g., octahydro-exo-4,7-methanoinden-5-al. Finally, the aldehyde can be converted into various unsaturated or saturated ketones, e.g., into (octahydro-exo-4',7'-methanoinden-5')-buten-1-one-3 by reaction with acetone or into the corresponding penten-1-one-3 derivative by reaction with methyl ethyl ketone. Saturated ketones can be obtained by suitable selective hydrogenation of such unsaturated ketones, e.g., in the presence of a palladium catalyst. The following example illustrates the process.

Example: Octahydro-Exo-4,7-Methanoinden-5-Ethyl Glycidate

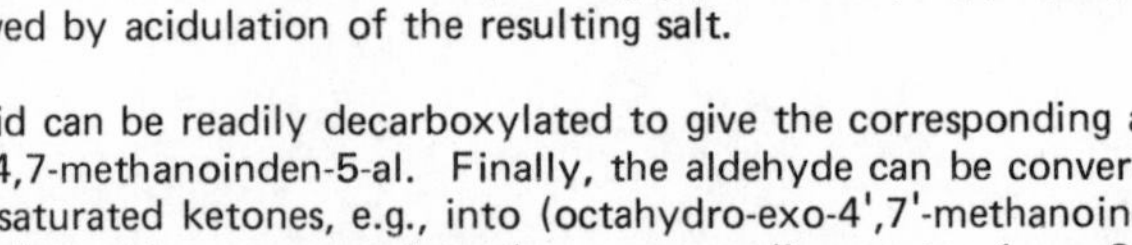

To a solution of 270 grams (1.8 M) octahydro-exo-4,7-methanoinden-5-one and 245.2 grams (2 M) ethyl chloroacetate in 900 ml anhydrous toluene, was added 96 grams (2 M) of 50% sodium hydride dispersion in mineral oil at 30° to 35°C over a three hour period. The reaction was exothermic and was controlled with an ice-alcohol bath. The mixture was stirred with cooling at 30° to 35°C for an additional hour. After this time the internal temperature dropped and no hydrogen gas evolved. The mixture was stirred overnight without further cooling. Then 50 ml methanol was added to react with excess sodium hydride. The mixture was diluted with 500 ml water and made acid to litmus with 15 ml acetic acid. The aqueous layer was extracted with 150 ml toluene. The organic layers were combined and washed with water, then bicarbonate solution, and finally with water to neutral.

The solvent was stripped on the steam bath at approximately 27" of Hg and the residue distilled through a 7" Vigreux column to yield 308.5 grams of product with a BP of 123°C/0.4 mm to 137°C/1.2 mm. This glycidate was 100% pure by saponification value and represented at 73% yield of theory. The glycidate derivative described in this example is an aromatic material possessing olfactory characteristics of the smooth floral type. It blends well in many floral perfume combinations and can be used to impart a floral-like quality to other perfumes, e.g., to woody ones. Its addition to such perfume oils in concentrations from about 1 to about 20%, imparts warmth and persistence to basic perfume oil formulations that otherwise lack these characteristics. A perfume oil which pleasingly simulates the fragrance of acacia can be formulated as follows:

Acacia

Novel glycidate derivative	15.0
Yara-yara (methyl naphthyl ether)	12.5
Aldehyde C–12, 10%	10.0
Fleur d'Oranger	1.5
Methyl anthranylate	2.5
Geraniol extra	10.0
Hydroxy citronellal	17.5
Phenyl ethyl alcohol	20.0
Benzyl benzoate	10.0
Linalool Ex Bois de Rose	15.0
Hydroxy citronellal methyl anthranylate	
condensation product	1.0
Oil Orange Florida	0.2
	115.2

OTHER FRAGRANCES

FRUIT-LIKE

Unsaturated Carbonyl Compounds from Tertiary Alcohols

R. Marbet and G. Saucy; U.S. Patent 3,453,317; July 1, 1969; assigned to Hoffman-La Roche Inc.; and U.S. Patent 3,574,715; April 13, 1971; assigned to Givaudan Corporation describe processes for the preparation of γ,δ-unsaturated aldehydes and ketones of the formula

$$(1) \qquad \underset{R^1-C=C-CH_2-CH-C=O}{\overset{R^2 \quad R^3 \qquad\quad R^4 \quad R^5}{}}$$

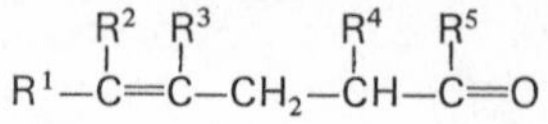

where R^1 is a saturated or unsaturated hydrocarbon group, an aralkyl group, preferably a phenyl lower alkyl group, or an aryl group, preferably phenyl, and where the group is other than aryl, it can also carry an oxygen-containing substituent attached to an aliphatic carbon atom; R^2 is a lower aliphatic hydrocarbon group, preferably a lower alkyl group; R^3, R^4, and R^5 are hydrogen atoms or a lower aliphatic hydrocarbon group, preferably a lower alkyl or lower alkenyl group; and R^1 taken together with R^2, and R^4 taken together with R^5 can form a closed ring.

The process is carried out by reacting a tertiary allyl alcohol, particularly, one of the formula

$$(2) \qquad \underset{\overset{\displaystyle R^1-C-C=CH_2}{\displaystyle OH}}{\overset{R^2 \quad R^3}{}}$$

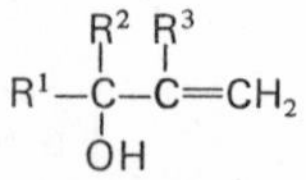

where R^1, R^2, and R^3 have the meaning given above for Formula (1), in the presence of an acidic catalyst, with either (a) an enol ether of an aliphatic aldehyde or ketone, especially with an enol ether of the formula

$$(3) \qquad \underset{HC=C-OR^6}{\overset{R^4 \quad R^5}{}}$$

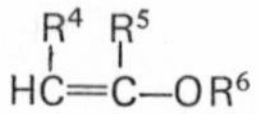

or (b) an acetal or ketal of an aliphatic aldehyde or ketone, especially with an acetal or ketal of the formula

$$(4) \qquad \underset{\overset{\displaystyle H_2C-C-OR^6}{\displaystyle OR^6}}{\overset{R^4 \quad R^5}{}}$$

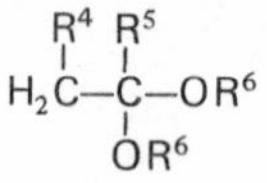

where in Formulas (3) and (4) R^6 is an alkyl group, preferably a lower alkyl group, and R_4 and R_5 have the meaning given above for Formula (1). The following examples illustrate the process.

Example 1: 86 grams of dry 3-methyl-1-buten-3-ol are mixed with 0.46 gram of phosphoric acid and 151 grams of isopropenyl methyl ether in a 400 ml pressure-vessel. Thereupon a gauge pressure of 2 atm is produced in the pressure-vessel by the introduction of nitrogen and the mixture heated to 125°C (inside temperature) during the course of one-half to one hour. The gauge pressure rises first to about 7.5 atm. During the course of the reaction it falls to about 5 atm. The reaction mixture is held for 13 to 15 hours at 125°C.

After cooling to room temperature, the reaction mixture is subjected to distillation after the addition of 1.25 grams of powdered sodium acetate. With bath temperatures of 90° to 160°C (without vacuum) crude acetone dimethyl ketal (containing some acetone and isopropenyl methyl ether) first distills over. After continuing the distillation under a water-jet vacuum, there is obtained 6-methyl-5-hepten-2-one; $n_D^{20} = 1.4392$; BP 59°C/10 mm.

The reaction of 3-methyl-1-buten-3-ol with isopropenyl methyl ether to obtain 6-methyl-5-hepten-3-one can also be undertaken continuously by forcing the mixture of the starting materials under pressure through a tube heated at 180° to 200°C, and thereafter condensing the reaction mixture in a condenser.

Example 2: 86 grams of dry 3-methyl-1-buten-3-ol are mixed with 300 ml of ligroin (BP 130° to 135°C) and 150 mg of p-toluenesulfonic acid (dissolved in 0.5 ml of methanol) in a flask. 172 grams of isopropenyl ethyl ether are added to this mixture while stirring and the mixture is boiled under reflux for 14 hours (bath temperature 100°C). Thereafter, the mixture is treated with 150 mg of p-toluenesulfonic acid (dissolved in 0.5 ml of methanol) and 86 grams of isopropenyl ethyl ether and again boiled under reflux of 8 hours (bath temperature 120°C, inside temperature about 100°C).

Then the p-toluenesulfonic acid is neutralized with 1.5 grams of sodium acetate and the reaction mixture is subjected to fractional distillation. Excess isopropenyl ethyl ether, followed by acetone diethyl ketal together with ligroin, and finally 6-methyl-5-hepten-2-one distills over; BP = 59°C/10 mm; $n_D^{20} = 1.4392$.

Example 3: 86 grams of 3-methyl-1-buten-3-ol are mixed with 0.5 gram of phosphoric acid and 181 grams of propenyl ethyl ether ($CH_3-CH=CH-O-CH_2-CH_3$) in a pressure-vessel. After the introduction of 5 atm of nitrogen, the mixture is held for one hour at 150°C (inside temperature). It can be determined gas-chromatographically that the methyl-butenol has disappeared completely after this time. The same results are achieved without the use of gauge pressure when the above reaction mixture is heated under reflux (bath temperature 100°C) for 48 hours.

After having completed the reaction, the phosphoric acid is neutralized with 2 ml of triethyl amine and then the resulting propionaldehyde diethyl acetal is first distilled off at 100 mm and a bath temperature of 100°C. By distillation at 17 mm, 2,5-dimethyl-4-hexen-1-al is subsequently obtained as a strongly smelling liquid. Odor characteristics: strongly fruit-like, slightly fatty; in the line of octyl alcohol and octyl aldehyde; lingering smell, delicately grassy. BP = 59°C/17 mm; $n_D^{20} = 1.4393$; melting point of the 4-phenylsemicarbazone = 89°C (from methanol).

Example 4: 154 grams of linalool are held in a pressure-vessel with 0.6 gram of phosphoric acid and 151 grams of vinyl ethyl ether under a nitrogen gauge pressure of 5 atm for 17 hr at a temperature of 120°C. (One can also heat at 150°C for 3 hours with approximately the same result.)

Thereafter, the phosphoric acid is neutralized with 2.4 ml of triethyl amine and then the resulting acetaldehyde diethyl acetal is first distilled off on the steam-bath. The residue is fractionally distilled in a high vacuum. There is obtained pure 5,9-dimethyl-4,8-decadien-

1-ol as a colorless liquid of individual, very clinging smell. Odor characteristics: mellow, fatty, somewhat fruit-like smoky smell which is reminiscent of lauric and tetradecyl alde-hyde. This compound completes the series of the fatty aldehydes which are so important in perfumes and allows the production of cloudy effects; moreover, this compound is useful as an intermediate for the manufacture of synthetic costus-root, tuber rose or jasmine oils, and has excellent clinging quality. BP = 69°C/0.04 mm; n_D^{20} = 1.4678; melting point of the 4-phenylsemicarbazone = 58°C (from methanol).

1,1-Dialkoxy Substituted Alkenes

R. Marbet; U.S. Patents 3,428,694; February 18, 1969 and 3,381,039; April 30, 1968; both assigned to Hoffmann-La Roche Inc. describes derivatives produced by the acetalization and/or catalytic hydrogenation of γ,δ-unsaturated aldehydes having the general formula

$$(1) \qquad R_1 - \underset{\underset{R_2}{|}}{C} = \underset{\underset{R_3}{|}}{C} - CH_2 - \underset{\underset{R_4}{|}}{CH} - CHO$$

in which R_1 represents a hydrocarbon residue or an oxygen-containing hydrocarbon residue; R_2 represents a lower alkyl group; and wherein R_1 and R_2, taken together, represent a carbo-cyclic radical; R_3 represents a hydrogen atom or a lower alkyl group and R_4 represents a hydrogen atom or a lower hydrocarbon residue.

The starting aldehydes of Formula (1) are, in a first step of the process, either acetalized to produce an γ,δ-unsaturated acetal of the following formula

$$(2) \qquad R_1 - \underset{\underset{R_2}{|}}{C} = \underset{\underset{R_3}{|}}{C} - CH_2 - \underset{\underset{R_4}{|}}{CH} - \underset{\underset{OR_5}{|}}{CH} - OR_5$$

or hydrogenated to yield an aldehyde having the following formula

$$(3) \qquad R_1 - \underset{\underset{R_2}{|}}{CH} - \underset{\underset{R_3}{|}}{CH} - CH_2 - \underset{\underset{R_4}{|}}{CH} - CHO$$

In a subsequent step of the process, the acetals of Formula (2) are hydrogenated or the aldehydes of Formula (3) are acetalized to yield a compound having the formula

$$(4) \qquad R_1 - \underset{\underset{R_2}{|}}{CH} - \underset{\underset{R_3}{|}}{CH} - CH_2 - \underset{\underset{R_4}{|}}{CH} - \underset{\underset{OR_5}{|}}{CH} - OR_5$$

In Formulas (2), (3) and (4), the symbols R_1, R_2 and R_3 have the same meaning as in Formula (1). The symbol R_5, which appears in Formulas (2) and (4) represents a lower alkyl group, e.g., an alkyl group having from 1 to 6 carbon atoms or a lower alkenyl group, e.g., an alkenyl group having from 2 to 6 carbon atoms; taken together, the two symbols R_5 represent a lower alkylene group.

The preferred compounds of Formula (4) contain as the R_5 substituents, lower alkyl groups, such as, methyl, ethyl, propyl, butyl, etc. groups. The lower alkylene group, which is re-presented by the symbols R_5 and R_5 includes ethylene, trimethylene, tetramethylene, etc. radicals. The following examples illustrate the process.

Example 1: A solution of 140 mg of p-toluenesulfonic acid in 280 ml of methanol was added to a mixture of 28 grams of 5-methyl-4-hexen-1-al and 37 grams of orthoformic acid ethyl ester. The reaction was exothermic, the temperature of the reaction mixture reaching 33°C. After standing for a period of two hours, the reaction mixture was treated with 1.4 grams of sodium acetate and concentrated in a 50°C-bath at 35 mm. Distillation of the residue, in vacuo, yielded 1,1-dimethoxy-5-methyl-4-hexene, boiling point at 89°C at 35 mm; n_D^{20} = 1.4294. The compound has a characteristic fruit-like green odor.

Example 2: A mixture of 112 grams of 5-methyl-4-hexen-1-al, 62 grams of ethylene glycol and 0.2 gram of p-toluenesulfonic acid was distilled at 50 mm in a 100°C-bath. A major portion of water present therein was thus removed. Thereafter, the pressure was reduced to 12 mm and there was thus obtained 1,1-ethylenedioxy-5-methyl-4-hexene-[1-(1,3-dioxolan-2-yl)-4-methyl-3-pentene] as a colorless oil which was purified by repeated distillation. This compound had a BP at 80°C at 12 mm; n_D^{20} = 1.4512. The compound had an odor resembling 5-methyl-1-hexanal, but much finer.

Example 3: 63 grams of 2,5-dimethyl-4-hexen-1-al were mixed with 640 ml of methanol, 75 grams of orthoformic acid ethyl ester and 1.5 ml of boron trifluoride etherate. After 30 minutes the mixture was treated with 3 ml of triethylamine and a fore-run was first distilled off at 13 mm in a 50°C-bath. Thereafter, there was obtained from a 100°C-bath, 1,1-dimethoxy-2,5-dimethyl-4-hexene which was purified by redistillation. This compound, boiling point at 77°C at 13 mm and n_D^{20} = 1.4343, had a harsh, fruit-like green color.

WATERMELON

Benzoxepin-3-ones

A process described by *J.J. Berreboom, D.P. Cameron and C.R. Stephens, Jr.; U.S. Patent 3,799,892; March 26, 1974; assigned to Pfizer Inc.* relates to compounds of the formula

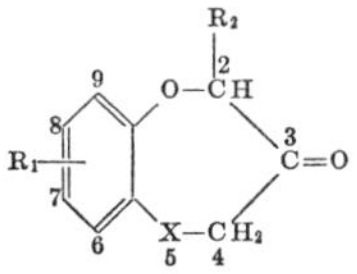

where R_1 and R_2 are each selected from hydrogen and alkyl having from 1 to 4 carbon atoms and X is oxygen or methylene. This process also relates to valuable intermediates of the formula

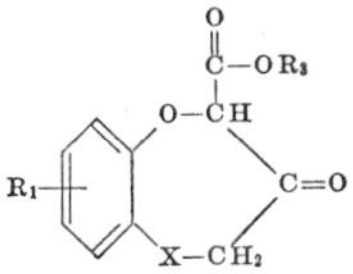

where R_1 and X are as above and R_3 is alkyl having from 1 to 4 carbon atoms.

The benzodioxepin compounds are prepared from substituted and unsubstituted catechol-O,O-diacetic acid esters which in turn are prepared according to the procedure of W. Carter and W. Trevor Lawrence, *J. Chem. Soc.,* vol. 77, page 1222 (1900).

The benzoxepin compounds are prepared from the corresponding 2-carbalkoxymethylphenoxyacetic acid esters which in turn are prepared from 2-hydroxy-phenoxyacetic acid esters by the procedure of Carter and Lawrence. These compounds are reacted in accordance with the following reaction scheme:

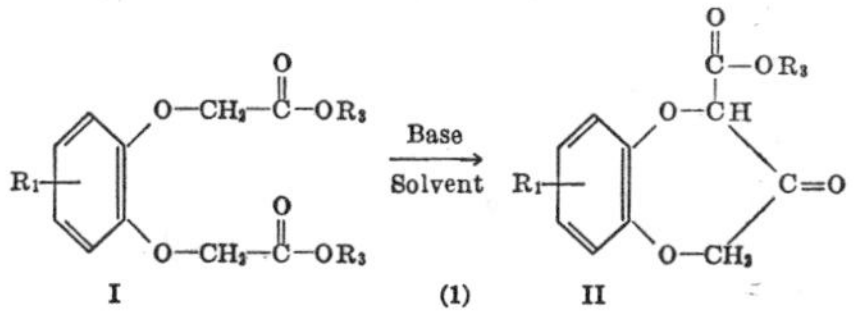

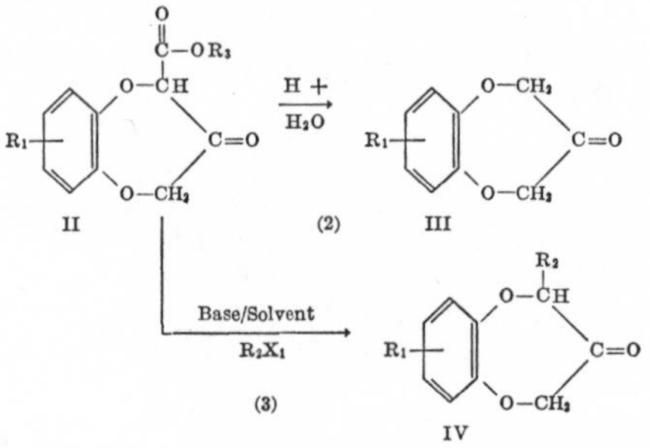

$$\text{II} \quad \xrightarrow[\text{H}_2\text{O}]{\text{H +}} \quad \text{III}$$

(2)

and

$$\text{Base/Solvent} \atop R_2X_1$$

(3) IV

$$\text{V} \quad \xrightarrow[\text{Solvent}]{\text{Base}} \quad \text{VI}$$

(4)

$$\text{VI} \quad \xrightarrow[\text{H}_2\text{O}]{\text{H+}} R_1 \quad \text{VII}$$

(5)

$$\text{Base/Solvent} \atop R_2X_1$$

(6) VIII

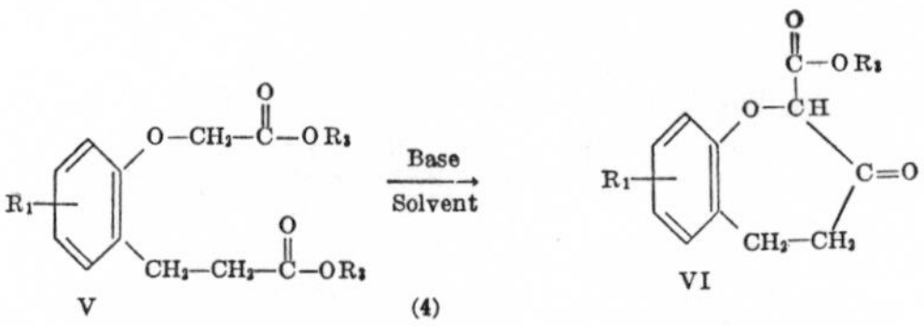

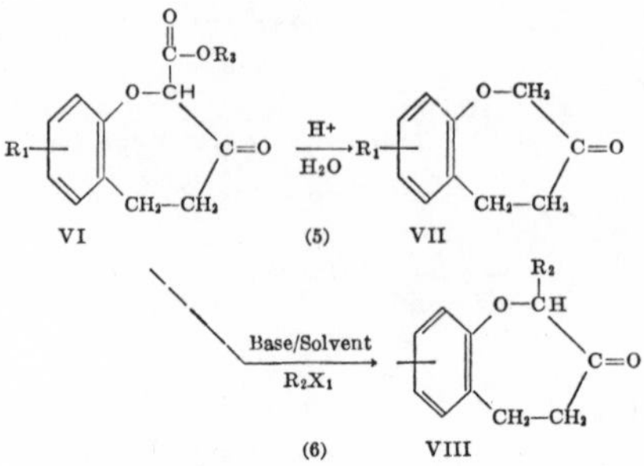

Example 1: 7-Methyl-3,4-Dihydro-2H-1,5-Benzodioxepin-3-one — To a stirred suspension of 31.7 grams (1.32 mols) of sodium hydride in 900 ml dry ethylene glycol dimethyl ether is added under a nitrogen atmosphere, a solution of 161 grams (0.6 mol) of dimethyl 4-methyl-catechol-O,O-diacetate in 900 ml of dry ethylene glycol dimethyl ether over a 3 hour period. As the addition proceeds, the reaction temperature rises and is held at reflux by adjusting the rate of addition. At the end of the addition, the reaction is refluxed for 30 minutes, cooled to room temperature and poured into 6 liters of ice water. The resulting suspension is acidified to pH 2.5 and extracted with four liter portions of ether.

The combined ether layers are washed with 500 ml of water and dried over anhydrous sodium sulfate. Evaporation of the ether in vacuo provides 134.5 grams (95%) of the crude esters; BP 141° to 143°C (1 mm Hg).

A solution of 126 grams (0.534 mol) of the crude esters, 7- and 8-methyl-2-carbomethoxy-3-oxo-3,4-dihydro-2H-1,5-benzodioxepin in 325 ml of ethanol and 325 ml of 5% hydrochloric acid is stirred at reflux temperature for 8 hours. The solution is poured into one liter of water and extracted with five 200 ml portions of ethyl ether. Evaporation of the ether followed by distillation provides 88 grams (93%) of 7-methyl-3-oxo-3,4-dihydro-2H-1,5-benzodioxepin; BP 88° to 91°C (0.7 mm Hg).

Example 2: The products of the following table are prepared by the procedure of Ex. 1 from the appropriate starting material.

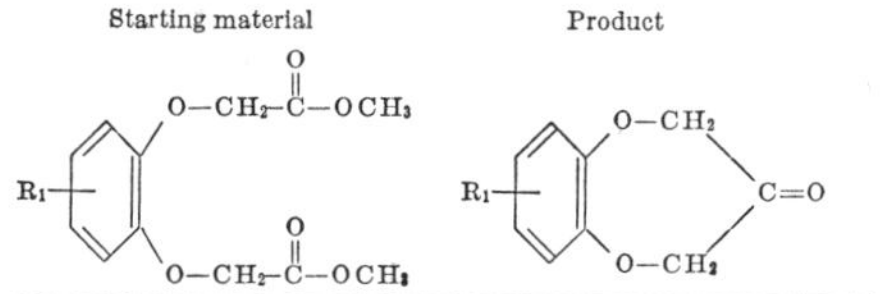

R_1	Substituted-3,4-dihydro-2H-1,5-benzoxepin-3-one
4-methyl or 5-methyl	7-methyl.
4-ethyl or 5-ethyl	7-ethyl.
4-isopropyl or 5-isopropyl	7-isopropyl.
4-tertiarybutyl or 5-tertiarybutyl	7-tertiarybutyl.
4-n-butyl or 5-n-butyl	7-n-butyl.
H—	H—.
3-methyl	6-methyl.
3-isopropyl	6-isopropyl.

Example 3: *7-Methyl-3,4-Dihydro-2H-1,5-Benzoxepin-3-one* — To a stirred suspension of 50.8 grams (1.3 mols) of sodamide in 900 ml of dry tetrahydrofuran is added, under a nitrogen atmosphere, a solution of 150 grams (0.6 mol) of 2-(2-carbomethoxymethyl)-4-methylphenoxyacetic acid methyl ester in 900 ml of tetrahydrofuran over a three hour period. The reaction temperature rises and is held at reflux.

At the end of the addition, the reaction is refluxed for an additional 30 minutes, then cooled to room temperature and poured into 6 liters of ice water. The resulting suspension is acidified to pH 2.5 and extracted with four 1 liter portions of ether. The combined ether layers are washed with 500 ml of water and dried over anhydrous sodium sulfate. Evaporation of the ether provides 7-methyl-2-carbomethoxy-3,4-dihydro-2H-1,5-benzoxepin-3-one.

The crude ester mixture is stirred for 8 hours in a mixture of 325 ml of ethanol and 325 ml of 5% aqueous hydrochloric acid at reflux. The solution is poured into 1 liter of water and extracted with five 200 ml portions of ethyl ether. Evaporation of the ether followed by distillation provides 7-methyl-3,4-dihydro-2H-1,5-benzoxepin-3-one.

Example 4: A synthetic, watermelon flavor was prepared with a watermelon ketone from those in the following table. Each of the ketones was formulated with the auxiliary chemicals to obtain the watermelon-flavored extract at a level of 0.001 and at 0.1 weight percent. The extracts gave a fruitful watermelon flavor at a level of 200 ppm when added to a non-carbonated soft drink, made from 14 grams sugar, 0.05 gram citric acid and 100 grams water.

Watermelon ketone:

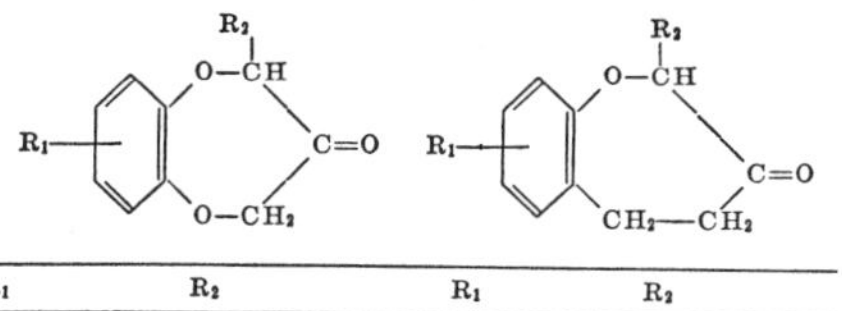

R_1	R_2	R_1	R_2
H	H	H	H
H	CH_3	H	CH_3
H	C_2H_5	H	C_2H_5
H	$n-C_3H_7$	H	$n-C_3H_7$
H	$n-C_4H_9$	H	$n-C_4H_9$
H	$iso-C_3H_7$	H	$iso-C_3H_7$
H	$iso-C_4H_9$	H	$iso-C_4H_9$
H	$tert.-C_4H_9$	H	$tert.-C_4H_9$
7-CH_3	H	7-CH_3	H
7-CH_3	$n-C_4H_9$	6-C_2H_5	$n-C_4H_9$
7-,8-CH_3	$iso-C_3H_7$	7-$n-C_3H_7$	$iso-C_3H_7$
7-,8-C_2H_5	CH_3	7-$iso-C_3H_7$	H
7-,8-$n-C_4H_9$	CH_3	7-$tert.-C_4H_9$	H
6-,9-CH_3	CH_3	9-CH_3	$n-C_4H_9$
6-,9-$iso-C_3H_7$	$iso-C_2H_7$	8-C_2H_5	$iso-C_2H_7$
6,9-CH_3	H	6-CH_3	CH_3

	Weight (grams)
Auxillary chemicals:	
Methyl ionone	0. 010
Neofoline	0. 010
Methyl heptine carbonate	0. 002
Benzaldehyde	0. 020
Diacetyl	0. 040
Ethyl butyrate	0. 060
Propylene glycol	8. 790
Watermelon ketone	0. 060
Total	10. 0

APPLE

Allyl Phenylpropionates

A process described by *M. Dunkel; U.S. Patent 3,745,130; July 10, 1973; assigned to Universal Oil Products Company* relates to perfume compositions containing allyl esters of beta-phenylpropionic acids as olfactory ingredient. The allyl phenylpropionates have the following general structural formula:

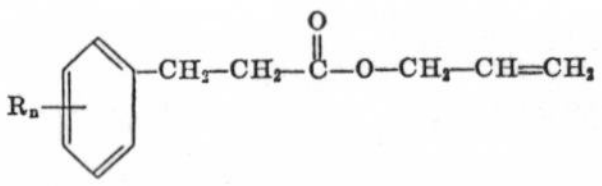

$$R_n \text{—} \bigcirc \text{—} CH_2\text{—}CH_2\text{—}\overset{\overset{\displaystyle O}{\|}}{C}\text{—}O\text{—}CH_2\text{—}CH{=}CH_2$$

where R is a lower alkyl group and n is an integer of from 0 to 3. Compounds having this general formula have desirable odor properties which render them highly valuable for perfumery use.

The allyl phenylpropionates are prepared in general by transesterifying a lower alkyl ester of a beta-phenylpropionic acid with allyl alcohol in the presence of a transesterification catalyst. The lower alkyl esters of a beta-phenylpropionic acid used in the reaction may be readily prepared by hydrogenating a corresponding alkyl cinnamate such as methyl or ethyl cinnamate in the presence of a suitable hydrogenation catalyst.

Examples of alkyl esters of beta-phenylpropionic acids which may be used in the reaction include lower alkyl, such as methyl or ethyl, esters of phenylpropionic acid, methylphenyl-propionic acid, dimethylphenylpropionic acid, ethylphenylpropionic acid and (p-ethyl-o-methylphenyl) propionic acid.

The transesterification catalyst used in the reaction comprises a wide class of materials and includes, for example, sodium methylate or an aluminum alkoxide such as aluminum iso-propylate. Examples of compounds having highly desirable perfume properties prepared according to the process by reacting allyl alcohol with an alkyl ester of a beta-phenyl-propionic acid of the above illustrated class include allyl beta-phenylpropionate, allyl beta-(methylphenyl) propionate; allyl beta-(p-isopropylphenyl) propionate; or allyl beta-(p-ter-tiary-butylphenyl)propionate.

Allyl beta-phenylpropionate imparts an apple-apple cider odor and an undertone of berry. This odor is especially useful in perfume compositions to be incorporated in sprays, lotions, cologne, soaps, creams, shaving creams and other toiletry articles used by the male species. The following examples illustrate the process.

Example 1: Allyl beta-phenylpropionate was prepared by the following procedure. About 164 grams (1 mol) of methyl beta-phenylpropionate, about 116 grams (2 mols) of allyl alcohol and 4.9 grams of sodium methylate catalyst were charged to a reaction flask equipped overhead with a short packed column with a reflux splitter. The mixture was heated to reflux temperature starting at about 66°C and rising up to 75°C in about 4 hours.

During this period about 24 grams of distillate containing mostly methyl alcohol were recovered. An additional 2.0 grams of the sodium methylate catalyst was then added and the refluxing was continued for about 2 hours to complete the reaction with temperature ultimately rising up to about 95°C. An additional 28.5 grams of distillate were recovered during this period. About 8.5 grams of acetic acid were then added to neutralize the sodium methylate catalyst prior to removing the excess allyl alcohol from the reaction mixture by distillation at a temperature up to about 165°C.

After removing about 31 grams of the allyl alcohol, the reaction mixture was then cooled to about 50°C and mixed with about 100 grams of water and about 100 grams of toluene. The resulting organic layer was separated from the aqueous mixture, washed with water and fractionated to recover about 163 grams of allyl beta-phenylpropionate boiling at 150°C at 10 mm Hg and having a refractive index n_D^{20} = 1.5031.

Example 2: Allyl beta-(p-tertiarybutylphenyl) propionate is prepared by the following procedure. About 234 grams (1 mol) of ethyl beta-(p-tertiarybutylphenyl) propionate, about 116 grams (2 mols) of allyl alcohol and 5.0 grams of aluminum isopropylate catalyst are charged to a reaction flask equipped overhead with a short packed column with a reflux splitter. The mixture is then heated to reflux temperature and maintained thereat for 6 hours. The ethyl alcohol which forms during the reaction is continuously removed from the reaction mixture as a distillate.

Acetic acid is then added to neutralize the aluminum isopropylate catalyst prior to removing the excess allyl alcohol from the reaction mixture by distillation. After removing the allyl alcohol, the reaction mixture is cooled to about 50°C and mixed with water and toluene. The resulting organic layer is separated from the aqueous mixture, washed with water and fractionated to recover the allyl beta-(p-tertiarybutylphenyl) propionate.

Example 3: An illustrative perfume composition comprises the following.

	Parts by Weight
Allyl beta-phenylpropionate	150
Wood complex	100
Terpineol	100
Phenylethyl alcohol	100
Resinodour benzoin	90
Linalol	60
Benzyl acetate	90
Patchouli oil	20
Isoeugenol	55
Artemisia oil (Moroccan)	40
Geraniol	90
Ionone	45
Oak moss absolute	5
Isobutyl salicylate	20
Coumarin	50
Heliotropin	100
Resinodour tonka	35

4-Methyl-2-Pentanol Crotonate

F. Exner and T. Leidig; U.S. Patent 3,709,929; January 9, 1973; assigned to Haarmann & Reimer Gesellschaft mit beschrankter Haftung, Germany describe 4-methyl-2-pentanol crotonate and a process for its production whereby 4-methyl-2-pentanol is esterified with crotonic acid.

4-methyl-2-pentanol crotonate has a very pleasant, pure fruit-like note reminiscent in particular of plum and apple preserves. It differs from conventional fruit-like odorants not only in its type of odor but also in the fact that it can be used more easily and more widely.

Example 1: The following formulation is given as an example of the preparation of a perfume with a plum-like odor which is a suitable fragrance for dishwashing detergents:

	Parts by Weight
β,γ-hexanol isobutyrate, 10%	5
Bergamot oil, Reggio	10
Geraniol	100
Geranyl acetate	170
Citronellyl acetate	40
Citronellyl isobutyrate	50
Citronellol	50
Phenylmethyl glycidic acid ethyl ester, 1%	5
Terpineol	20
Phenylethyl isobutyrate	50
4-methyl-2-pentanol crotonate	500

4-methyl-2-pentanol crotonate produces a pleasant full-fruit plum note without being found
to be overdosed in this concentration as is often the case with conventional plum odorants.
A diswashing detergent scented with this formulation can have the following composition
for example:

	Parts by Weight
Sodium alkyl sulfonate or sodium alkyl benzosulfonate	200
Fatty alcohol ether sulfate	70
Coconut fatty acid diethanolamide	30
Sodium chloride	20
Water, coloring and skin preservative	677
Perfume oil	3

Example 2: The following formulation is given as an example of the preparation of a
flower bouquet with a freshening fruit nuance which is suitable for perfuming creams:

	Parts by Weight
Cuminyl propionaldehyde	15
Linalool	50
Linalyl acetate	30
Terpinyl acetate	25
Terpineol	60
Geraniol	150
Phenylethyl alcohol	100
Phenylethyl dimethyl carbinol	100
Hydrocinnamic alcohol	30
Farnesol	100
Hydroxycitronellal	170
α-Amylcinnamic aldehyde	100
α-Ionone	20
Coumarin	20
Ethylene brassylate	10
4-methyl-2-pentanol crotonate	20

The somewhat flat, harmless, phantasy bouquet is distinctly freshened and aesthetically improved by the small addition of 4-methyl-2-pentanol crotonate. The fruit nuance introduced
gives the perfume more freshness and a natural character. A skin cream perfumed with
this composition can be prepared as follows.

Phase A: 50 grams of oleic acid decyl ester, 125 grams of glycerine monostearate (self-
emulsifying), 50 grams of paraffinum per liquidum, 20 grams of cetaceum DAB 7, 1 gram
of p-hydroxybenzoic acid propyl ester. Phase B: 720 grams of distilled water, 1 gram of

p-hydroxybenzoic acid methyl ester, 30 grams of sorbitol, 3 grams of perfume oil. Phase A and Phase B are heated to 75°C, after which Phase B is stirred into Phase A, cooled with stirring to 40°C and perfumed.

PEACH

2-Methyl-6-(4'-Methyl-3'-Cyclohexen-1'-yl)-5-Hepten-2-ol

A process described by *W. Kimel and R. Propper; U.S. Patent 3,492,360; January 27, 1970; assigned to Givaudan Corporation* relates to 2-methyl-6-(4'-methyl-3'-cyclohexen-1'-yl)-5-hepten-2-ol having the structure:

(1)

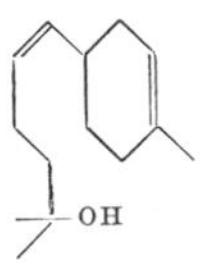

The compound of Formula (1) has a unique soft, mellow slightly sweet, fruity peach-like sesquiterpene odor. This compound of Formula (1), because of its fine fragrance, is extremely useful as an odorant in the preparation of perfumes and in the preparation of other scented compositions. The compound of Formula (1) above is prepared from a compound of the formula:

(2)

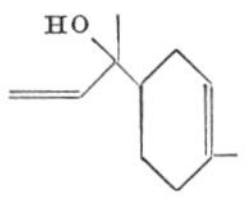

by first treating the compound of Formula (2) with diketene to produce a compound of the formula:

(3)

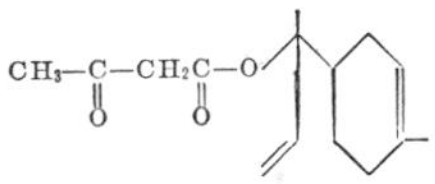

The compound of Formula (3) is then heated in the presence of aluminum tri(lower alkoxide) to form a compound of the formula:

(4)

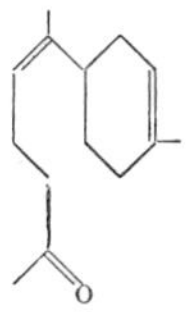

The compound of the Formula (4) above is converted to the compound of the Formula (1) above by treating the compound of the Formula (4) with an organometallic methyl compound. The following examples illustrate the process.

Example 1: This example is directed to the preparation of 3-(4'-methyl-3'-cyclohexen-1'-yl)-

1-buten-3-yl acetoacetate. To 1,113 grams (6.7 mols) of 3-(4'-methyl-3'-cyclohexen-1'-yl)-1-buten-3-ol in 1,115 cc pentane were added 13.4 cc acetic acid. To this mixture, 618 grams (7.37 mols) of diketene was added during 6 hours at 20° to 30°C. After stirring an additional two hours at room temperature, the reaction mixture was stored in a refrigerator at 0 to 10°C overnight. It was then transferred to a separatory funnel and washed two times with cold water, two times with saturated sodium bicarbonate solution and one time with saturated sodium chloride solution. The pentane solution was dried over anhydrous sodium sulfate, filtered and concentrated in vacuo at a maximum temperature of 50°C at 1 mm, giving 3-(4'-methyl-3'-cyclohexen-1'-yl)-1-buten-3-yl acetoacetate.

Example 2: This example is directed to the preparation of 6-(4'-methyl-3'-cyclohexen-1'-yl)-5-hepten-2-one. 1,677 grams (6.7 mols) of 3-(4'-methyl-3'-cyclohexen-1'-yl)-1-buten-3-yl acetoacetate was placed in a dropping funnel attached to a three-liter flask equipped with a thermometer, stirrer, reflux condenser and an outlet at the top of the condenser, leading to a Dry Ice trap and a gas meter.

To the flask were added 25.2 grams of aluminum isopropoxide and one quarter of the contents of the dropping funnel. Heat was applied and evolution of carbon dioxide was measured when the temperature reached 130°C. The temperature was raised to 175° to 190°C at which point carbon dioxide evolution was vigorous. After 20 minutes, gas evolution began to subside. The remaining contents of the dropping funnel were then added at such a rate as to maintain a steady vigorous rate of carbon dioxide evolution at 175° to 190°C. This required 3½ hours. Heat at the same temperature was continued until gas evolution ceased. 142.5 liters of carbon dioxide was evolved which is equal to 87% of theory. After cooling, the reaction mixture was distilled through a Vigreaux column. The fraction boiling at 93° to 97°C at 0.3 mm was collected. This material was identified as 6-(4'-methyl-3'-cyclohexen-1'-yl)-5-hepten-2-one.

Example 3: This example is directed to the preparation of 2-methyl-6-(4'-methyl-3'-cyclohexen-1'-yl)-5-hepten-2-ol. A solution of methyl magnesium iodide was prepared in ethyl ether by addition of 374.7 grams (2.64 mols) of methyl iodide in 1,350 cc ethyl ether during seven hours at 20° to 25°C under nitrogen.

After stirring overnight at room temperature, the solution was cooled to 0°C, and 495.2 grams (2.4 mols) of 6-(4'-methyl-3'-cyclohexen-1'-yl)-5-hepten-2-one in 500 cc of ethyl ether was added during eight hours at 0°C. The reaction mixture was then allowed to warm to room temperature while stirring overnight. It was then quenched by pouring into 129.3 grams (2.64 equivalents) of sulfuric acid in 3.5 kg of ice. The ether layer was separated and the aqueous layer was extracted twice with ethyl ether.

All ether layers were combined and washed twice with 2% sodium thiosulfate solution, once with cold water, once with saturated sodium bicarbonate solution and finally once with saturated sodium chloride solution. The ether solution was dried over sodium sulfate, filtered and concentrated at 50°C and 20 mm. The residue of 528.0 grams was distilled through a Vigreaux column. The fraction boiling at from 103.5° to 105.5°C at 0.15 mm was collected. This fraction was identified as pure 2-methyl-6-(4'-methyl-3'-cyclohexene-1'-yl)-5-hepten-2-ol.

CITRUS

7-Methyl-2,6-Octadienenitriles

P.W.D. Mitchell and J.H. Blumenthal; U.S. Patent 3,553,110; January 5, 1971; assigned to International Flavors & Fragrances, Inc. describe methods for the preparation and isolation of a variety of 7-methyl-2,6-octadienenitriles by condensation of cyanoacetic acid with 2-methyl-hept-2-ene-6-one in the presence of an amine or an acid addition salt of an amine at a temperature of from about 40° to 180°C. A mixture of nitriles is produced in the condensation reaction. The relative proportion of each nitrile in the mixture can be controlled by control of the alkalinity of the reaction medium. The compounds and mixtures are useful as olfactory agents.

The mixtures obtained by the process or the components of the mixture may be utilized alone, for example, in sachets for use in bureaus and in closets, or they may be utilized as olfactory components in detergents, cosmetics, soaps, space deodorants and other formulations. When so used they contribute a fresh, citrusy, lemon-like odor similar to that obtained with citral.

Cyclic Acetals of 2,4-Hexadienal

W.M. Easter, Jr. and R.F. Taveres; U.S. Patent 3,769,303; October 30, 1973; assigned to Givaudan Corporation describe compounds which have the following general formulas:

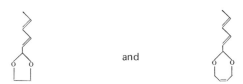

and

In accordance with the process, 2,4-hexadienal is reacted with the appropriate diol in the presence of an acid. The reaction may be illustrated as follows:

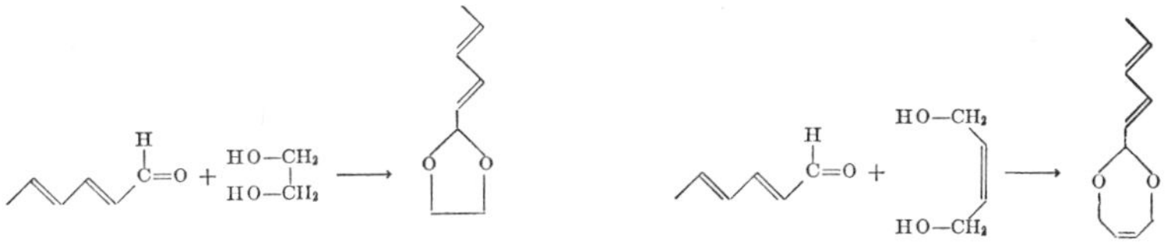

The compounds are useful odorants having a fruity or floral citrus type of odor. The following examples illustrate the process.

Example 1: Preparation of 2-(1,3-Pentadien-1-yl)-4,7-Dihydro-1,3-Dioxepin — Into a one liter flask equipped with heating jacket, agitator and a condenser fitted with a Dean-Stark trap was charged 96 grams of 2-butene-1,4-diol, 1 gram of citric acid and 160 grams cyclohexane. With vigorous agitation the mixture was refluxed until the collection of water in the Dean-Stark trap was completed. The reaction mixture was cooled and washed neutral. The solvent was removed and the oil vacuum distilled. There was recovered 147 grams of 2-(1,3-pentadien-1-yl)-4,7-dihydro-1,3-dioxepin.

Example 2: Preparation of 2-(1,3-Pentadien-1-yl)-1,3-Dioxolane — Into a one liter flask equipped with heating jacket, agitator and a condenser fitted with a Dean-Stark trap was charged 96 grams 2,4-hexadienal, 93 grams of ethylene glycol, 1 gram citric acid and 175 g toluene. With agitation the mixture was refluxed until collection of water-ethylene glycol mixture was completed. After 7 hours there was collected 50.5 grams of a water-ethylene glycol mixture. The reaction mixture was cooled and washed neutral. The solvent was removed and the oil vacuum distilled. There was recovered 111 grams of 2-(1,3-pentadien-1-yl)-1,3-dioxolane.

Example 3: The following citrus type odorant base formulation was used to demonstrate the use of 2-(1,3-pentadien-1-yl)-4,7-dihydro-1,3-dioxepin. The dioxepin imparted a neutral citrus quality and contributed to the bouquet of the perfume base. Without the dioxepin the base seemed unfinished and of inferior quality. All of the parts in the example are by weight.

	Parts by Weight
Linalool synthetic	8
Citral synthetic	12
Geranyl acetate extra	20
Linalool acetate	300
Orange oil, CP	100
Petigran, SA	20
Triethyl citrate	125
Terpinyl acetate extra	155
Lemon terpenes	160
2-(1,3-pentadien-1-yl)-4,7-dihydro-1,3-dioxepin	100

Extractive Distillation of Citrus Limonene

K.A. Kubitz and A.F. Wicke, Jr.; U.S. Patent 3,819,737; June 25, 1974; assigned to Reichhold Chemicals, Inc. have found that crude citrus linomene can be distilled safely and without destroying the contained flavor and fragrance values by adding a minor amount of an inert, high-boiling liquid, with which the oxygenated components of the crude citrus linomene are compatible, to the stillpot prior to distilling out limonene. By this extractive distillation process, the valuable flavor and fragrance components are sealed in the high boiling inert liquid medium while the limonene is removed by vacuum distillation.

After removal of the limonene, the flavor and fragrance concentrate is isolated from the high boiling liquid by any convenient method, such as by steam distillation or extraction with a volatile solvent immiscible with the high-boiling liquid. The flavor and fragrance concentrate can then be recovered as an oil, as by separating and discarding the water layer in the case of steam distillation, or by evaporation of the volatile liquid in the case of extraction. The following examples illustrate the process.

Example 1: The feed stock for this example was a crude citrus limonene obtained as a by-product from orange peels after removal of the juice from whole oranges. The crude material was found to contain 1.26% aldehydes and ketones by the hydroxylamine method, 0.86% alcohols by acetylation, and 0.45% esters by saponification.

Separate 500 ml portions of the crude material were subjected to simple distillation at about 20 mm pressure, during which 90% of the starting material was taken overhead and condensed as limonene. The still residue comprised 10% of the starting material, plus any additive employed.

The first portion contained no additive, and was distilled without incident even though no caustic was employed. It was considered that the explosion hazard was not great on the laboratory scale experiment. To a second portion, several sodium hydroxide pellets were added prior to distillation. To a third portion, a few grams of calcium hydroxide were added prior to distillation. To a fourth portion, about 50 ml of USP white mineral oil were added prior to distillation. To a fifth portion, about 50 ml of alpha-pinene dimer oil were added prior to distillation. The results of the analyses of the still residues are summarized in the following table.

Additive to still	Percent aldehydes and ketones, hydroxylamine methods	Percent alcohols, by acetylation	Percent esters by saponification
None	6.6	3.9	(1)
NaOH	0	4.1	0
Ca(OH)₂	2.8	4.0	(1)
Mineral oil	9.6	10.8	3.5
Terpene dimer oil	7.2	(1)	(1)

1 Not determined.

The results from Example 1 illustrate that distillation in the presence of sodium hydroxide destroyed all of the valuable aldehydes, ketones, and esters. When the weaker base, calcium hydroxide, was used a minor quantity of the aldehydes and ketones were preserved. In the absence of either base, but in the presence of mineral oil or terpene dimer oil, significantly larger quantities of oxygenated materials were preserved.

Example 2: Limonene resulting from the distillation of crude citrus limonene in Example 1 was used to prepare limonene homopolymers having a ball and ring softening point of 135°C. Polymerization was carried out using aluminum chloride as a catalyst, by a conventional method well-known in the art.

The limonene obtained by distillation in the presence of sodium hydroxide and the limonene obtained by distillation in the presence of USP white mineral oil each gave a resin having a ball and ring softening point of 135°C, in an overall yield of 68% based on the initial weight of crude citrus limonene.

By way of contrast, a homopolymer resin was prepared from the starting crude citrus limonene which had not been subjected to distillation. The overall yield of resin having a ball and ring softening point of 135°C was only 57%.

Example 3: The concentrate of oxygenated materials in the USP white mineral oil from Example 1 was liberated from the still residue by steam distillation, and used to prepare orange drinks and orange gelatin dessert. Both were found to be indistinguishable from commercially available orange drinks and orange gelatin in flavor, aroma, and general palatability.

CAMPHOR, MINTY

3,3,5-Trimethylcycloheptanol and Esters

J.H. Blumenthal; U.S. Patent 3,546,279; December 8, 1970; assigned to International Flavors & Fragrances Inc. describes a process for the conversion of 5,7-dimethyl-1,6-octadiene to a lower alkanoyl ester of 3,3,5-trimethylcycloheptanol, by cyclization of the diene with an acid such as formic or acetic acid in the presence of a strong acid catalyst, preferably at the reflux temperature of the mixture. The esters can be hydrolyzed to the alcohol, which in turn can be converted to the ketone. The compounds are useful as ingredients in perfume compositions. The alcohol prepared has a minty, camphoraceous, rosemary-like odor; the ketone is minty, camphoraceous, cedarleaf and tansy-like; the esters have a woody, piney odor.

Example 1: To a mixture of 2,900 grams of 5,7-dimethyl-1,6-octadiene (84%) and 2,100 g of 90% formic acid was added 264 grams of BF_3-etherate over a period of thirty minutes. The mixture was stirred at 50°C for five hours. After cooling 150 grams of sodium acetate was added and the mixture stirred for ten minutes. After separation, the lower (acid) layer was diluted with an equal volume of water and extracted with benzene. After stripping off the benzene the residue was combined with the original oil layer. The combined crude product weighed 3,804 grams and contained 49.8% formate ester (49% conversion).

One-third (1,291 grams) of the above crude ester was rushed-over to give 882 grams of distilled material testing 65.9% ester. Fractionation of the distilled ester yielded 3,3,5-trimethylcycloheptyl formate (mixture of two isomers). BP 80°C/55 mm.

Example 2: Two-thirds of the crude ester (2,540 grams from Example 1) was washed once with water and then saponified by refluxing with 1,560 grams of methyl alcohol, 624 grams of 50% sodium hydroxide and 180 cc of water for 1.5 hours. After workup, the crude alcohol weighed 1,590 grams and tested 68.7% (46.5% conversion based on diene). Rush-over of 779 grams of the crude alcohol yielded 565 grams of distilled product testing 81.5% (42% conversion based on diene). Fractionation of the distilled alcohol yielded 3,3,5-trimethylcycloheptanol (mixture of isomers). BP 90°C/9mm.

1-Methyl-2-Hydroxy-3-Oxatricyclononane

T.W. Gibson; U.S. Patent 3,522,276; July 28, 1970; assigned to Procter & Gamble Company describes the synthesis of 1-methyl-2-hydroxy-3-oxatricyclo[5.2.0.0^{4,9}] nonane which has an odor characterized as strong green-pithy camphoraceous and is useful in the perfume arts. This compound can be readily oxidized to 1-methyl-2-oxo-3-oxatricyclo[5.2.0.0^{4,9}] nonane, a compound that is also useful in the perfume art.

The synthesis of 1-methyl-2-hydroxy-3-oxatricyclo[5.2.0.0^{4,9}] nonane comprises nitrosylating cis-nopinol to form cis-2-nopinyl nitrite; irradiating the nitrite with ultraviolet light to form 8-nitroso-cis-nopinol dimer; pyrolyzing the dimer to form 8-oximino-cis-nopinol; and hydrolyzing the oxime to form 1-methyl-2-hydroxy-3-oxatricyclo[5.2.0.0^{4,9}] nonane. An optional step in this process comprises oxidizing this compound to form 1-methyl-2-oxo-3-oxatricyclo-[5.2.0.0^{4,9}] nonane.

Example: To a solution of 15.4 grams cis-nopinol in 200 ml dry pyridine was added 11.0 g NOCl by flask distillation, at 0°C. After another hour at 0°C, the mixture was allowed to warm to room temperature, poured into 1.5 liters water, and extracted with ether. The ether solution was washed with water, cold dilute HCl, and again with water. After drying over MgSO$_4$, filtration and removal of solvent gas, 18.6 grams of cis-2-nopinyl nitrite was left.

18.6 grams of the nitrite was dissolved in 430 ml cyclohexane, placed in a photochemical reaction flask equipped with a Vycor immersion well, and irradiated at room temperature with a 450 watt mercury lamp for 6 hours to yield, after removal of solvent, 14.2 grams of 8-nitroso-cis-nopinol dimer.

14.2 grams of the dimer was dissolved in 400 ml isopropyl alcohol and refluxed for 36 hours at 82°C. Under these conditions the dimer pyrolyzes to 8-oximino-cis-nopinol. Removal of solvent gave 10.5 grams which solidified on standing. Recrystallization from pentane-ether gave 8-oximino-cis-nopinol with MP 121° to 122°C. Analysis is calculated for C$_9$H$_{15}$NO$_2$ (%): C, 63.88; H, 8.94; N, 8.28. Found (%): C, 63.95; H, 8.96; N, 8.16.

9.5 grams of the 8-oximino-cis-nopinol was dissolved in 570 ml 80% acetone-water containing 2% concentrated HCl and stirred overnight at room temperature. The solution was poured into water, extracted with ether, and the ether solution washed with saturated NaHCO$_3$ and saturated NaCl, dried over MgSO$_4$, filtered and stripped to 5.0 grams of 1-methyl-2-hydroxy-3-oxatricyclo[5.2.0.0^{4,9}] nonane. Continuous extraction of the aqueous phase gave an additional 2.69 (87% total yield) of the product. Formation of a 2,4-dinonyl phthalate derivative, MP 177° to 178°C, was carried out in H$_3$PO$_4$-ethanol solution. Analysis is calculated for C$_{15}$H$_{18}$N$_4$O$_5$, percent: C, 53.88; H, 5.43; N, 16.76. Found, percent: C, 53.99; H, 5.51; N, 17.29.

Oxidation of 0.409 gram of 1-methyl-2-hydroxy-3-oxatricyclo[5.2.0.0^{4,9}] nonane with 0.2 g CrO$_3$ in 25 ml acetone at 70°C gave 0.350 gram of 1-methyl-2-oxo-3-oxatricyclo[5.2.0.0^{4,9}]-nonane, BP 83° to 84°C. A perfume composition was prepared by intermixing the following components.

Component	Percent by Weight
1-methyl-2-hydroxy-3-oxatricyclo-[5.2.0.0^{4,9}] nonane	5.00
Benzyl acetate	22.00
Cassia	0.50
Cinnamic alcohol	4.50
Clove buds	8.00
Coumarin	4.00
Hydroxycitronellal	2.00
Lavender 40/42	11.00
Patchouli	4.00
Spike Lavender	22.00
Rosemary Spanish	17.00

Photochemical Reactions of 4-Caranone

P.J. Kropp; U.S. Patent 3,560,571; February 2, 1971; assigned to The Procter & Gamble Company describes the photochemical reaction of 4-caranone to obtain the compounds, 2-(2'-methyl-2'-but-3'-enyl)-4-methylcyclobutanone and 2,2,5-trimethyl-3-vinylcyclopenta-none, and the process of converting 3-carene to 4-caranone by epoxidizing 3-carene and, subsequently, treating that product with a Lewis acid catalyst. The process comprises the steps of (1) treating 3-carene having the general formula:

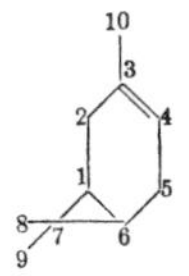

with a peracid having the structural formula, RCO_3H, where R is any alkyl group containing from 1 to 20 carbon atoms or any aryl group containing from 6 to 18 carbon atoms to obtain 3,4-epoxycarane having the general formula:

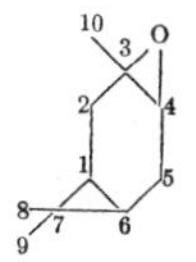

(2) Treating the 3,4-epoxycarane with a Lewis acid catalyst to obtain 4-caranone having the general formula:

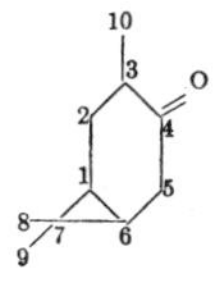

(3) Subjecting 4-caranone, which is obtained by the above method or conventional techniques, to ultraviolet irradiation to form a mixture of 2-(2'-methyl-2'-but-3'-enyl)-4-methyl-cyclobutanone having the general formula:

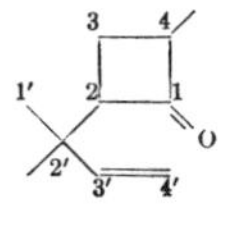

and 2,2,5-trimethyl-3-vinylcyclopentanone having the general formula:

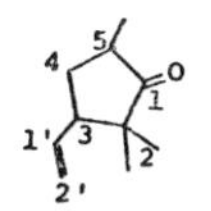

The ketone compounds prepared by the photochemical reaction both have highly desirable and useful odors. The odor of the mixture of the two ketones is characterized as a camphoraceous note being somewhat dry and minty.

P.J. Kropp; U.S. Patent 3,686,097; August 22, 1972; assigned to The Procter & Gamble Company describes additional work with irradiation of 4-caranone to give perfume compositions containing 4-caranone, 2-(2'-methyl-2'-but-3'-enyl)-4-methylcyclobutanone and 2,2,5-trimethyl-3-vinylcyclopentanone, para-menth-3-en-2-one.

Bicyclo[3.3.1] Nonyl Compounds

H.C. Kretschmar; U.S. Patent 3,524,884; August 18, 1970; assigned to The Procter & Gamble Company describes the intramolecular cyclization of cis-4-cyclooctene-1-carboxylic acid chloride to form bicyclo [3.3.1] nonyl compounds which are useful in perfume and flavor compositions.

The intramolecular cyclization process comprises: heating cis-4-cyclooctene-1-carboxylic acid chloride to form bicyclo[3.3.1] non-2-en-9-one, 2-exo-chlorobicyclo[3.3.1] nonan-9-one, and 2-endo-chlorobicyclo[3.3.1] nonan-9-one.

Cis-4-cyclooctene-1-carboxylic acid chloride, the starting material for the reaction, can be readily prepared from the corresponding cis-4-cyclooctene-1-carboxylic acid. This acid can also be easily prepared in three steps from the commercially available material cyclooctadiene according to the method of K. Ziegler and H. Wilms as described in *Ann. 567,* 1 (1950). The compounds have an odor defined as a grassy-weedy camphoraceous note with a musty-woody background.

Unsaturated Bicyclic Cyclobutanones Using Irradiation

H.C. Kretschmar; U.S. Patent 3,417,143; December 17, 1968; assigned to The Procter & Gamble Company describes a photochemical process which comprises irradiating a β,γ-unsaturated bicyclic-cyclohexenone compound of the formula:

$(CH_2)_n$

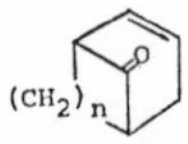

with ultraviolet light to produce a β,γ-unsaturated bicyclic-cyclobutanone compound of the formula:

$(CH_2)_n$

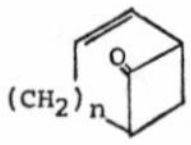

where n is an integer of 2 or 3.

The specific compounds (n is 2 or 3) prepared by the above described process are illustrated in the following table. Bicyclo[3.2.1] oct-2-en-8-one and bicyclo[3.3.1] non-2-en-9-one, the β,γ-unsaturated bicyclic-cyclohexenone starting materials in the photochemical process can be prepared by a multi-step synthesis starting with cyclopentanone or cyclohexenone respectively. More specifically, the process for the preparation of these starting materials is disclosed by Foote and Woodward in *Tetrahedron* 20, 687 (1964).

In carrying out the photochemical rearrangement of the starting material to the β,γ-unsaturated bicyclocyclo-butanone product, any convenient source of ultraviolet radiation can be used, i.e., a light source that emits photo-energy at wavelengths between 250 mμ and 500 mμ. The wavelength of irradiation is preferably concentrated about the maximum absorption line of the starting material, i.e., at wavelengths between about 280 and 320 mμ.

	β,γ-Unsaturated Bicyclic-cyclohexenone	$\xrightarrow[\longleftarrow]{h\nu}$	β,γ-Unsaturated Bicyclic-cyclobutanone (Product)
	$(CH_2)_n$		$(CH_2)_n$
n = 2	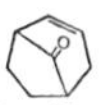 bicyclo[3.2.1]oct-2-en-8-one		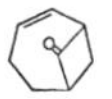 bicyclo[4.1.1]oct-2-en-8-one
n = 3	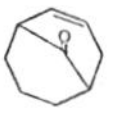 bicyclo[3.3.1]non-2-en-9-one		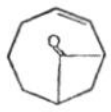 bicyclo[5.1.1]non-2-en-9-one

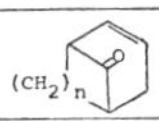

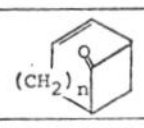

Tricyclo[3.2.1.0^{2,7}]Oct-3-en-8-ones

H. Schmid and J. Zsindely; U.S. Patent 3,711,553; January 16, 1973; assigned to Hoffmann-La Roche Inc. describe compounds of the formula:

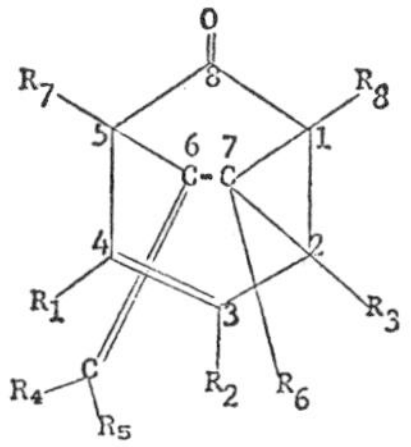

where R_1, R_2 and R_3 are independently selected from the group consisting of hydrogen, halogen, hydroxy, lower alkyl, lower alkyloxy, lower alkylamino, amino, di(lower alkyl)-amino, mercapto and lower alkyl mercapto; R_4 and R_5 are independently selected from the group consisting of hydrogen, lower alkyl and lower alkoxy; R_6 is hydrogen or lower alkyl and R_7 and R_8 are independently selected from the group consisting of hydrogen, lower alkyl and lower alkoxy with the proviso that at least one of R_7 and R_8 is lower alkyl or lower alkoxy; and acid addition salts.

These compounds and their acid addition salts have a camphor-like odor. The compounds and their acid addition salts because of their fragrance, are useful in the preparation of perfumes, colognes and other scented compositions. The compounds can be prepared by heating ethers of the formula:

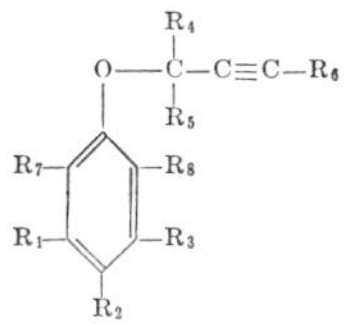

where R_1, R_2, R_3, R_4, R_5, R_6, R_7 and R_8 are as above, or cyclohexadienones of the formula shown on the following page.

(1)

$$\begin{array}{c} O \\ R_7 - \overset{\|}{C} - R_8 \\ R_1 - \underset{}{\bigcirc} - R_3 \\ R_2' \quad \overset{R_4}{\underset{R_5}{C}} - C \equiv C - R_6 \end{array}$$

R_1, R_3, R_4, R_5, R_6, R_7 and R_8 are as described above and R_2 is selected from the group consisting of halogen, hydroxy, lower alkyl, lower alkyloxy, lower alkylamino, amino, di-(lower alkyl)amino, mercapto and lower alkyl mercapto. The ethers are heated to a temperature of from 50° to 200°C. The following examples illustrate the process. In the examples, all temperatures are in degrees centigrade and the ether utilized is diethyl ether.

Example 1: One gram of 2,6-dimethylphenyl propargyl ether in 2 grams of n-decane are heated at 185°C for 9 hours in a degassed, evacuated bomb-tube. After this period, the reaction mixture is chromatographed on 45 grams of silica gel with a hexane-benzene mixture (1 to 1 parts by volume). In this manner, the n-decane and unreacted starting ether are separated off. For further purification, the product is chromatographed on 30 grams of silica gel with a pentane-ether mixture (19:1 parts by volume) and distilled in a bulb-tube. Tricyclo[3.2.1.0^{2,7}]-1,5-dimethyl-6-methylidene-oct-3-en-8-one is obtained. BP 90° to 93°C (air-bath)/10 mm Hg; 35° to 40°C (air-bath)/0.01 mm Hg.

Example 2: 61 grams of 2,6-dimethylphenol (0.5 mol), 71.9 grams of propargyl bromide (0.6 mol) and 76 grams of freshly ignited and powdered potassium carbonate (0.55 mol) in 115 ml of acetone are heated at reflux for 14 hours. The inorganic salts are thereupon filtered off. The acetone and the excess propargyl bromide are distilled off via a column and the oily residue is dissolved in pentane. The resulting solution is washed with Claisen's lye (35 grams of caustic potash, 25 ml of water and 65 ml of methanol) and water, dried over sodium sulfate, filtered, evaporated and distilled. 2,6-Dimethylphenyl propargyl ether is obtained. BP 50° to 51°C/0.02 mm Hg.

Example 3: One gram of 2,6-dimethylphenyl 2'-butynyl ether in 2 grams of n-decane is heated at 185°C for 14 hours in a bomb-tube. After this period, the reaction mixture is chromatographed on 45 grams of silica gel with a hexane-benzene mixture (1 to 1 parts by volume). In this manner, n-decane and the unreacted starting ether are separated off. For further purification, the product is chromatographed on 30 grams of silica gel with a pentane ether mixture (19 to 1 parts by volume) and distilled in a bulb-tube. Tricyclo-[3.2.1.0^{2,7}]-6-methylidene-1,5,7-trimethyl-oct-3-en-8-one is obtained. BP 40° to 45°C (air-bath)/0.01 mm Hg.

2-Methylenecycloalkane Carboxylic Acids

Y. Bonnet; U.S. Patent 3,455,991; July 15, 1969; assigned to Rhone-Poulenc SA, France describes the preparation of 2-methylenecycloalkane carboxylic acids, esters and amides of the formula:

$$R \overset{\displaystyle CH-CO-Z}{\underset{\displaystyle C=CH_2}{\Big\langle}}$$

where R is an optionally substituted polymethylene radical of formula $-(CH_2)_n-$, where n is 3 to 15, Z is $-OR^1$ or $-NR^2R^3$, where R^1 is hydrogen or alkyl of 1 to 4 carbon atoms and R^2 and R^3, which are the same or different, represent alkyl, alkenyl, cycloalkyl, cyclo-alkylalkyl, aryl or aralkyl radicals, and R^2 may also represent hydrogen, or R^2 and R^3 are linked together to form a saturated or unsaturated divalent organic radical, optionally containing one or more hetero atom, such as O, S or N.

The process for the preparation of the compounds of Formula (1) comprises (a) halogenating an aminomethyl-cycloalkanone of formula:

(2)

$$\begin{array}{l} \text{—CH}_2 \\ \text{R} \quad \text{CO} \qquad \qquad \text{R}^2 \\ \text{—CH—CH}_2\text{—N} \\ \qquad \qquad \qquad \text{R}^3 \end{array}$$

R, R^2 and R^3 being as defined above so as to produce a halo-compound of formula:

(3)

$$\begin{array}{l} \text{—CHX} \\ \text{R} \quad \text{CO} \qquad \qquad \text{R}^2 \\ \text{—CH—CH}_2\text{—N} \\ \qquad \qquad \qquad \text{R}^3 \end{array}$$

where X is halogen, e.g., chlorine or bromine, and then (b) reacting the halo-compound with a mineral alkaline substance in an alcohol of formula R'—OH (where R' is alkyl of 1 to 4 carbon atoms) so as to produce a mixture of compounds of Formula (1) in which Z is OR' and —NR^2R^3.

It is known that when a compound containing an N-substituted-aminomethyl substituent is heated in the presence of an alkaline agent, decomposition occurs which gives rise to a compound containing a methylene group with the liberation of a secondary amine in accordance with the equation:

$$>\text{CH—CH}_2\text{N}< \longrightarrow >\text{C}=\text{CH}_2 + \text{HN}<$$

It is also known that, by the action of an alkaline agent, α-mono halogenated-cycloalkanones are converted, in accordance with Favorskii's reaction into cycloalkanecarboxylic acids having in their nucleus one carbon atom less than the treated ketone, the hydracid corresponding to the halogen being liberated.

It has been found that, by reacting one molecule of a compound of the Formula (2) with one molecule of a halogen, or an equivalent quantity of another halogenating agent, an N-substituted-α'-monohalogeno-α-aminomethylcycloalkanone of the Formula (3) is obtained, and that when this compound is subjected to the action of an alkaline agent in an alcoholic medium, a mixture of ester and amide of Formula (1) is obtained in which the ring contains one carbon atom less than the ring of the starting material of Formula (2).

These compounds may be used as intermediates in organic synthesis. In addition methyl 2-methylenecycloundecane carboxylate has a pleasant odor, and is useful in perfumery, as it imparts to compositions containing it a delicate and balanced woody, camphor like and minty scent. The following examples illustrate the process.

Example 1: Preparation of 12-Bromo-2-Dimethylaminomethylcyclododecanone — Into a 500 cc three-necked, round-bottomed flask provided with a reflux condenser, a dropping funnel and a stirring system, 17.8 grams (0.074 mol) of 2-dimethylaminomethylcyclodo-decanone, 130 grams of glacial acetic acid and 40 grams of acetic anhydride are introduced.

12.7 grams of a 48% aqueous hydrobromic acid solution are then added with stirring in ten minutes. At the end of the addition, the temperature in the mixture reaches 60°C. It is then raised to boiling point and 12.8 grams of bromine in solution in 25 cc of glacial acetic acid are added in fifteen minutes and the boiling is then maintained for 30 minutes. The acetic acid is removed by distillation in vacuo, and the solid residue obtained is finely ground and then taken up in 60 cc of diethyl ether.

After filtration, the solid product is dried in an oven in vacuo and 29.5 grams of crystals of pale beige color are obtained, MP 133° to 134°C, identified by nuclear magnetic resonance as 12-bromo-2-dimethylaminomethylcyclododecanone hydrobromide. The yield is 99%. From the hydrobromide thus obtained, the amine is liberated as follows. 25.5 grams of the hydrobromide, 135 cc of diethyl ether, and 135 cc of water are introduced into an apparatus identical with that previously described, and 7.7 cc of an aqueous 10% ammonia solution are added with stirring at normal temperature. Stirring is continued until the hydrobromide has completely dissolved. The ethereal layer is separated, washed to neutrality with water and then dried over anhydrous sodium sulfate, and the solvent is driven off. 16.8 grams of a white crystalline product, MP 65° to 69°C, are thus collected which, after recrystallization from a mixture of diethyl ether and pentane (10.90 percent by volume), has a melting point of 73° to 73.5°C, and is identified by nuclear magnetic resonance as 12-bromo-2-dimethylaminomethylcyclododecanone.

2-Dimethylaminomethylcyclododecanone was prepared by the reaction of cyclododecanone with dimethylamine hydrochloride and trioxymethylene, by the process described in Belgian Patent 601,671.

Preparation of Methyl 2-Methylenecycloundecane Carboxylate — Into a 1,000 cc three-necked, round-bottomed flask provided with a reflux condenser and a stirring system, 63.6 g of 12-bromo-2-dimethylaminomethylcyclododecanone, 34 grams of sodium bicarbonate and 600 cc of methanol are introduced. Stirring is started and the mixture is raised to the boiling point and maintained at this temperature for 20 hours. By distillation, followed by evaporation under the vacuum of a water jet pump, the methanol is removed and the residue is then taken up in 200 cc of diethyl ether and 100 cc of water. To the separated ethereal layer 100 cc of a 10% aqueous hydrochloric acid solution are added and the ethereal solution is then washed to neutrality with water and dried over anhydrous sodium sulfate.

On evaporation of the ether, 37 grams of a yellow oil are obtained, which is saponified with 40 grams of caustic potash in 400 cc of methanol with heating under reflux for six hours with stirring. The methanol is driven off in a vacuum and 200 cc of water are then added. The organic layer is extracted with 200 cc of diethyl ether and separated. The ethereal layer is then washed to neutrality with water and dried over sodium sulfate.

After elimination of the ether, 20.4 grams of an oily product are collected which, on distillation in vacuo, gives 16.8 grams of a colorless product, BP 121° to 121.5°C/0.1 mm Hg, identified as 1-dimethylcarbamoyl-2-methylenecycloundecane.

The aqueous layer of the saponified reaction mass, which has been separated from the organic layer, is combined with the washing liquors of the ethereal extract of this layer. The mixture is acidifed to a pH of 1 by adding 270 cc of a 10% aqueous hydrochloric acid solution. The solution is then extracted with 100 cc of diethyl ether, and the ethereal layer is washed to neutrality with water and dried over anhydrous sodium sulfate.

By evaporation of the ether, 15.3 grams of a solid product are isolated, MP 50° to 53°C which, after recrystallization from a mixture of diethyl ether and pentane (50:50 by volume), has a melting point of 60°C. This product, which is identified by nuclear magnetic resonance, is 2-methylenecycloundecane carboxylic acid. Esterification of this acid with methanol gives methyl 2-methylenecycloundecane carboxylate, which is a colorless product, BP 100° to 101°C/0.1 mm Hg, having a pleasant woody odor.

TOBACCO

Alkyl Ethers of Dihydrocaryophyllene Alcohol

J.D. Grossman; U.S. Patent 3,531,532; September 29, 1970; assigned to International Flavors & Fragrances Inc. describes lower alkyl ethers of dihydrocaryophyllene alcohol and dihydroisocaryophyllene alcohol and their use in perfume and fragrance compositions.

Caryophyllene is a naturally occurring material found in oil of cloves, as obtained from the flower-heads of *Eugenia caryophyllata*. It is a sesquiterpene material which is also found in certain species of the genus Pinus. The elucidation of the caryophyllene structure has received attention, and Ramage & Whitehead show the structure of both normal (β-caryophyllene) and isocaryophyllene (γ-caryophyllene) in *J.Chem. Soc.* Part IV, 4336 et seq. (1954). It is known to obtain epoxides of both the abovementioned caryophyllenes by treatment of these materials with peracids and then to reduce the epoxides to the corresponding alcohols.

This process provides two preferred ethers, namely: 6-methoxy-2,6,10,10-tetramethyl[7.2.0]-undecane having the formula:

(1)

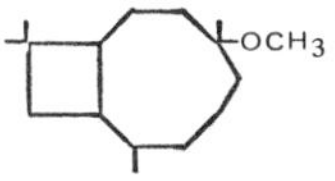

and 5-methoxy-2,6,10,10-tetramethyl[7.2.0] undecane having the formula:

(2)

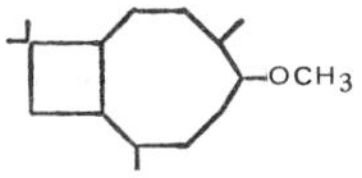

The starting materials used in the preparation of the ethers are the two dihydro alcohols which can ultimately be derived from caryophyllene or isocaryophyllene. The ethers are obtained from the alcohols by treatment with a metal hydride followed by treatment with an alkyl sulfate or halide.

The starting material can be either caryophyllene having the formula:

(3)

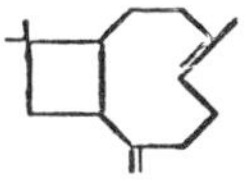

or isocaryophyllene having the formula:

(4)

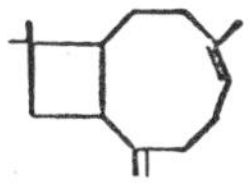

The caryophyllene or isocaryophyllene ultimate starting material is treated with a peracid to form epoxides. After epoxidation the unsaturated epoxides are hydrogenated to obtain the corresponding saturated alcohol. After suitable purification, the dihydro alcohol is esterified.

The ethers are desirably prepared by treating the dihydro alcohols with an alkali-metal hydride to form the alcoholate and then treating the alcoholate with an alkyl sulfate or halide. Alkali-metal hydrides such as lithium hydride, sodium hydride, potassium hydride, and the like can be used. A preferred hydride is sodium hydride. The amount of hydride should be about stoichiometric. The following examples illustrate the process.

Example 1: Alcohol Preparation — Dihydrocaryophyllene alcohol is prepared by hydrogenating 2 kg of epoxidized caryophyllene in the presence of 200 grams of Raney nickel and 200 grams of isopropyl alcohol as a solvent. The hydrogenation is carried out at 500 to 1,000 psig and 50° to 90°C for five hours. The catalyst is removed by filtration and the solvent is stripped off. The product is then purified by fractional distillation at reduced pressure (0.5 to 0.9 mm Hg). The product has a boiling point of 39° to 117°C at 0.65 to 0.9 mm Hg and is of sufficient purity for conversion to the lower alkyl ether.

Ether Preparation — A suspension of 310 grams of commercial sodium hydride (52% in mineral oil) is heated in 2,200 cc of toluene under a nitrogen atmosphere. At reflux temperature a solution of 1,386 grams of dihydrocaryophyllene alcohols produced above and 1,100 cc of toluene is introduced into the refluxing mass with efficient stirring. Reflux of the mixture and the stirring are continued until the theoretical amount (136 liters) of hydrogen is evolved.

The reaction mass is maintained at reflux while 860 grams of dimethyl sulfate is added over two hours. After addition is complete reflux is continued for another fifty minutes. The reaction mixture is cooled to 25°C and poured into two liters of cold 10% aqueous sodium hydroxide. The upper layer of ether product in toluene is washed with an equal volume of saturated aqueous sodium chloride. Toluene is recovered under a pressure of 50 mm Hg, and the remaining 1,400 grams of crude product is purified by fractional distillation utilizing 15 grams of triethanolamine in the distillation flask. The product obtained from the distillation has a fine woody, tobacco aroma. The liquid has a boiling point of 84° to 88°C at 0.5 mm Hg.

Example 2: Alcohol Preparation — Isocaryophyllene epoxides (883 grams) are hydrogenated using 90 grams of Raney nickel catalyst and 225 grams of isopropyl alcohol as solvent. The hydrogenation is carried out at 500 to 1,100 psig and 35° to 95°C for five hours. The catalyst is thereupon removed by filtration and the product is purified by fractional distillation after the solvent has been stripped off. The product has a boiling point of 96° to 110°C at 1.0 to 0.9 mm Hg.

Ether Preparation — A suspension of 110 grams of sodium hydride (52% in mineral oil) in 700 cc of toluene is heated to reflux. At reflux a solution of 493 grams of dihydro-isocaryophyllene alcohol, produced above, in 400 cc of toluene is added. The mixture is then refluxed for ten hours. The reflux is continued while 302.3 grams of dimethyl sulfate is added over two hours. After an additional thirty minutes of reflux, the reaction mixture is cooled and poured into 2 liters of cold 10% aqueous sodium hydroxide. The top layer containing toluene and product is separated and washed with an equal volume of sodium chloride solution. The toluene is evaporated from the product at 50 mm Hg to obtain 530 grams of crude material which is then purified by fractional distillation.

The finished product is a mixture of ethers (1) and (2) with a boiling point of 80° to 84°C at 0.15 to 0.3 mm Hg. The mixtures of ethers produced above can be separated into individual isomers, and these individual isomers are also useful in the preparation of perfume and fragrance materials.

Example 3: A perfume composition is prepared with the following ingredients:

Ingredient	Parts
Vetivert oil	40
Methyl ether obtained from Example 1	85
Sandalwood oil	100
Rose geranium oil	200
Musk ambrette	25
Benzyl-iso-eugenol	100
Coumarin	100
Heliotropin	50
Bois de rose oil	200
Benzoin resin	100

The perfume composition exhibits an excellent woody fragrance. When the process ether is omitted, the composition lacks the woody fulness. In comparison with caryophyllene alcohol and dihydrocaryophyllene alcohol, the process ether is found to have a much stronger, richer woody, tobacco odor character which renders it highly useful in the preparation of fragrances and perfumes.

Lactones from 2-Substituted Aldehydes Using Lead Dioxide

J.C. Leffingwell; U.S. Patent 3,658,849; April 25, 1972; assigned to R.J. Reynolds Tobacco Company describe a process for producing substituted γ-lactones and substituted alkenoxy-alcohols from 2-substituted aldehydes using lead dioxide. The following example illustrates the process.

Example 1: A mixture of 55 grams (0.76 mol) isobutyraldehyde, 255 grams (1.07 mols) lead dioxide and 300 cubic centimeters dioxane was prepared and stirred at reflux under a nitrogen atmosphere for a period of 24 hours, then cooled and filtered. The lead oxides were washed with diethyl ether and the combined filtrates stripped of solvent and any un-reacted starting material to give 51.6 grams (94%) crude products. The material was ana-lyzed by vapor-phase chromatography on a 6 foot, ¼ inch, 15% Carbowax column and the there major components purified and isolated by preparative gas chromatography.

The first major compound eluting comprised 23% of the volatile components and was iden-tified as 2-methyl-2-(2'-methyl-1'-propenoxy)-propanol from its spectral characteristics com-pared to those of an authentic sample prepared from the lithium aluminum hydride reduc-tion of 2-methyl-2-(2'-methyl-1'-propenoxy)-propionaldehyde.

The second major product, comprising 14% of the volatile components was identified as tetramethylsuccinaldehyde by comparison with an authentic sample.

The third major component, which accounted for 40% of volatile components, was a white crystalline solid with a marked camphoraceous odor. This material, melting point 97° to 101°C, was identified as the lactone of 2,2,3,3-tetramethyl-4-hydroxybutyric acid by com-parison of its spectra with that of an authentic sample. The substitued γ-lactones find utility as odorants in perfumes and as tobacco flavorants.

Bicyclic Dehydropiperazines

A.O. Pittet, R. Muralidhara and E.T. Theimer; U.S. Patent 3,705,158; December 5, 1972; assigned to International Flavors & Fragrances, Inc. have found that bicyclic dehydropiper-azines are capable of imparting a wide variety of flavors to various consumable materials. The process contemplates altering the flavors of such consumable materials by adding there-to a small but effective amount of at least one bicyclic dehydropiperazine having the for-mula:

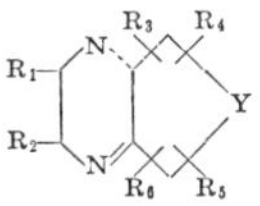

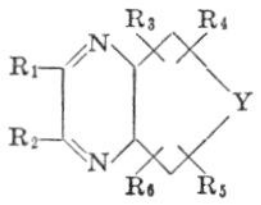

where Y is $(-CH_2-)_n$; n is an integer from one to six, inclusive; one dashed line represents a double bond and the other represents a single bond; and R_1, R_2, R_3, R_4, R_5, and R_6 re-present hydrogen or alkyl and are the same or different.

A particularly preferred bicyclic piperazine is 5-methyl-3,4,6,7-tetrahydro-2(H)-cyclopenta-pyrazine having the structure

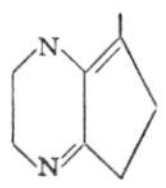

This is a crystalline solid having a melting point of 117° to 121°C. It has a roasted nut, burnt aroma.

Another material according to the process is 5-methyl-3,5,6,7-tetrahydro-2(H)-cyclopenta-pyrazine having the structure

The bicyclic dehydropiperazines can be obtained by a number of reaction routes, as by reacting diaminocycloalkane or monoalkyl- or polyalkyl-substituted diaminocycloalkane with glyoxal (a dioxoalkane) or 1-alkyl or 1,2-dialkyl derivatives thereof, e.g., 2,3-butan-dione, under ring closing conditions, or by reacting ethylenediamine or an alkyl or 1,2-dialkyl derivative thereof with a 1,2-cycloalkadione or a mono- or polyalkyl derivative there-of. The following examples illustrate the process.

Example 1: A five liter Morton flask equipped with an agitator, thermometer, reflux con-denser, addition funnel, and gas sparging tube is charged with a solution of 114.2 grams (1.0 mol) of 1,2-diaminocyclohexane in 2,700 ml of 95% ethanol. The flask contents are cooled to -20°C, and 159.8 grams (1.1 mol) of 40% aqueous glyoxal is added during ten minutes. About 2 to 3 minutes after the addition is complete, the reaction mixture as-sumes a milky, heterogenous appearance. The mixture is then stirred for two hours at -20°C. The resulting mixture is found to have an intense popcorn aroma. The mixture is found by mass spectroscopy to contain the 4a,5,6,7,8,8a-hexahydroquinoxaline.

Example 2: A reaction mixture is prepared by dissolving 12.4 grams 3-methyl-2-hydroxy-2-cyclopenten-1-one (the enol form of 3-methyl-1,2-cyclopentadione) in 10 grams of eth-ylenediamine. The mixture is then stirred at room temperature (23°C) and an exothermic reaction takes place. The mixture thickens and after two hours forms a solid crystalline mass.

The solid mass is dissolved in 50 ml of methylene chloride and washed with 10 ml of water. The water layer is back-washed with an equal volume of methylene chloride, and the com-bined methylene chloride solutions are evaporated to dryness to yield 15.2 grams of a crystalline mass having a bready, nut-like aroma. The product is purified by sublimation.

The product obtained is 5-methyl-3,4,6,7-tetrahydro-2(H)-cyclopentapyrazine. Infrared (IR) analysis indicates an NH band, and mass spectroscopy shows a molecular weight of 136. The material has a good nut-like aroma suggestive of tobacco and burns well with natural tobacco. The odor is also similar to that of fresh baked goods in a one percent solution in 95% ethanol. The taste in water at 5 ppm is near the threshold level with a pleasant, sweet, light roasted, buttery note. A 20 ppm aqueous solution has a melted butter flavor character; a 50 ppm solution, a bread-crust character. A 50 ppm solution in sugar water has a flavor like fresh sugar cookies or fresh corn flakes. In salt water at 50 ppm it has a taste reminiscent of fresh baked pretzels, with a bread-crust flavor note.

Example 3: The preparation of 2,3-dimethyl-4a,5,6,7,8,8a-hexahydroquinoxaline is as follows. A Morton flask equipped with agitator, thermometer, condenser, addition funnel, gas dispersion tube, and cooling means is charged with 11.40 grams of 1,2-diaminocyclo-hexane in 200 cc of 95% ethanol. During a 20 minute period a solution of 816 grams of 2,3-butanedione is added dropwise. The temperature rises from 25° to 37°C and the flask contents turn milky-white upon such addition. The reaction mixture turns clear after fif-teen minutes.

The ethanol is removed by evaporation under reduced pressure and the residue is distilled under vacuum yielding 16.1 grams of product boiling at 72° to 76°C at 1.4 to 1.7 mm Hg. Gas chromatographic (GC) analysis shows a mixture of the cis and trans isomers, and the material has a broad melting range of 60° to 110°C. Initially a white solid, the product discolors on storage. The material has a clear wood, tobacco, buttery odor. In chocolate beverages it imparts a bitter character without the addition of any foreign flavor note. In a soap bouquet perfume composition, the compound can be used to replace natural cedarwood. Other 2,3-dialkylhexahydroquinoxalines or 2-alkylhexahydroquinoxalines can be similarly prepared by utilizing other 1,2-dialkyl glyoxals or 1-alkylglyoxals instead of 2,3-butanedione.

Example 4: The preparation of 5,7,7-trimethyl-2,3,4,6,7,8-hexahydroquinoxaline is as follows. A mixture of 6 grams (0.1 mol) of ethylenediamine and 15.4 grams (0.1 mol) of 2-hydroxy-3,5,5-trimethyl-2-cyclohexen-1-one (the enol form of 3,5,5-trimethyl-1,2-cyclohexandione) is refluxed for five hours in one liter of benzene in a three liter flask fitted with a Bidwell-Sterling distillation receiver. During the refluxing, 3.5 ml of water is collected. After refluxing is completed, the solvent is stripped off. The resulting trimethyl substituted reduced bicyclic pyrazine has a tobacco, nougat aroma in a 0.2% solution in 95% ethanol. In aqueous solution at 0.4 ppm it has a fruity taste with tobacco leaf and cedarwood notes. It is suitable for honey, nougat, and tobacco flavors.

Dihydroisocaryophyllene Epoxide

A process developed by *J.D. Grossman; U.S. Patent 3,620,982; November 16, 1971; assigned to International Flavors & Fragrances, Inc.* provides dihydroisocaryophyllene epoxide, which has a superior woody fragrance note with a very desirable tobacco-like quality. This compound also denominated 5,6-epoxy-2-cis-6,10,10-tetramethylbicyclo[7.2.0] undecane, has the formula:

(1)

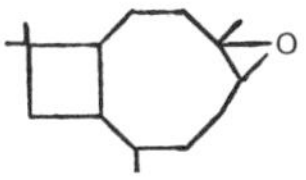

The starting material for use in the process can be either caryophyllene having the formula:

(2)

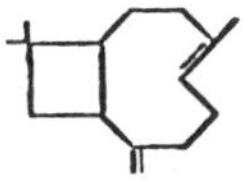

or isocaryophyllene having the formula:

(3)

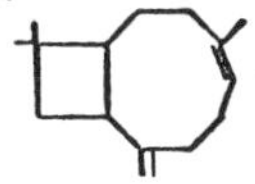

When the starting material is caryophyllene, it is first converted to isocaryophyllene by well-known methods, such as photochemically by the method of Schulte-Elte et al, *Helv. Chem. Acta,* Vol. 51, Fasc. 3, pp 494-505 (1968) or by treatment with nitrous acid. It is preferred that the isocaryophyllene utilized in the process be refined to a purity of at least 90% to minimize the formation of undesired by-products which complicate recovery and reduce the odor intensity of finished epoxide (1). The isocaryophyllene starting material containing little or no caryophyllene is treated with a peracid to form the epoxide.

After oxidation the isocaryophyllene epoxide isomers so produced are hydrogenated to add a mole of hydrogen to the oxide molecule. The hydrogenation is carried out under mild conditions which will hydrogenate the methylene group without reducing the epoxide linkage.

It is preferred to carry out this hydrogenation with metallic catalysts, especially precious metal catalysts such as palladium, platinum, rhodium, and the like. A preferred catalyst is palladium on calcium carbonate. The amount of catalyst used is from 0.1 to 10% of the isocaryophyllene oxide.

After hydrogenation is substantially completed, the reaction product is separated from the catalyst by suitable means such as settling, centrifugation and filtering. Fractional distillation is a preferred method of purifying epoxide (1). The dihydro epoxide (1) so produced has a BP of 85° to 86°C at 0.2 mm Hg, a refractive index of 1.4795, and a specific rotation in sodium D light of –4.24° at 20°C. The purified product has an intense, persistent woody odor with a very fine tobacco-like character.

Example 1: Isocaryophyllene is prepared from caryophyllene by treatment of the latter with nitrous acid, as shown in *Annalen,* 1907, 356, 1. Into a 12 liter flask equipped with a stirrer, thermometer, condenser, and dropping funnel are charged 2,250 grams of such isocaryophyllene and 298 grams of anhydrous sodium acetate, and the contents of the flask are cooled to 0°C with a Dry Ice bath. Forty percent peracetic acid (2,182 grams) is added to the flask very slowly with rapid stirring. The reaction is strongly exothermic, and the rate of addition is controlled to maintain the temperature at from 0° to 5°C. A 2.5 hour time is necessary for the peracetic acid addition, after which the flask contents are maintained at 0° to 5°C for 3 hours, during which interval the course of the reaction is monitored via gas/liquid phase chromatography (GLC) to 90% of completion.

At the end of this interval, the flask contents are poured into five liters of water, and one liter of toluene is added to aid in the separation. The toluene extract so obtained is washed with a saturated aqueous sodium chloride solution, then with sodium bicarbonate until alkaline, and finally with saturated aqueous sodium chloride; dried over magnesium sulfate, and filtered, and the toluene is removed by evaporation.

The isocaryophyllene epoxide is flash-distilled and then redistilled at 128° to 205°C and 0.2 mm Hg. Prior to the distillation, 100 grams of Primol mineral oil, 20 grams of triethanolamine, and 5 grams of Ionol 2,6-di-t-butyl-p-cresol antioxidant are added.

The purified isocaryophyllene epoxide so obtained in the amount of 1,816 grams (6.64 mol) is then placed into a hydrogenation bomb, and 500 grams of isopropyl alcohol and 25 g of 5% palladium on calcium carbonate catalyst are added. Hydrogen is introduced in stoichiometric amount at a pressure of 250 psig and a temperature from 33° to 47°C over an interval of 4.5 hours. The hydrogenated material so produced is filtered, combined with 100 grams of Primol mineral oil, 20 grams of triethanolamine and 5 grams of Ionol antioxidant, and distilled at 128° to 205°C and 0.2 mm Hg to obtain about 1,364 grams of dihydroisocaryophyllene epoxide (1). The material has an excellent woody, tobacco-like fragrance, and the boiling point, refractive index, and specific rotation indicated above.

A perfume composition is prepared with the following ingredients:

Ingredient	Parts
Vetivert oil	40
Epoxide	85
Sandalwood oil	100
Rose geranium oil	200
Musk ambrette	25
Benzyl-iso-eugenol	100
Coumarin	100
Heliotropin	50
Bois de rose oil	200
Benzoin resin	100

The perfume composition exhibits an exceptional tobacco-woody fragrance character. When the dihydro oxide is omitted, the composition lacks this quality. In comparison with caryophyllene epoxide and dihydrocarophyllene epoxide, the novel dihydro epoxide (1) is found to have much stronger, richer and more persistent woody plus the tobacco-like odor which renders it highly useful in the preparation of fragrances and perfumes.

PEPPERMINT

2-Substituted Cyclohexanones from Phenols

A process described by *L.J. Dankert and D.A. Permoda; U.S. Patent 3,124,614; March 10, 1964; assigned to The Dow Chemical Company* pertains to the preparation of such 2-substituted cyclohexanones by direct catalytic hydrogenation of o-substituted monohydric phenols where the ortho-substitutent is an alkyl group having at least three carbon atoms or is a cyclohexyl group and wherein only one of the positions ortho to the phenolic hydroxyl group is substituted.

Specific examples of useful o-substituted phenols are o-isopropylphenol, o-sec-butylphenol, o-tert-butylphenol, o-tert-amylphenol and o-cyclohexylphenol. From such phenolic starting materials and in accordance with this process there are obtained 2-substituted cyclohexanone products, for example, 2-isopropylcyclohexanone, 2-sec-butylcyclohexanone, 2-tert-butylcyclohexanone.

The catalyst employed is one containing elemental palladium in extremely fine state of subdivision, preferably supported in and on adsorbent charcoal although other solid supporting materials can be employed such as calcium carbonate, barium sulfate, magnesia, diatomaceous earth, pumice, or kieselguhr.

6-Halo-2,5-Dimethylhexanone-3

H.A. Stansbury, Jr. and H.R. Guest; U.S. Patent 3,122,587; February 25, 1964; assigned to Union Carbide Corporation describe the preparation of halogenated aliphatic ketones and their derivatives by a rearrangement of 2,5-dimethyltetrahydropyran-2-methanol.

The process by which the halogenated aliphatic ketones may be produced is illustrated by the following equation:

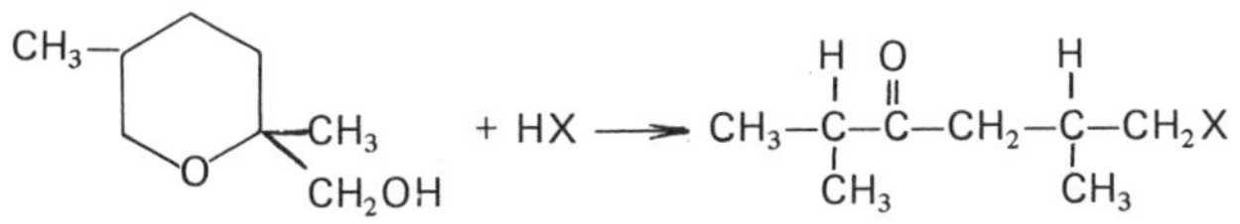

where X is a halogen.

The 6-halo-2,5-dimethylhexanone-3 may also be reacted with a strong base such as sodium hydroxide or potassium hydroxide to produce isopropyl 2-methylcyclopropyl ketone. This reaction may be conducted at temperatures of about 20° to 150°C. The preferred temperature range being 80° to 110°C. This ketone is a useful resin solvent. It has a fragrant odor reminiscent of both menthol and peppermint and thus has utility as an odorant. Such odorants are useful when formulated in soaps, perfumes and lotions. They also may be placed in open or wick-type containers to give rooms a fragrant odor.

The isopropyl 2-methylcyclopropyl ketone may be reduced with compounds such as lithium aluminum hydride, aluminum isopropoxide and sodium borohydride to produce isopropyl-2-methylcyclopropyl carbinol. This fragrant alcohol has utility as an odorant and may be placed in open or in wick type containers to give rooms a fragrant odor.

CARAMEL

Ethyl 2,4-Dioxyhexanoate

Z.G. Hajos and D.R. Parrish; U.S. Patent 3,760,087; September 18, 1973; assigned to Hoffmann-La Roche, Inc. have found that ethyl 2,4-dioxohexanoate has a high odor value and desirable blending properties so as to be useful in perfume compositions. The following examples illustrate the process.

Example 1: The preparation of ethyl 2,4-dioxohexanoate is as follows. 236 grams of anhydrous ethyl alcohol is distilled directly into a 1,000 ml three-necked flask equipped with a fast agitator, water-cooled condenser, addition funnel, thermometer and gas inlet-outlet tube. The reaction is conducted under a nitrogen atmosphere. Anhydrous sodium ethoxide (68 grams) is added with agitation and the mixture refluxed for 1 hour.

The mixture is then cooled to a range of 0° to 5°C whereupon a mixture of 72 grams of 2-butanone and 146 grams of diethyl oxalate is slowly added through the addition funnel over a 30 minute period and under a nitrogen atmosphere at 0° to 5°C. The resulting mixture was then further cooled and agitated for 3 hours at 0° to 5°C.

After cooling to 0°C, 168 ml of a 1:1 hydrochloric acid:H_2O (6N) solution was added and the temperature of the resultant solution was maintained below 10°C. The acidified solution was extracted twice, each time with 300 ml of toluene. The organic phase was then successively washed twice with 600 ml water, once with 600 ml of a 10% Na_2CO_3 solution and once with 400 ml of a saturated sodium chloride solution.

The toluene layers were then separated from the aqueous layers, combined, dried over magnesium sulfate and filtered. The toluene was removed by distillation under 25 mm/Hg pressure yielding ethyl 2,4-dioxohexanoate. Purity (VPC) about 91%. Optional and further purification was effected by fractional distillation through a 6 inch glass Helix packed column at 0.2 mm/Hg. Distillation yielded:

Fraction	Vapor	Pot	Pressure
1	80° to 85°C	95° to 104°C	2.0 mm
2	85°C	104°C	2.0 mm
3	86°C	112°C	2.0 mm
4	89°C	122°C	2.0 mm
5	85°C	165°C	2.0 mm

Vapor phase chromatography (VPC) analysis (125°C/SE-30) showed Fraction 1 to be the desired product plus a small amount of unreacted diethyl oxalate. Fractions 2 to 4 were shown to be 97 to 99% of the desired product and were accordingly combined to give a fraction of about 98% pure ethyl 2,4-dioxohexanoate. Fraction 5 was shown to contain the desired product plus about 5 to 6% of unknown by-product.

Example 2: The preparation of Cassia absolute perfume composition is as follows. A perfume composition containing the following ingredients and having a Cassia absolute odor was prepared (10,000 ml) by combining the ingredients in the order as listed below, and adequately mixing each ingredient into the resulting mixture in order to ensure a homogenous dispersion of each ingredient.

Ingredients	Amount	Ingredients	Amount
n-nonyl aldehyde	560 ml	Ethyl 2,4-dioxohexanoate 10%	500 ml
Methyl n-nonyl acetaldehyde	392 ml	Benzopyrrole (indol) 10% in	
Anisic aldehyde	280 ml	triethanolamine	280 ml
Anisyl aldehyde	280 ml	2-nonenal, pure 1%	112 ml
Benzyl alcohol (PG)*	2,240 ml	Beta-ionone	560 ml
Citronellol extra	168 ml	Hydroxycitronellal	1,120 ml
Cuminic aldehyde	56 ml	Linalool coeur	280 ml
Dipropylene glycol	148 ml	Methyl salicylate (syn)	560 ml
Methyl 2-octynoate	560 ml	p-methyl acetophenone, 10%	112 ml
Geraniol	560 ml	Styrax soluble resin	560 ml
Geranyl butyrate	392 ml	Terpineol extra	280 ml

*PG is perfume grade.

Polyene Ketones

R. Marbet; U.S. Patent 3,456,015; July 15, 1969; assigned to Hoffmann-La Roche Inc. describes allene ketones of the formula:

$$R'CH{=}C{=}CH{-}\underset{\underset{R^2}{|}}{CH}{-}\overset{\overset{O}{\|}}{C}{-}CH_2R^3$$

where R', R^2 and R^3 are hydrocarbon groups. These compounds are prepared by heating a ketal of the formula:

$$CH{\equiv}C{-}\underset{\underset{}{\overset{\overset{R'}{|}}{}}}{CH}{-}O{-}\underset{\underset{CH_2R^3}{|}}{\overset{\overset{CH_2R^2}{|}}{C}}{-}OR$$

where R is a lower alkyl group and R', R^2 and R^3 are as defined above, at temperatures from about 80° to 200°C in the presence of an acid catalyst.

These ketones are characterized by especially valuable odor properties which differ from those of structurally closely related compounds. Thus, for example, 7,10-dimethyl-4,5,9-undecatrien-2-one within the scope of the process has a pleasant caramel-like odor, while 6,10-dimethyl-4,5,9-undecatrien-2-one, which is isomeric thereto, differing only in the position of a methyl group, has an unpleasant metallic, ozone-like odor.

Just as significant a qualitative difference exists, for example, between the odor notes of 7,10-dimethyl-3,5,9-undecatrien-2-one obtainable in accordance with the process and 6,10-dimethyl-3,5,9-undecatrien-2-one (pseudoionone) in that the first shows a dry wood-like odor without a balsamic note. The latter, however, as is known, shows a fatty balsamic somewhat cinnamon-like odor. The ketals primarily resulting by reaction of the starting materials also have odorant character and can accordingly find use for the manufacture of perfumes or perfumed products. In the following example the temperatures are given in degrees centigrade.

Example: (a) Preparation of Acetone (1-Butyn-3-yl) Methyl Ketal and Acetone Di(1-Butyn-3-yl) Ketal — To 70 grams of 1-butyn-3-ol there are added 20 mg of p-toluenesulfonic acid and thereafter at 0° to 10°C, 170 grams of isopropenyl methyl ether. As soon as the evolution of heat has died away, the reaction mixture is neutralized with 0.5 ml of triethyl amine and then shaken with 250 ml of petroleum ether and 250 ml of 10% sodium bicarbonate solution. The petroleum ether solution is dried over anhydrous sodium bicarbonate and then distilled, whereby, after removal of the solvent, two fractions are obtained:

(1) Fraction: acetone (1-butyn-3-yl) methyl ketal of boiling point 41°C/14 mm. Harsh, fruit-like odor with nut and Russian leather-like side notes.

(2) Fraction: acetone di(1-butyn-3-yl) ketal of boiling point 75°C at 15 mm. Odor: very fresh and green fruity.

(b) Preparation of 4,5-Heptadien-2-one —1-Butyn-3-ol can be converted with isopropenyl methyl ether into 4,5-heptadien-2-one without isolation of the ketal intermediate product as follows.

To a solution of 20 mg of p-toluenesulfonic acid in 70 grams of 1-butyn-3-ol there are added with stirring and cooling 170 grams of isopropenyl methyl ether. The reaction mixture is thereupon enclosed in a pressure vessel. After the impressing of 5 atm of nitrogen, the reaction mixture is heated at 180°C for 3 hours, thereafter cooled and twice washed with 250 ml of 5% sodium bicarbonate solution, whereupon first the acetone dimethyl ketal and then the 4,5-heptadien-2-one (90 grams) is distilled off. Pure 4,5-heptadien-2-one has the following properties: BP = 56°C/mm. Odor: reminiscent of 6-methyl-5-hepten-2-one, but harsher and slightly fatty. Melting point of the phenyl-semicarbazone = 117° to 119°C.

(c) Preparation of 3,5-Heptadien-2-one —70 grams of 1-butyn-3-ol are allowed to react between 0° and 30°C with 200 grams of isopropenyl ethyl ether in the presence of 20 mg of p-toluenesulfonic acid. Thereupon the mixture is heated at 150°C for 30 minutes in the autoclave. The cooled mixture is then allowed to flow at 0° to 10°C into a solution of 30% aqueous caustic soda in 200 ml of methanol for the purpose of isomerization of the allene ketone.

After 15 minutes the mixture is neutralized with glacial acetic and the excess isopropenyl ethyl ether and the acetone diethyl ketal produced are evaporated off at 100 mm pressure in a 60°C bath. Thereafter the 3,5-heptadien-2-one is separated at 15 mm pressure in a 100°C bath as a pale yellow colored liquid. Yield: 89 grams; BP = 68° to 69°C/15 mm.

On the basis of the NMR spectrum, an isomer mixture is obtained in which the isomer with the trans-configuration in the 3,4- and cis-configuration in the 5,6-position is the main product. Odor: harsh fruity and bitter almond-like.

The isomeric 3,5-heptadien-2-one with cis-configuration in the 3,4- and trans-configuration in the 5,6-position can be obtained as follows. To 70 grams of 1-butyn-3-ol there are added 200 mg of p-toluenesulfonic acid and 2 ml of pyridine. After addition of 170 grams of isopropenyl methyl ether the mixture is heated in the autoclave under 2 atm of nitrogen first of all to 100°C, whereby a sudden exothermic reaction commences (increase of the internal temperature to 158°C) (no reaction takes place at room temperature). After this reaction fades away, the reaction mixture is heated at 180°C for ½ hour.

A product is thus obtained which, in the gas chromatogram, shows a peak which is almost completely missing with the 3,5-heptadien-2-one described above, directly behind the position of the 4,5-heptadien-2-one. After working up and distillation through a column, there is obtained pure 3,5-heptadien-2-one of boiling point 55°C/13 mm in a yield of 77 grams.

MISCELLANEOUS SPECIFIC FRAGRANCES

Oximes—Green Leaf, Earthy

A process described by *R.T. Dahill, Jr.; U.S. Patent 3,637,533; January 25, 1972; assigned to Givaudan Corporation* relates to perfume-containing compositions containing certain oximes as olfactory agents. The oximes which have been found useful are those of 7 to 10 carbon atom branched-chain ethylenic unsaturated hydrocarbyl aldehydes and ketones. Among specific oximes found to be suitable are citral oxime; citronellal oxime; 2,6-dimethyl-5-heptenal oxime; 3-methylheptan-5-one oxime; octan-3-one oxime; 3,7-dimethyl-octanal oxime; 2-methylheptan-6-one oxime; heptan-2-one oxime; nonan-3-one oxime; octan-2-one oxime and 2-methyl-2-hepten-6-one oxime. All parts and percentages are by weight, the percentages being based on the total composition, unless otherwise stated in the following examples.

Example 1: 3-Methylheptan-5-one oxime was prepared as follows. Into a 2 liter, 3-necked flask fitted with a mechanical stirrer, dropping funnel and condenser was charged 82.1 g of hydroxylamine sulfate and 100 ml of water. To this solution was added dropwise 118.5 g of 33.7% sodium hydroxide at 30°C. When the addition was complete a solution of 128 g of 3-methyl-5-heptanone in 300 ml of ethyl alcohol was added dropwise at 30°C. The resulting mixture was refluxed for one hour at 80° to 85°C. The mixture was poured on a large volume of water. The organic material was separated and the water phase extracted several times with toluene. The combined organic phases were washed once more with water. The solvent was removed under 20 mm of mercury pressure and the product distilled through a 37 mm column packed with glass helices: BP 70°C (0.7 mm).

The oxime has an intense green-leaf odor quite suggestive of crushed fig leaves. It is useful as a base for the synthetic reconstruction of the odor of natural fig leaves absolute, as illustrated by the following formulation:

Coumarin	30
Heliotropin	20
Benzyl valerianate	20
Estragole	60
3-Methylheptan-5-one oxime	485
Linalool	80
Nonadienal	5
Raldeine gamma	300
Total	1,000

Raldeine is the registered trademark of Givaudan Corporation for methylionones. The oxime of this example can be used as a total or partial substitute for natural fig leaves absolute. It has the following advantages over the natural products:

Lower cost
Readily available
Constant in odor (the natural product varies
   from crop to crop)
Colorless (the natural product imparts an in-
   tense green color)
Nonirritant (natural fig leaves absolute has been
   reported as an irritant when in contact with the
   the skin)
Stable in soap, cosmetics, and aerosols.

Trimethyloctene Nitriles—Grass

J.H. Blumenthal; U.S. Patent 3,531,510; September 29, 1970; assigned to International Flavors & Fragrances, Inc. describes methods for the preparation and isolation of a variety of 5,7,7-trimethyl-2-octenyl nitriles and 5,7,7-trimethyl-3-octenyl nitriles.

The process involves the condensation of cyanoacetic acid with 3,5,5-trimethyl hexanal in the presence of an amine or an amine salt at a temperature of from 40° to 180°C. A mixture of nitriles is produced in the condensation reaction.

The relative proportion of each nitrile in the mixture can be controlled by control of the alkalinity of the reaction medium. The compounds and mixtures are useful as olfactory agents.

The trimethyl-octenenitriles contribute a fresh, green, cut grass odor having a fully carroty earthy note. The trimethyl-octenenitriles possess a clover, sweet-grass, and orris-like fragrance.

Alkadienyl Pyridines—Seashore

J.B. Hall; U.S. Patent 3,669,908; June 13, 1972; assigned to International Flavors & Fragrances, Inc. describes alkadienyl-substituted heterocyclic nitrogen compounds, particularly pyridines and pyrazines having the general formulas:

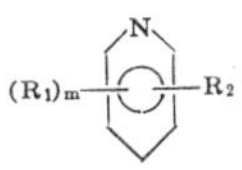

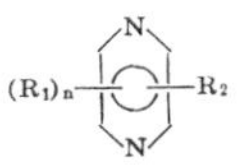

where R_1 and R_2 are substituents on the carbon atoms of the heterocyclic rings; where R_1 is either H or lower alkyl; where m is 1, 2, 3 or 4; where n is 1, 2 or 3 and where R_2 is a C-11 nonallenic alkadienyl moiety.

The heterocyclic compounds are obtained by processes involving the reaction of a picoline (α-, β-, or γ-methylpyridine) or a methylpyrazine with a C-10 alkadienyl halide, tosylate, mesylate or similar sulfonic acid esters. The process encompasses

> 2-(4,8-dimethyl-3,7-nonadienyl)pyridine
> 3-(4,8-dimethyl-3,7-nonadienyl)pyridine
> 2-(4,8-dimethyl-3,7-nonadienyl)pyridine
> 2-(4,8-dimethyl-3,7-nonadienyl)-5-ethylpyrazine
> 2-(4,8-dimethyl-3,7-nonadienyl)-5-n-propylpyrazine

Even small percentages of the compounds will alter, improve, modify or vary the odor impression so as to impart either such seashore or nut-like notes. The following examples illustrate the process.

Example 1: The preparation of α-(C_{11}-alkadienyl)pyridine is as follows. Into a 5 liter three-neck flask equipped with stirrer, thermometer, condenser, addition funnel, drying tube and gas bubbler were placed the following ingredients: 465 grams 2-methylpyridine (5 mols) and 500 grams benzene.

At room temperature, with stirring 200 grams of sodium amide were added. The temperature of the reaction mass was allowed to rise to 80° to 85°C. 807 grams of myrcene hydrochloride (3.5 mols) was added to the reaction mass over a period of one hour while maintaining the temperature at 80°C. The reaction mass was then stirred for 3 hours at 80°C.

On cooling, 100 cc of water was slowly added. The reaction mass was subsequently poured into one liter of water and the organic layer was separated and washed first with a 300 cc quantity of 5% aqueous sodium hydroxide and then with two 300 cc volumes of water. The solvent was stripped off the organic layer and the reaction product was rushed over at 2 mm Hg pressure and 130° to 140°C. The reaction product was then distilled in a fractionation column at a temperature in the range of 110° to 113°C and a pressure of 0.7 mm Hg. The resulting 2-(4,8-dimethyl-3,7-nonadienyl)pyridine had a distinct nut-like aroma. The following formula was confirmed by NMR, mass spectral and IR analyses:

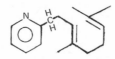

Using the foregoing procedure, when 2-methylpyridine was replaced by 2-methylpyrazine, as a starting reactant, the compound: 2-(4,8-dimethyl-3,7-nonadienyl)pyrazine was synthesized.

Example 2: The preparation of a γ-(C_{11}-alkadienyl)pyridine is as follows. Into a 22 liter reaction flask equipped with stirrer, thermometer, addition funnel, reflux condenser and gas bubbler were added the following materials: 4,185 grams 4-methylpyridine (45 mols) and 3,600 grams benzene.

Through an addition tube over a period of 25 minutes, 1,802 grams (45.9 mols) of sodium amide were added, the temperature of the reaction mass remaining at 24° to 30°C. The reaction mass was then heated slowly to reflux (pot temperature of 84°C) and maintained at reflux until gas evolution ceased (4½ hours). Over a period of 2½ hours while continu-

ing reflux, 6,291 grams of myrcene hydrochloride was added. The reaction mass was refluxed for 3 hours, maintaining the temperature thereof at 90° to 94°C. At the end of the
reaction the mass was cooled and poured slowly over 9,000 grams of ice and water. The
aqueous phase was extracted with a 2½ liter volume of benzene and the organic phases
were combined and washed with two 3.0 liter volumes of water. The solvent was then
stripped off at 100 mm Hg pressure. The reaction product was rushed over at a vapor
temperature of 52° to 159°C (1 to 15 mm Hg pressure). The reaction product was then
fractionally distilled on a 12 inch Goodloe column at a temperature range of 123° to 150°C
and a pressure of 2.4 mm Hg (reflux ration 1:1). Mass spectral analysis indicated that the
reaction product included a compound having the structure:

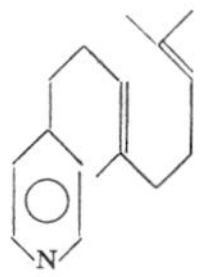

The product had a highly desirable seashore aroma reminiscent of ocean spray.

Example 3: The following composition is prepared:

Ingredient	Parts by Weight
Linalyl acetate	135
Bergamot oil	275
Citronellol	135
Lavandulol	135
Portugal oil	135
Neroli oil	40.5
Jasmin oil	20.5
Jasmin absolute	20.5
Neroliol, bigarade	28.0
Rosemary oil	28.0
4-(4,8-dimethyl-3,7-nonadienyl)pyridine prepared by the process of Example 2	13.5
Rose absolute	13.5
Hydroxy citronellol	13.5
Cyclopentadecanolide 10%	7.0

The addition of the 4-(C_{11}- alkadienyl)pyridine in the quantity given adds a distinct seashore aroma to the fragrance. When the compound 4-(4,8-dimethyl-3,7-nonadienyl)pyridine
is replaced with 2-ethyl-4-(4,8-dimethyl-3,7-nonadienyl)pyridine or mixtures of these pyridine
compounds, the same results as mentioned above are obtained.

Pyrazine Derivatives—Cooked Potato

*B.D. Mookherjee, C. Giacino, E.A. Karoll and M.H. Vock; U.S. Patent 3,711,482; Jan. 16,
1973; assigned to International Flavors & Fragrances* have found that a certain pyrazine,
2-acetyl-3-ethylpyrazine, having the formula:

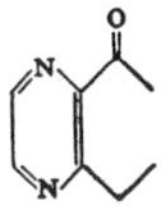

has a strong raw or cooked potato aroma and fragrance.

This pyrazine can be produced by the reaction of a 2,3-diethylpyrazine with N-halosuccinimide to form 2-(1-haloethyl)-3-ethylpyrazine and then treating the halogenated derivative with an alkali metal and 2-nitropropane. It has been found that the reaction is a general one which can be utilized to produce 2-acetyl-3-alkylpyrazines by utilizing 2-ethyl-3-alkyl-pyrazine as the starting material. The alkyl group is desirably a lower alkyl group such as one having from 1 to 6 carbon atoms in the molecule, and the alkyl group preferably contains one or two carbon atoms.

8-Camphene Carbinol and Patchouli Oil—Spicy

J.F. Janes, B.G. Jaggers and A.J. Curtis; U.S. Patent 3,673,120; June 27, 1972; assigned to Bush Boake Allen Limited, England describe a compounded perfumery composition which comprises natural Patchouli oil with which there has been incorporated from 1 to 200 parts of 8-camphene carbinol per 100 parts of the Patchouli oil.

8-Camphene carbinol has the chemical structure (represented in conventional terpene symbolism)

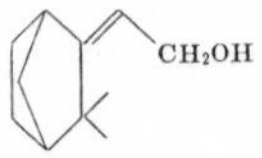

This compound has also been described as $\Delta^{3,\beta}$-camphenilane ethanol or 3,3-dimethyl-$\Delta^{2,\beta}$-norbornane ethanol, as obtained by a Prins type reaction between camphene and formaldehyde.

Thus to prepare 8-camphene carbinol camphene may be treated with formaldehyde in the presence of an acid. Often acetic acid is used and the product is then a mixture of 8-camphene carbinol and the acetate ester thereof. This mixture is then subjected to saponification and the free alcohol purified by distillation under vacuum.

The Patchouli oil is obtained from natural sources by steam distillation of the leaves of *Pogostemon Patchouli,* which grows in such countries as Indonesia, Seychelle Islands, Malaya and China. It is used as produced or after having undergone some purification technique such as redistillation. In the following examples all quantities are expressed on a weight basis.

Example 1: Patchouli oil (80 parts) obtained from the Seychelle Islands was blended with 8-camphene carbinol (20 parts). The carbinol was found to act as an extender for the Patchouli oil in that the characteristic odor effect of the latter was only slightly modified.

Example 2: The extended Patchouli oil as prepared in Example 1 was successfully incorporated into a compounded composition of the chypre type by blending the following ingredients.

	Parts		Parts
Cinnamic aldehyde	1	Hydroxycitronellal	40
Ethyl methyl phenyl glycidate	1	Isoeugenol	40
Methyl nonyl acetaldehyde	2	Extended Patchouli oil (Ex. 1)	40
Oak moss (absolute)	20	Coumarin	50
Sandalwood oil (East Indian)	20	Musk ketone	50
Vetiveryl acetate	20	Amyl salicylate	60
Ylang oil No. 1	20	Cedarwood oil (American)	60
Benzoin resoin (Sumatra)	30	Citronellol	60
Ionone (100%)	30	Benzyl acetate	80
Clove stem oil (Zanzibar)	36	Phenyl ethyl alcohol	150
Bergamot oil	40	Terpinyl acetate	150

Example 3: A Patchouli oil extender base was prepared by blending the following ingredients.

	Parts
8-Camphene carbinol	38
Guaioxide	27
Isolongifolene oxidate	20
ω-Hydroxymethyl longifolene	10
Cedrol	3
Sandalwood oil (East Indian)	2

This mixture (46 parts) was then blended with natural Patchouli oil (Seychelles) (60 parts) to provide a satisfactory extended Patchouli oil.

Example 4: The extended Patchouli oil prepared in Example 3 was incorporated into a compounded perfumery composition of the Fougere type containing the following ingredients.

	Parts
Balsam (Peru)	30
Labdanum resoin	30
Oak moss (absolute)	30
Sandalwood oil (East Indian)	30
Linalyl acetate	40
Terpinyl acetate	40
Geranium oil (Bourbon)	50
Musk ambrette	50
Coumarin	60
Amyl salicylate	60
Methyl ionone	70
Cedarwood oil (American)	80
Clove stem oil (Zanzibar)	80
Vetivert oil (Bourbon)	80
Extended Patchouli oil (Ex. 3)	130
Lavandin oil	140

α-Methyl-γ-Isobutylbutyrolactone—Herbaceous

A process described by *A. Flecchi; U.S. Patent 3,530,149; September 22, 1970; assigned to Collins Chemical Co., Inc.* concerns a flavoring agent of the empirical formula $C_9H_{16}O_2$ and of the structural formula:

(1) $(CH_3)_2CH-CH_2-\underset{\diagdown O \diagup}{\overset{CH_2-CH-CH_3}{CH \quad CO}}$

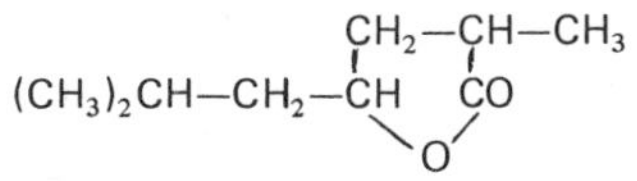

referred to as α-methyl-γ-isobutyl-butyrolactone. It could also be referred to as the lactone of the 2,6-dimethyl-4-hydroxyheptanoic acid.

This lactone is a colorless liquid, distillable in vacuum preferably below 20 mm Hg and it typically boils at 65°C at 0.5 mm Hg. Its infrared spectrum exhibits the sharp band peculiar to γ-lactones at 1,775 cm^{-1}. The lactone is soluble in alcohols, such as ethanol, methanol, glycols, benzyl alcohol, in aprotic dipolar solvents such as acetone, acetonitrile, dimethyl-formamide, in ethers such as ethyl ether, in esters such as triacetin, in aliphatic, aromatic and chlorinated hydrocarbons, in vegetable oils, in fats and in glycols. It is slightly soluble in water and solutions of alkali bicarbonates, but dissolves in aqueous solutions of alkali metal hydroxides.

This lactone has a very pleasant, penetrating and persistent smell, of a herbaceous-creamy nature. It may be employed alone or combined, for a large variety of purposes. The α-methyl-γ-isobutyl-butyrolactone is very effective in reinforcing and fixing. Also, since the lactone withstands high temperatures it can be used in aromatic compositions which are subjected to high temperature processing.

Thus the process also includes flavoring compositions containing α-methyl-γ-isobutyl-butyro-lactone. In these compositions the lactone is substantially dissolved in one or a plurality of the above solvents and/or aromatic mixtures. Solutions of the lactone in vegetable oils, such as palm nut oil, coconut oil, olive oil and other oils, in natural or synthetic fats, such as cocoa butter, and in glycols were found just as useful, particularly in the cosmetic, perfume and foodstuff industries.

Alternatively, the lactone may be absorbed onto a solid carrier, such as starch, gums, baking powders, or mineral powders such as talcum. The proportion of lactone in all such compositions is a matter of choice, so that it is not thought advisable to set particular limits herein. Impregnation of a solid carrier may be very easily effected by dissolving the lactone in a volatile solvent, such as ethanol, acetone or ethyl ether, impregnating the carrier by means of this solution and evaporating the solvent employed.

A similar technique may be adopted for homogeneously dispersing the lactone, for instance in a fat of a more or less high consistency. Alternatively, conventional milling or kneading machines can be employed, such as the type known in the cosmetic industry.

By this process α-methyl-γ-isobutyl-butyrolactone can be obtained through well defined intermediates by very simple reaction steps. In the reaction 2-morpholino-4-methyl-1-pentene

$$(CH_3)_2CH-CH_2-C{=}CH_2$$

(2)

$$
\begin{array}{c}
N \\
CH_2 \quad CH_2 \\
CH_2 \quad CH_2 \\
O
\end{array}
$$

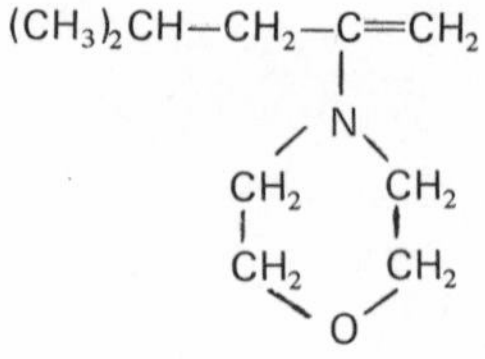

reacts with methyl- or ethyl-2-bromopropionate:

$$CH_3CHBrCOOR$$

(where R is $-CH_3$ or $-C_2H_5$) in the presence of a tertiary amine NR'_2R'' (where R' is $-CH_3$ or $-C_2H_5$; and where R'' is $-CH_3$, $-C_2H_5$ or $-C_6H_5$) in an aprotic dipolar solvent, typically at a temperature of 50° to 150°C. This reaction generally takes 10 to 30 hours. Subsequently, by mixing the reaction mixture with a dilute aqueous solution of a mineral acid (typically hydrochloric or sulfuric acid), a neutral oily phase is separated which essentially comprises the methyl or ethyl ester of the 2,6-dimethyl-4-keto-heptanoic acid:

(3) $(CH_3)_2CH-CH_2COCH_2-CH(CH_3)COOR$

where R is methyl or ethyl.

By saponifying this ester with NaOH or KOH the corresponding 2,6-dimethyl-4-heptanoate of the alkali metal is obtained:

(4) $(CH_3)_2CH-CH_2COCH_2-CH(CH_3)COOMe$

where Me is Na or K, from which reduction of the keto-group to the alcoholic group yields the 2,6-dimethyl-4-hydroxyheptanoate of sodium or potassium:

(5) $(CH_3)_2CH-CH_2CHOHCH_2-CH(CH_3)COOMe$

which on acidification with a dilute aqueous solution of a mineral acid (typically hydro-chloric or sulfuric acid) is converted to the desired lactone (1).

The 2-morpholino-4-methyl-1-pentene and the method of preparing it were described by R. Fusco et al (*Gazz. Chim. Ital.* 92, 382, 1962). For the purposes of this method it is dissolved together with the bromopropionate and tertiary amine mentioned above in at least substantially equimolar proportions in the aprotic dipolar solvent. Trimethylamine, triethylamine or dimethylaniline is preferably employed as the tertiary amine. The solvent preferably consists of acetonitrile, dimethylformamide, dimethylacetamide, dimethylsulfoxide, N-methyl-2-pyrrolidone, tetrahydrothiophene-dioxide, nitrobenzene or mixtures thereof. The reaction is promoted by stirring throughout the reaction period (10 to 30 hours). On completion of the reaction a mixture containing a crystalline precipitate is obtained and is allowed to cool at room temperature.

Admixture thereto of a sufficient quantity of a dilute aqueous solution of a mineral acid, such as hydrochloric or sulfuric acid, will cause the crystalline phase to dissolve, leaving two liquid phases, namely an aqueous heavy phase and an oily light phase essentially com-prising the ester (3).

The ester (3) in pure state is a colorless actually water-insoluble liquid which dissolves in conventional organic solvents, such as ethyl ether, benzene and chloroform. It is recovered from the reaction mixture by separating the oily phase from the aqueous phase by extrac-tion with one of the above mentioned solvents. The extraction step is preferably carried out three times, whereupon the three extracts are brought together and the solvent is re-moved by distillation, usually at atmospheric pressure. The oily residue is rectified in vacuum, preferably below 20 mm Hg and the ester (3) is thus obtained (boiling point 85°C at 0.5 mm Hg).

Saponification of the ester is effected by conventional methods. Typically, the ester is admixed with ethyl alcohol (in which it is highly soluble) and a molar excess (about twice as much) of a concentrated aqueous solution of sodium or potassium hydroxide and re-fluxed about 2 hours. The solution is then concentrated (preferably at a reduced pressure of 300 to 500 mm Hg) in order to remove the organic solvent.

The liquid residue which contains the salt (4) is then dissolved in water, in which the salt is soluble, and admixed with a slight excess of sodium borohydride ($NaBH_4$) which has been previously dissolved in water. This reagent quantitatively reduces the keto-group of the salt (4) to an alcohol group, whereby the oxyheptanoate (5) is obtained. The reduction reaction takes 8 to 24 hours.

After this period has elapsed, the resulting solution is acidified to a pH of between 1.5 to 3.5 by means of a dilute aqueous solution of a mineral acid (typically sulfuric or hydro-chloric acid) till a heavy aqueous phase and an oily organic light phase appear, the latter essentially comprising the lactone (1). The oily phase is separated from the aqueous one, the latter being then extracted by means of a water-immiscible organic solvent (typically ethyl ether) till practically complete removal from the aqueous phase of the peculiar strong odor of the lactone (1).

The organic extracts are mixed with the oily phase and distilled (usually at room pressure) in order to remove the solvent. Finally, the residue is distilled in vacuum, preferably at 0.5 mm Hg, and the fraction boiling at 65°C is collected. This is a liquid having the typical characteristics of α-methyl-γ-isobutyl-butyrolactone (1).

The preparation of the ethyl 2,6-dimethyl-4-ketoheptanoate is as follows. A solution was obtained by dissolving 114 grams (0.67 mol) of 2-morpholino-4-methyl-1-pentene in 250 ml acetonitrile. The solution was admixed with 120 grams (0.67 mol) of ethyl-2-bromopro-pionate and 67 grams (0.67 mol) of triethyl amine at room temperature.

The solution is maintained at 80°C during 24 hours and, upon cooling to room temperature, is mixed with 300 ml aqueous 10 weight percent hydrochloric acid (about 0.85 mol), whereby the mixture separates into two phases.

The mixture is then extracted three times using 200 ml of ethyl ether in each extraction. The ether solutions are then mixed, washed with an aqueous 2% by weight sodium bicarbonate solution, washed with water, and finally dried on sodium sulfate.

The resulting anhydrous extract is evaporated at room pressure until almost complete removal of ether. The liquid residue is rectified in vacuum and the colorless liquid fraction, boiling at 85°C at 0.5 mm Hg is collected. The product is ethyl 2,6-dimethyl-4-ketoheptanoate. Its infrared spectrum exhibits characteristic strong bands at 1,740 cm^{-1} (ester and 1,710 cm^{-1} (ketone).

The preparation of the lactone is as follows. 43 grams (0.215 mol) of ethyl 2,6-dimethyl-4-ketoheptanoate obtained as above were dissolved in a solution comprising 300 ml ethanol and 43.5 ml aqueous 30% sodium hydroxide solution (about 0.43 mol).

The resulting solution was refluxed for two hours, and concentrated at 450 mm Hg with most of the ethanol therein evaporating. On reduction of its volume to 80 ml, the solution was cooled, diluted with 200 ml water and admixed (at room temperature, and under cooling if necessary) with a solution of 2.3 grams (0.06 mol) of sodium borohydride in 10 ml water.

After 12 hours the mixture is acidified by adding 175 ml of aqueous 10% hydrochloric acid (about 0.5 mol), two phases being obtained. The organic upper phase is separated and the heavy aqueous phase extracted three times with 100 ml ethyl ether each time. The ether solutions are mixed with the organic phase and this extract is washed first with an aqueous 3 weight percent sodium bicarbonate solution, and then with water. Upon drying on sodium sulfate, the ether in the extract is almost fully evaporated therefrom, by first operating at atmospheric pressure, and then in vacuum.

From the residue, a colorless liquid is distilled at 65°C and at 0.5 mm Hg. The product is the α-methyl-γ-isobutyl-butyrolactone. Its infrared spectrum (obtained by operating on the liquid) exhibits a strong sharp band at 1,775 cm^{-1} (γ-lactone).

GENERAL PROCESSES

ESTERS

Unsaturated Ether Esters

W.H. Urry; U.S. Patent 3,201,456; August 17, 1965; assigned to Monsanto Company describes unsaturated ether esters of the structure

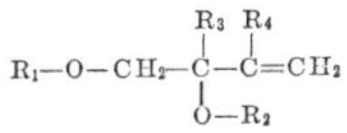

$$R_1-O-CH_2-\underset{\underset{O-R_2}{|}}{\overset{\overset{R_3}{|}}{C}}-\overset{\overset{R_4}{|}}{C}=CH_2$$

where R_1 is an alkyl group, R_2 is an acyl group and R_3 and R_4 are independently selected from the group consisting of hydrogen, a methyl radical and a halogen atom. The compounds are attained by reacting certain conjugated dienes with certain peroxide compounds in the presence of a cuprous salt. The dienes employed in the process conform to the formula set forth below

$$CH_2=\overset{\overset{R_3}{|}}{C}-\overset{\overset{R_4}{|}}{C}=CH_2$$

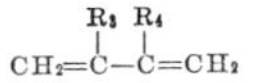

where R_3 and R_4 are independently selected from the group consisting of hydrogen, a methyl group and a halogen atom. The peroxides employed in the process conform to the formula set forth below

$$R_1-O-O-R_2$$

where R_1 is a tertiary alkyl group and R_2 is an acyl group selected from the group consisting of the acetyl group and the benzoyl group. In the process the product appears to arrive by the addition of the elements of the peroxide compound across the 1,2 position of the diene. This is an unusual reaction, since in most addition reactions involving conjugated dienes the addition takes place across the 1,4 position. The following examples illustrate the process. Unless otherwise noted, where parts or quantities are mentioned they are parts or quantities by weight.

Example 1: A suitable reaction vessel is charged with 170 grams (2.5 mols) of isoprene, 0.5 gram of cuprous bromide and 1,500 ml of glacial acetic acid. The reaction mixture is heated to reflux and 194 grams (1 mol) of t-butyl perbenzoate are added dropwise over a two-hour period. Heating is continued to maintain the reaction mixture at reflux and the reflux temperature increases from an initial value of 64°C to a final value of 83°C. The reaction mixture is maintained at reflux temperature for four hours after the addition of the t-butyl perbenzoate is completed. The reaction mixture turns a deep green in color with the first addition of t-butyl perbenzoate.

After cooling to room temperature, the reaction mixture is dissolved in 3 liters of ether and washed with sodium carbonate solution to remove virtually all of the acid from the organic layer. The ether solution is washed twice more with water and dried over anhydrous magnesium sulfate. After removing the ether by distillation, the product is distilled under reduced pressure to obtain the following fractions.

Fraction	Boiling Point	Weight, g
1	39° - 79°C (7 – 10 mm Hg)	29
2	77° - 86°C (7.5 - 10 mm Hg)	58
3	83° - 92°C (7.5 - 10 mm Hg)	14
4	83° - 120°C (7.5 - 10 mm Hg)	26

A small quantity of benzoic acid is recovered from the distillation pot. The four fractions set forth above are combined and fractionated under reduced pressure using a column rated at 90 plates. A compound (1) is isolated in the amount of 57 grams. This compound has a boiling point of 78° to 80°C at 10 mm Hg, a refractive index at 25°C at 1.42414 and a density at 25°C at 0.9180. The compound contains 65.8% carbon and 9.81% hydrogen.

This analysis corresponds closely with the theoretical analysis for a compound of the empirical formula $C_{11}H_{20}O_3$. A second compound (2) is obtained in the amount of 15 grams. This product has a boiling point of 85° to 86°C at 10 mm Hg, a refractive index at 25°C of 1.42759 and a density at 25°C of 0.9219. This compound analyzed 65.4% carbon and 9.77% hydrogen. This analysis again compares well with theory for a compound of the empirical formula:

$$C_{11}H_{20}O_3$$

Vapor phase chromatograms of compound (1) and (2) both show single peaks. Infrared spectra of both compounds show peaks corresponding to the following groups.

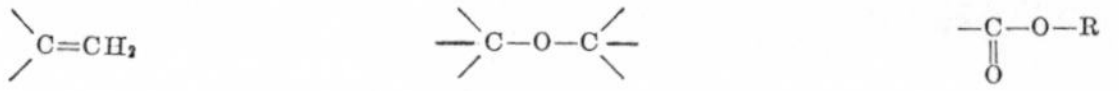

Nuclear magnetic resonance data establish the structure of compound (1) to be

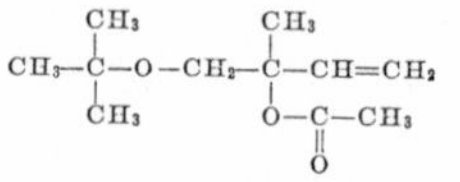

Nuclear magnatic resonance data establish the structure of compound (2) to be

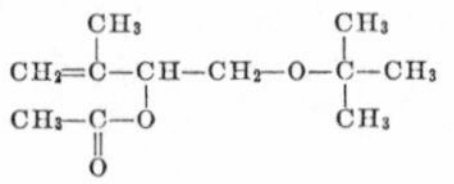

It will be noted that in the two formulas set forth immediately above the acid moiety of the ester group is derived from acetic acid. This is the result of ester interchange on the initially formed benzoate ester.

Example 2: Compound (1) is heated with a methanol solution of KOH to obtain compound (1a) which is an unsaturated ether alcohol as shown in the formula below.

$$
\underset{(1)}{\underset{\overset{\displaystyle |}{CH_3}}{\overset{\displaystyle \overset{CH_3}{|}}{CH_3-C}}-O-CH_2-\underset{\overset{\displaystyle |}{\underset{\overset{\displaystyle ||}{O}}{O-C-CH_3}}}{\overset{\displaystyle \overset{CH_3}{|}}{C}}-CH=CH_2} \quad \xrightarrow[\text{KOH}]{\text{CH}_3\text{OH}} \quad \underset{(1a)}{\underset{\overset{\displaystyle |}{CH_3}}{\overset{\displaystyle \overset{CH_3}{|}}{CH_3-C}}-O-CH_2-\underset{\overset{\displaystyle |}{OH}}{\overset{\displaystyle \overset{CH_3}{|}}{CH}}-CH=CH_2}
$$

Compound (1a) has a boiling point of 58° to 59°C at 10 mm Hg, a refractive index at 25°C of 1.4321 and a density at 25°C of 0.8669. A vapor phase chromatogram of this compound exhibits a single peak.

The compounds of the process are unsaturated ether esters which have a very pleasant odor. Consequently, they may be used in the formulation of perfumes or can be used as odor masking agents.

Esters of α-(C$_{10}$-Terpenyl)Alkanoic Acids

R.C. Kuder; U.S. Patent 3,637,801; January 25, 1972; assigned to General Mills, Inc. describes the preparation of certain α-substituted carboxylic acid compounds, and more particularly, esters produced from the combination of certain carboxylic acid anhydride reactants with certain ethylenically unsaturated reactants to effect α-substitution in such anhydride reactants which are esterified.

The unsaturated reactant contains an ethylenically unsaturated group through which one might expect to obtain olefinic addition polymerization in the presence of a typical polymerization catalyst, i.e., hydrogen peroxide, which is a preferred catalyst. Also, the carboxylic acid reactant is an organic acid anhydride which one might expect to function as a polymerization accelerator in combination with such hydrogen peroxide catalyst and/or as a coreactant therewith, e.g., to form a corresponding organic peroxide or hydroperoxide.

In contrast, the ethylenically unsaturated reactant (x) and the organic carboxylic acid reactant (a), in the presence of such a polymerization catalyst (b), hydrogen peroxide, are believed to undergo primarily a reaction according to the following oversimplified equation below

$$
\overset{\text{(x)}}{H_2C{=}CH_2} + \overset{\text{(a)}}{CH_3CO-} \quad \overset{\text{(b)}}{\longrightarrow} \quad \overset{\text{(P)}}{CH_3CH_2CH_2CO-}
$$

where it will be seen that anhydride reactant (a) is represented by an acyl group and so is the acid anhydride product (P). Reaction product (P) is substantially a 1:1 adduct of the specific unsaturated reactant (x) and the carboxylic acid anhydride (a), based on the acyl or acetyl equivalent thereof, vis-a-vis the unsaturation at the methylene group $=CH_2$ in (x).

The adducts are prepared by adding the olefin and a small amount of a peroxide initiator gradually, over a period of several hours, to a large excess of boiling acetic anhydride (reaction-temperature is usually 135° to 140°C). If the olefin is a solid (such as camphene), it may be predissolved in part of the acetic anhydride before adding it to the reaction mixture. It will be appreciated that this procedure provides for a very substantial molar excess of acetic anhydride at all times, beginning with the first incremental additions of the olefin and peroxy catalyst, and continuing to maintain the substantial molar excess of the acetic anhydride with subsequent incremental additions of the olefin and the catalyst. The following Examples 1 through 3, show adducts of about 2:1 in molar ratio of (a) to (x) [i.e., 1 acyl (a) equivalent to each

$$
\overset{\displaystyle |\quad|}{\underset{\displaystyle |\quad|}{C{=}C}}
$$

(x) equivalent] ; but the reaction mix should have an (a):(x) equivalent ratio within a practical range of about 10:1 to 1,000:1 (i.e., molar range of 5:1 to 500:1). Preferably, the (a):(x) equivalent ratio of at least about 25:1 (Example 2), or better about 50:1 (Example 3) to about 100:1 is preferred as the minimum. The maximum (a):(x) equivalent ratios of about 500:1 to 1,000:1 are determined essentially by practical considerations of plant capacity, etc.; and all such ratios are on an overall basis, in view of incremental additions of (x) and (b) to (a) which no doubt, maintain still higher ratios at the immediate reaction scene.

The primary product of the reaction is probably a mixed anhydride, which disproportionates during distillation of the excess acetic anhydride to give the symmetrical cycloaliphatic carboxylic anhydride and acetic anhydride.

Examples 1 through 3 illustrate the use of camphene as the olefin. A commercial grade of camphene is used containing 83% actual camphene; the remainder is chiefly tricyclene, a saturated isomer of camphene which is not understood to react with acetic anhydride under the conditions used.

Example 1: A solution of 136 grams commercial camphene (1.00 mol total, 0.83 mol actual camphene) and 22 grams t-butyl peroxide (0.15 mol) in 390 grams acetic anhydride is added incrementally over a period of eight hours to 2,160 grams acetic anhydride (total of 25 mols or 50 equivalents) maintained at the reflux temperature (138° to 139°C). The reaction mixture is then refluxed for 16 hours longer, then excess acetic anhydride is distilled off at atmospheric pressure until a pot temperature of 150°C is attained and only 304 grams of material remains.

Of this remainder, 300 grams is vacuum-stripped to a pot temperature of 150°C at 6 mm Hg pressure, leaving a residual liquid product of 155 grams. This product has a saponification number of 338.8, corresponding to 0.95 equivalent of combined acetic anhydride and 0.80 mol of combined camphene, or 96% of the actual camphene charged. This product comprises mostly the symmetrical anhydride of 3,3-dimethyl-2-norbornanepropionic acid

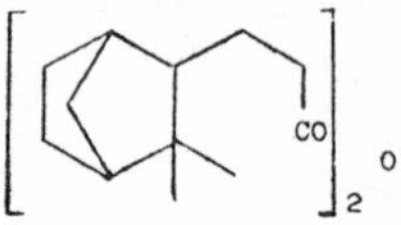

as shown by the acetic anhydride/camphene ratio of 1.19 and by the fact that the product when esterified with ethanol contains 82% of the corresponding ethyl ester (calculated saponification number, 251; found 252.1, 252.4). Further runs using camphene and acetic anhydride with tertiary butyl peroxide catalyst are summarized in Tables 1 and 2 below.

TABLE 1: REACTION OF CAMPHENE WITH ACETIC ANHYDRIDE*

Run No.	Camphene purity, percent	Mol ratio, Ac₂O: camphene	Reaction time, hr. Addn.	Reaction time, hr. Total	Max. stripping temp., °C.
A	90	25:1	5	6	144
B	83	25:1	5	6	150
C	83	25:1	8	24	150
D	83	25:1	8	24	150
E	83	25:1	8	24	158
F	88	25:1	8	24	162
a	83	14.4:1	8	24	150
b	83	12.5:1	6	7	100
c	83	12.5:1	4	7	100
d	83	12.5:1	8	24	100
e	83	12.5:1	8	24	101
f	83	12.5:1	8	24	151
G	83	12.5:1	8	24	152
g	83	12.5:1	8	24	160
H	83	12.5:1	8	24	164

*At reflux using 0.15 mol t-Bu₂O₂ per 136 g commercial camphene, except in D where 0.3 mol of H₂O₂ was used.

TABLE 2

Run No.	Product S.N.[1]	Ac₂O, equiv.[3]	Camphene Mol[2]	Camphene Percent	Percent 1:1 adduct in product[3]
A	367.0	1.115	0.812	90	85
B	333.1	0.798	.695	84	90
C	338.8	.949	.800	96	82
D	334.0	.571	.491	59	---
E	323.4	.880	.795	96	84
F	324.0	.943	.847	96	85
a	321.0	.855	.778	94	81
b	391.8	.910	.620	75	83
c	393.2	.940	.635	77	---
d	341.8	.947	.790	95	80
e	352.6	.965	.768	93	---
f	317.0	.825	.765	92	82
G	325.9	.858	.765	92	82
g	335.5	.903	.775	93	81
H	325.0	.855	.762	92	83

[1] Saponfication number.
[2] Per 136 g of commercial camphene charged.
[3] As determined by esterification.

Example 2: The preparation described in Example 1 is repeated except that twice as much camphene and t-butyl peroxide are used, keeping the amount of acetic anhydride the same; reaction temperature is 134° to 139°C and final stripping temperature is 164°C at 12 mm Hg. A product is obtained with saponification number of 326.0 corresponding to an acetic anhydride/camphene ratio of 1.12 equivalent per mol and a conversion of 92% of actual camphene charged. The butyl esters of the product contain 83% of the ester of the 1:1 adduct.

Example 3: A solution of 136 grams commercial camphene in 390 grams acetic anhydride is added from one addition funnel, and 34.2 grams 30% hydrogen peroxide (0.3 mol) is added separately but simultaneously from another addition funnel, incrementally over a period of eight hours, to 2,160 grams acetic anhydride maintained at the reflux temperature (134° to 138°C). The reaction mixture is then refluxed for 16 hours longer, then the excess acetic anhydride is distilled off at atmospheric pressure until a pot temperature of 150°C is attained and only 290 grams of material remains. Of this remainder, 288.5 grams is vacuum-stripped to a pot temperature of 150°C at 7.5 mm Hg leaving a residual liquid product of 95.5 grams. This product has a saponification number of 334.0, corresponding to an acetic anhydride/camphene ratio of 1.16 equivalent/mol and a conversion of 59% of actual camphene charged.

Carboxylic Esters of 3-Formylbuten-3-ol-1

W. Himmele, W. Aquila and R. Prinz; U.S. Patent 3,661,980; May 9, 1972; assigned to Badische Anilin- & Soda-Fabrik AG, Germany describe the production of carboxylic esters of 3-formylbuten-3-ol-1 by reacting bismonocarboxylic esters of buten-2-diol-1,4 with carbon monoxide and hydrogen in the presence of carbonyl complexes of rhodium at temperatures of 50° to 110°C and pressures of 300 to 1,000 atmospheres. The products are perfumes and intermediates for the manufacture of vitamin A. The following examples illustrate the process.

Example 1: 172 grams of butene-2-diol-1,4 diacetate, 5 mg of rhodium trichloride and 1 gram of dicobalt octacarbonyl are placed in a 700 ml stainless steel rolling autoclave and oxygen is expelled from the autoclave by rinsing three times with nitrogen at a pressure of 20 atmospheres. A mixture of carbon monoxide and hydrogen in equimolar amounts is then forced in up to a pressure of 200 atmospheres, the autoclave is heated to 110°C and the pressure is maintained at 700 atmospheres by repeated forcing in of the gas mixture. Four hours later the reaction is stopped and the reaction mixture is worked up as usual by fractional distillation. 3-formylbuten-3-ol-1 acetate is obtained in a yield of 54%; the boiling point is 77°C at 6 mm. The 2,4-dinitrophenylhydrazone prepared in acetic acid is orange-red and has a melting point of 134°C.

Example 2: A mixture of 200 grams of butene-2-diol-1,4 diacetate, 200 grams of benzene

and 5 mg of rhodium chloride is reacted at 700 atmospheres and 100°C in the manner described in Example 1. 3-formylbuten-3-ol acetate is obtained in a 72% yield.

Alkyl 2-Alkoxy-2-Cyclenecarboxylates

According to a process described by *Y. Bonnet; U.S. Patent 3,468,929; September 23, 1969;
assigned to Rhone-Poulenc SA, France* alkyl 2-alkoxy-2-cyclenecarboxylates, useful as intermediates in the production of cycloalkanones, are made by reacting an α,α,ω-trihalo-
genocycloalkanone with an alkali metal alkoxide.

The process for the preparation of alkyl 2-alkoxy-2-cyclenecarboxylates of the formula

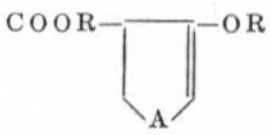

$$\text{COOR} - \boxed{} - \text{OR}$$
$$A$$

in which R is an alkyl radical of 1 to 4 carbon atoms and A is an alkylene radical of 4 to
11 carbon atoms which comprises reacting an α,α,ω-trihalogenocycloalkanone of the formula

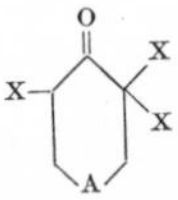

$$\begin{array}{c} O \\ X - \diagup\diagdown X \\ X - \diagdown\diagup X \\ A \end{array}$$

in which X is a halogen atom and A is as defined with an alkali metal alkoxide of 1 to 4
carbon atoms in an anhydrous alkanol at an elevated temperature. The process may be
represented by the following reaction

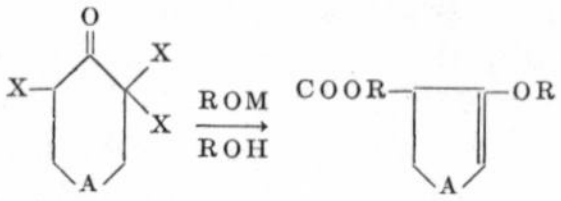

$$\begin{array}{c} O \\ X - \diagup\diagdown X \\ X - \diagdown\diagup X \\ A \end{array} \xrightarrow[\text{ROH}]{\text{ROM}} \text{COOR} - \boxed{} - \text{OR} \quad A$$

in which R and A are as defined, M is an alkali metal such as sodium, potassium or lithium
and X is a halogen atom such as chlorine or bromine. The starting material may be prepared by halogenating the corresponding cyclic ketones such as cyclononanone, cyclodecanone, cycloundecanone, cyclododecanone or cyclohexadecanone. This may be effected
either by the action of a halogen in the cold on the cycloalkanone in carbon tetrachloride
solution or by the action of a halogen at an elevated temperature on the cycloalkanone in
solution in a lower aliphatic acid solution such as acetic acid solution. The following examples illustrate the process.

*Example 1: Preparation of Cyclodecanone — (1) Preparation of 2,2,11-tribromocyclo-
undecanone:* 50 grams (0.298 mol) of cycloundecanone and 100 grams of anhydrous carbon tetrachloride were introduced into a three-necked round-bottomed 500 cc flask fitted
with a stirrer, a reflux condenser, a dropping funnel and a thermometer. This solution was
stirred with cooling to 0° to 5°C. Then 144.5 grams of anhydrous bromine in 62.5 grams
of carbon tetrachloride were added in one hour. The mixture was maintained at 0° to 5°C
for 8 hours and then allowed to return to ambient temperature.

The stirring was continued for 15 hours at this temperature. A white solid precipitated
which was separated by filtration and washed with 30 cc of carbon tetrachloride at 0°C.
After drying, 111.8 grams of solid matter, MP 74° to 80°C (82° to 83°C after recrystallization from a mixture of diethyl ether and pentane), identified by IR spectrography as 2,2,11-
tribromocycloundecanone (yield 92.7% of crude product), were collected.

(2) Preparation of 2-Methoxy-Cyclodec-2-ene-Carboxylic-Acid: (a) 910 cc of anhydrous methanol containing 35.4 grams of dissolved sodium (1.54 mols) were introduced into a 2,000 cc three-necked round-bottomed flask equipped as in part (1). 111.5 grams (0.257 mol) of 2,2,11-tribromocycloundecanone were then added with stirring, and the mixture refluxed for 48 hours.

(b) 450 cc of methanol were distilled off and the product was cooled to 20°C and 450 cc of water added. The whole was refluxed with stirring for 25 hours. The product was allowed to stand for 47 hours at ambient temperature to complete the saponification of the methyl 2-methoxycyclodec-2-ene-carboxylate. The alcohol was then distilled off in vacuo, and the residue taken up in 200 cc of diethyl ether to extract the unsaponified neutral portion. After decantation, the alkaline aqueous layer was acidified with 300 cc of 3N hydrochloric acid in the presence of 100 cc of diethyl ether to liberate the 2-methoxy-cyclodec-2-ene-carboxylic acid.

The ethereal layer was decanted, washed with 3 x 50 cc of distilled water and dried over anhydrous Na_2SO_4. After evaporation, 55.3 grams of a solid white product, MP 99° to 104°C, identified by IR spectrography as 2-methoxy-cyclodec-2-ene-carboxylic acid were obtained. After recrystallization from a mixture of diethyl ether and pentane, the MP was 113° to 114°C.

(3) Decarboxylation: 55.3 g of 2-methoxy-cyclodec-2-ene-carboxylic acid were introduced into a 250 cc round-bottomed flask equipped with a reflux condenser, a thermometer, a nitrogen inlet, a stirrer and a heating device, and the flask was purged with nitrogen and then gradually heated to 130°C and maintained at this temperature for 2 hours. After cooling, the contents of the flask were extracted with 200 cc of diethyl ether. The ethereal layer was twice treated with 40 cc of 3% by weight sodium hydroxide and then washed to neutrality with 3 x 100 cc of water and dried over anhydrous Na_2SO_4. After evaporation of the solvent, 39.85 grams of an orange-yellow mobile oil were collected containing at least 90% of 1-methoxycyclodecene (35.86 grams) and 10% of cyclodecanone.

(4) Hydrolysis: The oil obtained above (39.85 grams), 280 cc of methanol and 30 cc of 3N hydrochloric acid were introduced into a round-bottomed flask provided with a reflux condenser. The temperature was raised to 60°C over one hour and maintained at this temperature for a further hour. The methanol was then distilled off in vacuo. The heterogeneous liquid was extracted with 150 cc of diethyl ether and the ethereal layer washed to neutrality with water and then dried over anhydrous Na_2SO_4.

After evaporation of the solvent, 35.6 grams of yellow oil were collected which after distillation, gave 33.8 grams of a colorless oil, BP 97.5° to 98.5°C/9 to 10 mm Hg, and BP 100° to 102°C/11 mm Hg. This product was identified as cyclodecanone. Yield 74% calculated on the cycloundecanone. The melting point of the 2,4-dinitrophenylhydrazone was 161°C.

Example 2: Preparation of Cycloundecanone — (1) Preparation of 2,2,12-Tribromocyclo-Dodecanone: The procedure of Example 1 was followed with the following reactants and proportions: cyclododecanone = 4 grams (0.022 mol), anhydrous CCl_4 = 13 grams, anhydrous bromine = 10.7 grams (0.066 mol). After the usual treatments, 8.4 grams of a white solid, MP 104.5° to 105°C, identified as 2,2,12-tribromocyclododecanone (yield 91.1%) were isolated.

(2) Preparation of 2-Methoxy-Cycloundec-2-ene-Carboxylic Acid: (a) 41.9 grams (0.1 mol) of 2,2,12-tribromocyclododecanone were converted into methyl 2-methoxy-cycloundec-2-ene-carboxylate by heating under reflux in 330 cc of methanol containing 13.8 grams of sodium (0.6 gram atom).

(b) 170 cc of methanol were distilled off and replaced by distilled water and the mixture heated under reflux to saponify the ester. The acid was liberated by acidification and recovered by the usual treatments to give 22.25 grams of an oily acid identified as 2-methoxycycloundec-2-ene-carboxylic acid. After recrystallization from a mixture of diethyl ether and pentane, the product had a melting point of 102°C.

(3) Decarboxylation: The previously obtained acid (22.25 grams) was heated for 2 hours at 120° to 130°C under nitrogen and, after the usual treatments, gave 14.4 grams of a yellow mobile oil consisting of 1-methoxy-cycloundecene containing a little cycloundecanone.

(4) Hydrolysis: The oil previously obtained (14.4 grams) was treated with 10 cc of 3N hydrochloric acid in 100 cc of methanol. After the usual treatments, 13.4 grams of an oil which, on distillation, gave 12.8 grams of colorless fraction, BP 62° to 63°C/0.1 mm Hg, a solidification point 16° to 16.5°C were obtained. Yield = 69.4% calculated on the cyclododecanone. The melting point of the 2,4-dinitrophenylhydrazone was 149.5°C.

2,4,4-Trimethyl-2-Pentyl Acetate

A process described by *W.E. Wright and P.A. Immethun; U.S. Patent 3,484,386; December 16, 1969; assigned to Ethyl Corporation* relates to perfumes and perfumed products having the unique odor or odor component conferred by the compound 2,4,4-trimethyl-2-pentyl acetate.

(1)
$$H_2C-\underset{\underset{CH_3}{|}}{\overset{\overset{CH_3}{|}}{C}}-\underset{\underset{H}{|}}{\overset{\overset{H}{|}}{C}}-\underset{\underset{O-\overset{O}{\overset{||}{C}}-CH_3}{|}}{\overset{\overset{CH_3}{|}}{C}}-CH_3$$

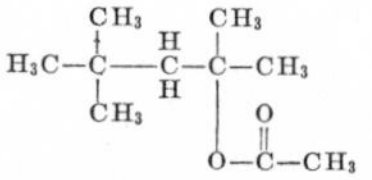

The compound itself and a mode of preparation have been reported in *J. Org. Chem.* 28, 55 to 64 (1963).

To illustrate the compositions of this process the following ointment, salve, and cream bases are described. According to this process, pleasantly scented bases are made by mixing the unscented bases described below with 0.001, 0.01, and 1.0% by weight of the compound of Formula 1, or the same weight of compound plus (based on the weight of compound) up to 30% of the parent alcohol.

Base 1: A mixture having the following ingredients is prepared. All parts are by weight.

	Parts
Cholesterol	10
Stearyl alcohol	30
White wax	80
Wool fat (anhydrous)	150
White petrolatum	730

The ingredients are melted together on a water bath and mixed thoroughly. Thereafter, the mixture is removed from the bath and stirred until it congeals. The table below further illustrates bases of this type. The numbers in the columns are parts by weight.

Ingredient	2	3	4	5	6	7	8	9	10	11	12
Lanolin (anhydrous)	5	5	15.6		10.4				5.5	7.5	16.8
Paraffin wax	15		26.1								
Petrolatum (white)	50	90	76.0	10.9	89.6	100			83.5		83.2
Mineral oil, U.S.P.	30			62.13			100				
White beeswax		5	8.3						11.0		
Carbowax 4000								40.5			
Carbowax 400								59.5			
Hydrogenated cotton seed oil									92.5		
Cetyl alcohol	5		31.2		4.16						
Stearyl alcohol			10.4								
Cholesterol							8.9				
Lanolin alcohols					66		2.2			7.5	0.67
Glyceryl monostearate									13.8		
Stearic acid									2.2		
Magnesium oleate						33.3					
1,2,6-hexanetriol								19			

Using the same percentages of the compound of Formula 1 as used in the above bases, and as well as 2, 4, and 8% of the compound of Formula 1, other pleasantly scented ointment bases are made from the following unscented base.

Base 13: A mixture having the following ingredients is prepared. All parts are by weight.

	Parts
Petrolatum	71.2
Lanolin	11.1
Mineral oil	16.7
Sorbitan monooleate	11.1
Glycerin	11.1

As apparent to a skilled perfumer, the compound of Formula 1 or perfume compositions containing same can be used to confer a pleasant odor to materials other than the above-described bases. For example, other bases which can be perfumed are those within Tables 2, 3, and 4 of U.S. Patent 3,250,677, May 10, 1966.

Esters of 2,2,4-Trimethyl-3-Ketopentanoic Acid

G.C. Kitchens and T.F. Wood; U.S. Patent 3,197,500; July 27, 1965; assigned to Givaudan Corporation describe a general method for making 2,2,4-trimethyl-3-ketopentanoates. The process involves the reaction of 2,2,4,4-tetramethyl-1,3-cyclobutanedione with alcohols, ROH, in the presence of strong alkaline material, to yield keto esters. The reaction may be represented as follows:

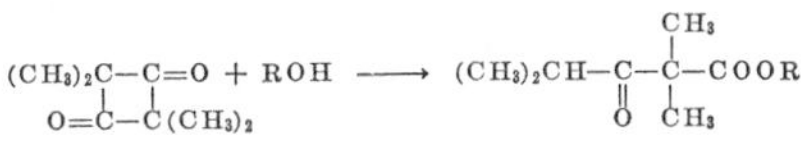

$$(CH_3)_2C-C=O + ROH \longrightarrow (CH_3)_2CH-\overset{CH_3}{\underset{O}{\overset{|}{C}}}-\overset{|}{\underset{CH_3}{C}}-COOR$$

$$O=\overset{|}{\underset{}{C}}-\overset{|}{\underset{}{C}}(CH_3)_2$$

2,2,4,4-tetramethyl
1,3-cyclobutanedione

2,2,4-trimethyl-
3-ketopentanoate ester

where R may be a C_3 to C_{10} branched chain alkyl group, a C_4 to C_{10} straight chain alkyl group, a C_3 to C_{10} mono- or di-unsaturated aliphatic hydrocarbon group, a phenyl group, a phenyl group substituted with a lower alkyl group, a lower alkyl group substituted with a phenyl group, or a lower alkenyl group substituted with a phenyl group.

ALDEHYDES

Unsaturated Aldehydes

A.F. Thomas; U.S. Patent 3,654,309; April 4, 1972; assigned to Firmenich & Cie, Switzerland describes a process for the preparation of α,β-olefinically unsaturated carbonyl compounds of the formula

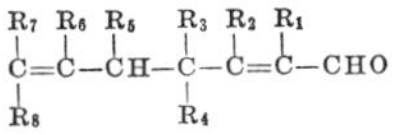

$$\overset{R_7}{\underset{R_8}{\overset{|}{C}}}=\overset{R_6}{\underset{}{\overset{|}{C}}}-\overset{R_5}{\underset{}{\overset{|}{CH}}}-\overset{R_3}{\underset{R_4}{\overset{|}{C}}}-\overset{R_2}{\underset{}{\overset{|}{C}}}=\overset{R_1}{\underset{}{\overset{|}{C}}}-CHO$$

by condensing, with a condensing agent at 60° to 400°C, a butadienyl ether (or a substance which generates such ether) of formula

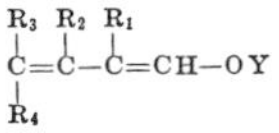

$$\overset{R_3}{\underset{R_4}{\overset{|}{C}}}=\overset{R_2}{\underset{}{\overset{|}{C}}}-\overset{R_1}{\underset{}{\overset{|}{C}}}=CH-OY$$

where Y is a linear or branched C_1-C_4 alkyl radical, or a benzyl, p-nitrobenzyl or furfuryl radical and R_1, R_2, R_3 and R_4 each is hydrogen or a linear or branched C_1-C_6 alkyl radical, with an allyl alcohol containing at least three carbon atoms and at least four carbon atoms less than the end product, of formula

$$\underset{R_8}{\overset{R_7 \ R_6 \ R_5}{C=C-CH-OH}}$$

where R_5, R_6, R_7 and R_8 each is hydrogen, or other radicals. In the following examples, certain conventional techniques are performed as described below.

(A) Column Chromatography: In a column having a diameter to length ratio of about 1:10, filled with silica (Merck, 0.008 mm), the mixture to be separated is charged in a weight proportion equal to or lower than $1/10$ of the weight of silica. The chromatogram is developed with benzene and the elution is carried out with benzene-chloroform solutions containing increasing amounts of chloroform.

(B) Vapor Phase Chromatography: This is performed on a 4 m Carbowax column, at temperatures from 100° to 250°C with a helium stream.

(C) Reduction of the Carbonyl to the Alcohol Function: Lithium aluminum hydride (0.1 to 0.2 mol) is suspended in ether (100 ml) under nitrogen protection and a solution of 0.2 mol of the aldehyde or ketone to be reduced in ether (100 ml) is added dropwise at room temperature. Thereafter, the excess of reducing agent is destroyed with water (5 to 10 ml), and the mixture is filtered, concentrated and distilled under reduced pressure. Temperatures are given in degrees centigrade.

Example 1: Preparation of α- and β-Sinensal — A mixture of 10 grams of 2-methyl-6-vinyl-2,6-heptadien-1-ol, 25 grams of methylbutadienyl ethyl ether, 6.6 grams of mercuric acetate and 2.7 grams of powdered sodium acetate is heated for 18 hours at 98°C under nitrogen protection. After cooling, the solid materials are filtered and the liquid phase is neutralized by stirring with anhydrous potassium carbonate. Then distillation is effected in a high vacuum, and the fraction distilling over at 80°C/0.001 torr is collected. This fraction comprises β-sinensal whose purity is higher than 90% according to gas-chromatographic analysis (yield 43%).

In the NMR the methyl group present in the portion of the field with the highest intensity has a resonance at $\delta = 1.60$ ppm (corrected value). The mass and IR spectra are in agreement with those of natural β-sinensal [cf *J. Org. Chem.* 30, 1690 (1965)], and the dinitrophenylhydrazone of synthetic β-sinensal (MP 80° to 81°C) does not show any depression of the MP in admixture with the dinitrophenylhydrazone of natural β-sinensal.

When using the same method and the same amounts of reactants but replacing the above vinylheptadienol by its isomer, 3,7-dimethyl-1,3,6-octatrien-8-ol, α-sinensal is obtained in a comparable yield, its dinitrophenylhydrazone melting at 96° to 98°C. The α- and β-sinensals prepared according to the above example have valuable flavoring properties and are useful in the flavor industry.

Example 2: Preparation of trans- and cis-2,7,11-Trimethyl-2,6,10-Dodecatrien-1-al — A mixture of 10 grams of geraniol, 25 grams of methylbutadienyl ethyl ether, 6.6 grams of mercuric acetate and 2.7 grams of sodium acetate is heated for 18 hours at 98°C under nitrogen protection. After cooling, the liquid phase is neutralized and separated as indicated in Example 1, then distilled in a high vacuum. 9.3 grams of distillate are obtained which is purified by chromatography on a silica column. The analytical sample of 2,7,11-trimethyl-trans-cis-2,6,10-dodecatrien-1-al thus obtained is again redistilled and converted into its dinitrophenylhydrazone, MP 83° to 84°C. Analysis—Calculated for $C_{21}H_{28}O_4N_4$ (percent): C, 62.98; H, 7.05; N, 14.0. Found (percent) C, 62.47; H, 7.29; N, 14.5.

When replacing in the above mixture geraniol by nerol and proceeding exactly under the same conditions, 11.5 grams of crude 2,7,11-trimethyl-trans-trans-2,6,10-dodecatrien-1-al are obtained, the dinitrophenylhydrazone of which melts at 102° to 104°C.

Analysis–Calculated for $C_{21}H_{28}O_4N_4$ (percent): C, 62.98; H, 7.05; N, 14.0. Found (percent): C, 63.6; H, 7.23; N, 14.8. The aldehydes prepared according to the above example have valuable odoriferous and flavoring properties and are useful in the perfume and flavor industry.

Example 3: Preparation of 2-Methyl-2,6-Octadien-1-al – A mixture of crotyl alcohol (20 grams), 2-methylbutadienyl ethyl ether (50 grams), mercuric acetate (6.6 grams) and sodium acetate (2.7 grams) is heated for 17 hours at 100°C under nitrogen. After cooling, anhydrous potassium carbonate (5 grams) is added, the mixture is vigorously stirred and filtered. The filtrate is distilled and filtered. The filtrate is distilled and the fraction distilling over at 78° to 80°C/10 torr is collected. There is thus obtained a yield of 40% of 2-methyl-2,6-octadien-1-al which is practically pure according to gas chromatography. The following derivatives are readily prepared by means of the usual methods: dinitrophenylhydrazone, MP 139° to 140°C, semicarbazone, MP 153° to 155°C. The aldehyde prepared according to the above example has valuable odoriferous and flavoring properties and is useful in the perfume and flavor industry.

β-Isobutoxypivalaldehyde

G.J. Mantell and C.S. Rondestvedt, Jr.; U.S. Patent 3,676,500; July 11, 1972; assigned to E.I. du Pont de Nemours and Company describe β-alkoxy aldehydes, such as β-isobutoxypivalaldehyde, which, being like most aldehydes, are odoriferous compounds useable as aids in the composition of perfumes. The β-alkoxy aldehydes are characterized by two distinguishing features:

(1) The aldehyde radical —CHO is attached to a tertiary carbon radical, and
(2) In a position β with respect to the —CHO group, the compound bears an ether radical of the form OR, where R is an organic radical free of hydroxy groups and ionizable radicals.

The β-alkoxy aldehydes can be monoaldehydes or bisaldehydes, and may be defined, respectively, by the two formulas:

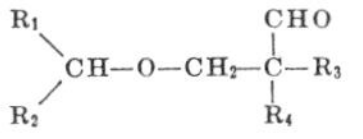

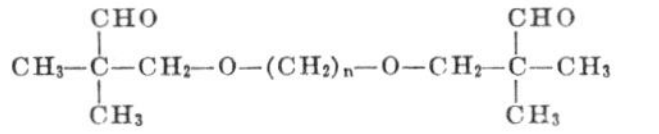

where R_1 is hydrogen, an alkyl group of 1 to 11 carbons, a vinyl group, cyclohexenyl, phenyl, isopropylphenyl, tolyl, trifluoromethylphenyl, chlorophenyl, dichlorophenyl, tetrahydrofuryl, 1,1,5-trimethyl-3-oxahexyl; R_2 is hydrogen, methyl or together with R_1, a divalent alkylene radical of 4 to 5 carbons; R_3 is an alkyl group of one to two carbons; R_4 is an alkyl group of 1 to 3 carbons, vinyl, allyloxymethyl or, together with R_3, a saturated or mono-olefinically unsaturated divalent aliphatic hydrocarbon radical of 5 carbons; and n is an integer of from 3 to 5.

The aldehyde compounds of this process can be prepared by a synthesis which involves splitting cyclic meta-dioxanes by the aid of certain specific mildly acidic solid catalysts. These catalysts are granular pumice and low-surface area silica gel. The meta-dioxanes mentioned above may be defined by the formulas:

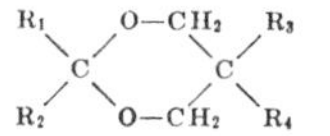

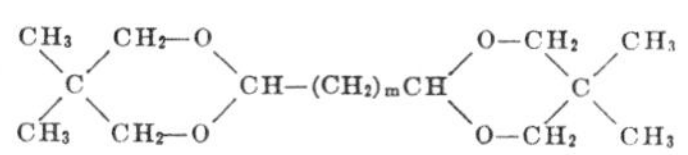

where R_1, R_2, R_3 and R_4 are as defined above, and m = 1 to 3.

The meta-dioxanes, which may also be designated as cyclic acetals or ketals, can be prepared from an aldehyde, ketone, acetal or ketal as typified by the following equations

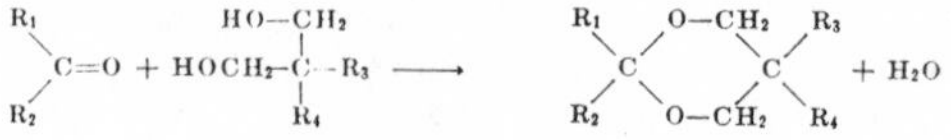

$$\begin{array}{l} R_1 \\ \quad \diagdown \\ \qquad C{=}O + HOCH_2{-}C{\cdot}{-}R_3 \longrightarrow \\ \quad \diagup \\ R_2 \qquad\qquad R_4 \end{array} \qquad \begin{array}{l} R_1 \quad O{-}CH_2 \quad R_3 \\ \quad \diagdown \diagup \quad\quad \diagdown \diagup \\ \qquad C \qquad\quad C \quad + H_2O \\ \quad \diagup \quad \diagdown \qquad \diagup \diagdown \\ R_2 \quad O{-}CH_2 \quad R_4 \end{array}$$

and

$$\begin{array}{l} R_1 \\ \quad \diagdown \\ \qquad C{-}(OCH_3)_2 + HOCH_2{-}C{-}R_3 \longrightarrow \\ \quad \diagup \\ R_2 \qquad\qquad\qquad R_4 \end{array} \qquad \begin{array}{l} R_1 \quad O{-}CH_2 \quad R_3 \\ \quad \diagdown \diagup \quad\quad \diagdown \diagup \\ \qquad C \qquad\quad C \quad + 2CH_3OH \\ \quad \diagup \quad \diagdown \qquad \diagup \diagdown \\ R_2 \quad O{-}CH_2 \quad R_4 \end{array}$$

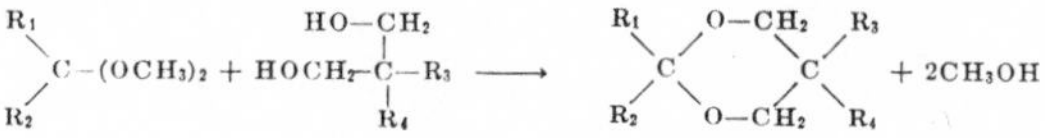

The above meta-dioxanes when heated at a temperature in the range of from 200° to 550°C in contact with mildly acidic solid catalyst undergo fission apparently according to the following scheme.

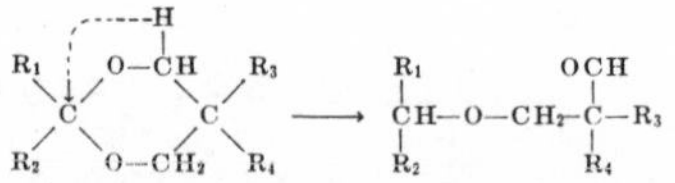

$$\begin{array}{l} \qquad\qquad\qquad {-}{-}{-}{-}H \\ R_1 \quad O{-}CH \quad R_3 \qquad\qquad R_1 \qquad OCH \\ \quad \diagdown \diagup \quad\quad \diagdown \diagup \qquad\qquad\quad | \qquad\qquad | \\ \qquad C \qquad\quad C \quad \longrightarrow \quad CH{-}O{-}CH_2{-}C{-}R_3 \\ \quad \diagup \quad \diagdown \qquad \diagup \diagdown \qquad\qquad\quad | \qquad\qquad | \\ R_2 \quad O{-}CH_2 \quad R_4 \qquad\qquad R_2 \qquad R_4 \end{array}$$

The operation of splitting is effected by conducting vapors of the selected initial material (cyclic acetal or ketal), preferably diluted with an inert gas such as nitrogen, argon or carbon dioxide, over the solid catalyst, heated to a temperature in the range of 200° to 550°C. The initial materials are generally volatile solids or liquids. The reaction products are usually liquids. Accordingly, the reaction is best arranged to proceed in a pipe or column containing the solid catalyst in a heated portion. The initial material, powder or liquid, may be swept into the receptacle at one end thereof by the aid of the carrier gas (e.g., N_2). It vaporizes as it approaches the reaction zone, undergoes splitting, and emerges as a gas, which cools to a liquid at the other end of the tubular reactor.

Allenic Aldehydes

A process described by *B. Thompson; U.S. Patent 3,225,102; December 21, 1965; assigned to Eastman Kodak Company* relates to compounds having two adjacent carbon-carbon double bonds such as are found in allene. The process is based on the discovery that when certain aldehydes having at least two carbon atoms per molecule are heated with an acetylenic alcohol in the presence of an acidic catalyst reaction occurs with an unexpected molecular rearrangement that results in the formation of a type of allenic aldehyde having a characteristic functional group,

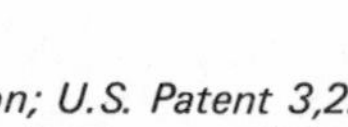

$$\begin{array}{l} \quad\quad | \qquad | \quad | \\ C{=}C{=}C{-}C{-}CHO \\ \quad | \qquad\qquad | \end{array}$$

The basic reaction of the process is applicable to a wide range of different aldehyde and acetylenic alcohol starting materials. The reaction has been demonstrated most extensively in preparing 3,4-dienaldehydes of the formula

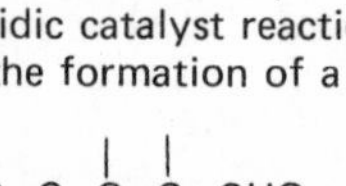

$$\begin{array}{l} R^4 \qquad\qquad R^3 \quad R^1 \\ \quad \diagdown \qquad\qquad | \qquad | \\ \qquad C{=}C{=}C{-}C{-}CHO \\ \quad \diagup \qquad\qquad\qquad | \\ R^5 \qquad\qquad\qquad R^2 \end{array}$$

where R^1 and R^2 are alkyl groups or cycloalkyl groups, and R^3, R^4 and R^5 are hydrogen or alkyl or cycloalkyl groups. The following examples illustrate the process.

Example 1: A solution of 280 grams (5 mols) of propargyl alcohol, 504 grams (7 mols) of isobutyraldehyde, 1.0 gram of p-toluenesulfonic acid, and 200 grams of diisopropyl benzene was heated in a fractionating still having means for removing water at the head. 95 grams of water was removed over a period of 30 hours. The charge was then fractionated. More than 220 grams of 2,2-dimethyl-penta-3,4-dien-1-al was recovered. BP 131°C, $n_D{}^{20}$ 1.4531. Infrared analysis showed that there was no conjugated unsaturation present but that allenic unsaturation was present (absorption at 5.1 microns). Nuclear magnetic resonance showed that there were the correct number and intensities of hydrogen protons present to agree with the structure CH_2:C:CH—C$(CH_3)_2$CHO.

Analysis—Theoretical: C, 76.32; H, 9.15; O, 14.53. Found: C, 75.85; H, 9.19; O, 14.96. Carbonyl equivalent weight 111 (theory 110.15). Reduction of the product, resulting in its taking up 3 molecules of hydrogen, gave 2,2-dimethylpentanol, BP 156°C, $n_D{}^{20}$ 1.4259.

Example 2: A solution of 1,720 grams of 2-methylbutyraldehyde, 1,120 grams of propargyl alcohol, 1 gram of methionic acid, 1 gram of hydroquinone, and 160 cc of benzene was boiled in a still topped by a reflux condenser and water separator. After 360 cc of water had separated, 1 gram of sodium bicarbonate was added. Fractionation at atmospheric and reduced pressure separated 2-ethyl-2-methyl-penta-3,4-dien-1-al, BP 92°C at 100 mm, $n_D{}^{20}$ 1.4603. Infrared analysis showed this aldehyde to have a strong absorption at 5.1 microns, which is characteristic of the C:C:C structure.

Example 3: Substituting equal mols of 2-ethylhexanaldehyde for 2-methylbutyraldehyde in Example 2 produced 2-butyl-2-ethyl-penta-3,4-dien-1-al, BP 210°C.

Example 4: Substituting 2-methyl-pentanaldehyde for 2-methylbutyraldehyde in Example 2 produced 2-methyl-2-propyl-penta-3,4-dien-1-al, BP 175°C.

sec-Butylcyclohexane Carboxaldehyde

S. Lemberg; U.S. Patent 3,514,489; May 26, 1970; assigned to International Flavors & Fragrances, Inc. describes derivatives of sec-butylcyclohexane having the structural formula

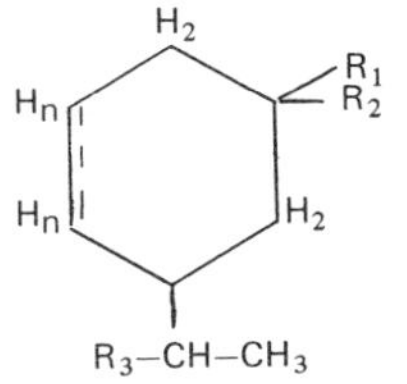

where R_1 is hydrogen or lower alkyl; R_2 is

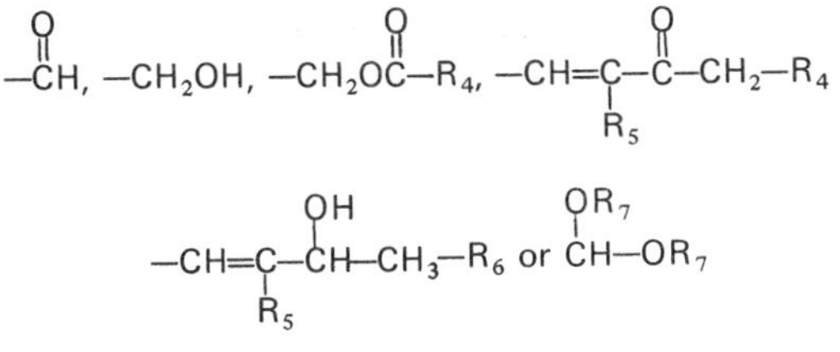

R_3 is ethyl or vinyl; R_4, R_5, and R_6 are hydrogen or lower alkyl; R_7 is lower alkyl; n is one or two; and the dashed line indicates that a single bond is present when n is two and a double bond is present when n is one.

They are prepared by the reaction of 5-methyl-1,3,6-heptatriene with an unsaturated aldehyde. Thus, this process provides 5-(3-buten-2-yl)-3-cyclohexene carboxaldehyde having the structural formula below.

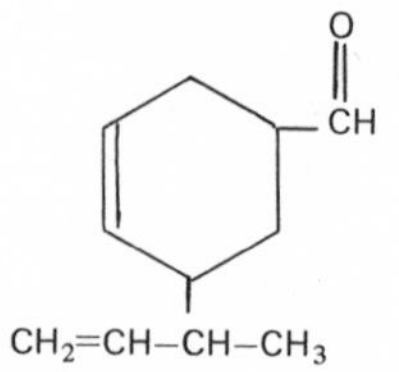

$$CH_2{=}CH{-}CH{-}CH_3$$

This material has a boiling point of 72°C at 3.0 mm Hg, an n_D^{20} of 1.4890 to 1.4892, and a good green twiggy odor which is relatively long-lasting and dries out cleanly. A second material is 5-(3-buten-2-yl)-1-methyl-3-cyclohexene carboxaldehyde having the formula

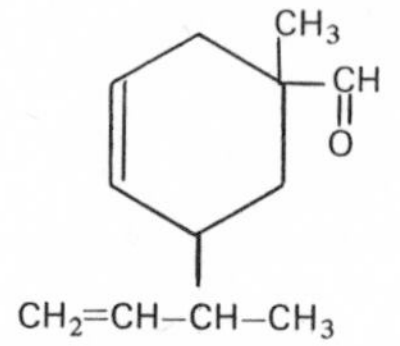

$$CH_2{=}CH{-}CH{-}CH_3$$

This material has a boiling point of 45°C at 0.20 mm Hg, an n_D^{20} of 1.4907 to 1.4909, and a camphoraceous, herbaceous piney odor.

Another carboxaldehyde produced according to the process is a 5-sec-butyl-3-cyclohexene carboxaldehyde having the formula

$$CH_3{-}CH_2{-}CH{-}CH_3$$

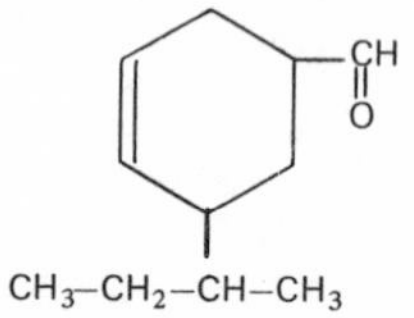

having an n_D^{20} of 1.4730 to 1.4745. It has a powerful rosy, green, floral odor.

The process to produce the materials described above involves the reaction of α,β-unsaturated aldehydes with alkyl-substituted heptatriene, preferably methyl-substituted heptatriene such as 5-methyl-1,3,6-heptatriene to produce an alkenylcyclohexene carboxaldehyde. While the heptatriene can be utilized in the commercially available form at about 80% purity, it is especially preferred in carrying out the process that the material be distilled substantially to 100% purity before use. The preferred unsaturated aldehydes are propenals such as acrolein and alkyl acroleins, especially lower 2-alkyl acroleins such as methacroleins. The following examples illustrate the process.

Example 1: Thirteen hundred and fifty grams of substantially pure 5-methyl-1,3,6-heptatriene, 700 grams of acrolein, and 50 grams of hydroquinone are introduced into an autoclave and the mixture is maintained at 100°C for 8 hours to form a reaction product. The reaction product so obtained is distilled in a fractionating column.

There is obtained 1,192 grams of 5-(3-buten-2-yl)-3-cyclohexene carboxaldehyde having the structural formula given above. This material is a clear liquid having a boiling point of 72°C at 3.0 mm Hg and an n_D^{20} of 1.4890 to 1.4892. Gas-liquid chromatographic (GLC) analysis shows that two components are present in equal amounts. Spectroscopic analyses utilizing nuclear magnetic resonance (NMR), mass, and infrared (IR) methods show that these are the cis and trans isomers of 5-(3-butene-2-yl)-3-cyclohexene carboxaldehyde. This material has a good green-twiggy odor which is long-lasting.

Example 2: About 1,080 grams of 5-methyl-1,3,6-heptatriene, 700 grams of methacrolein, and 50 grams of hydroquinone are introduced into an autoclave. The mixture is heated at 73°C for 12 hours and the product is fractionally distilled to obtain 1,450 grams of a clear liquid.

This clear liquid material is 5-(3-buten-2-yl)-1-methylcyclohexene carboxaldehyde having the structural formula shown above. This liquid has a boiling point of 45°C at 0.20 mm Hg and an n_D^{20} of 1.4907 to 1.4909. NMR and mass spectra support the given structure. The material has a camphoraceous, herbaceous piney odor.

Example 3: A hydrogenation unit is charged with 166 grams of the product of Example 1, 100 grams of ethanol, and 8 grams of Raney nickel. The flash is purged four times with hydrogen, and the contents are then hydrogenated at a pressure of 14 to 45 psig and a temperature of 25° to 30°C for slightly over 4 hours. The product is filtered, the alcohol is recovered, and the product is distilled under vacuum. The product is chiefly 5-sec-butyl-3-cyclohexene carboxaldehyde. It is a liquid having an n_D^{20} of 1.4730 to 1.4745. It has a powerful rosy, green, floral odor.

α-Substituted Pinoacetaldehyde

J.B. Hall; U.S. Patent 3,716,498; February 13, 1973; assigned to International Flavors & Fragrances Inc. describes pinane derivatives, α-alkyl and α, α-dialkyl-6,6 dimethyl bicyclo-[3.1.1] hept-2-ene-alkanals (referred to as α-substituted pinoacetaldehydes) having the formulas

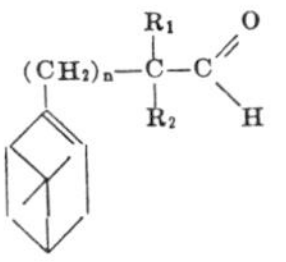

where R_1 is hydrogen or lower alkyl, R_2 is lower alkyl, and n is 1 or 2; as well as the corresponding lower alkyl acetals having the structure

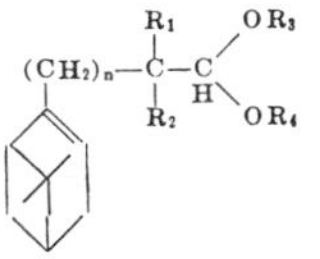

where R_3 and R_4 are the same or different lower alkyl groups, and wherein n is 1 or 2; and lower alkylene cyclic acetals having the structure

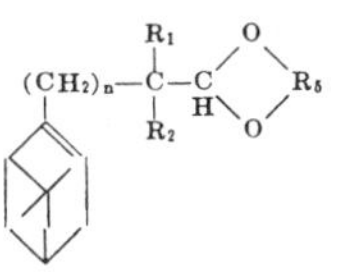

where R_5 is lower alkylene. The materials found to be useful in the process are produced by several methods. One such method involves reacting pinocarveol with a substituted or unsubstituted ethyl vinyl ether in the presence of a protonic acid such as phosphoric acid with or without a suitable additional inert reaction vehicle. When ethyl vinyl ether is used, the reaction product is pinoacetaldehyde. When the vinyl group is alkyl or dialkyl substituted in the β-position, the reaction product is one of the products of this process. The reaction can be represented as follows.

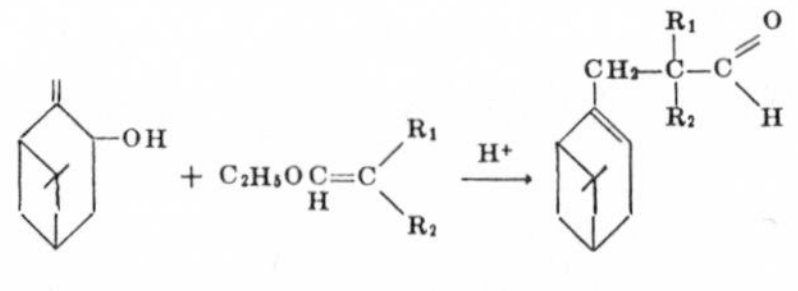

Dialkyl acetals of the abovementioned aldehydes can be formed by reaction thereof with ethyl orthoformate or alcohols in the presence of an acid catalyst. Alkylene cyclic acetals of the abovementioned aldehydes can be produced by reaction thereof with a lower alkylene glycol such as ethylene glycol or propylene glycol. The following examples illustrate the process.

Example 1: Preparation of Pinoacetaldehyde by Reaction of Pinocarveol with Ethyl Vinyl Ether — Into a one-liter autoclave the following ingredients were placed: 250 grams pino-carveol, 250 grams ethyl vinyl ether and 0.5 gram 85% phosphoric acid. The contents of the autoclave were heated at a temperature range of 150° to 155°C over a period of 2½ hours. The pressure within the autoclave was in the range of 70 to 80 psig.

At the termination of the reaction the contents of the autoclave were removed and the organic phase was washed with an equal volume of 5% of sodium bicarbonate and then with an equal volume of water. The excess ethyl vinyl ether was stripped off and the re-sulting crude product was distilled at 84° to 88°C on a 12" Goodloe column (pressure: 2.8 to 3.2 mm Hg; reflux ratio 9:1). Infra red, NMR and mass spectral analysis confirmed the following structure of the product

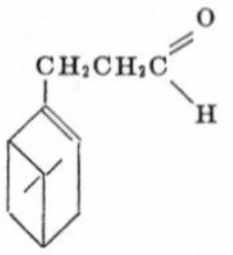

The pinoacetaldehyde thus formed had a highly persistent, very fresh, pungent, flowery, woodsy, ozone-like odor reminiscent of early morning dew-laden vegetation.

Example 2: Preparation of Pinoisobutyraldehyde — (a) Formation of Schiff Base: 396 grams (4.0 mols) of cyclohexylamine was placed in a flask. Over a period of 1 hour, while maintaining the temperature at 20°C, 292 grams of isobutyraldehyde was added. At the end of the addition period, the aqueous and organic phases were separated and the organic phase consisting of the Schiff base N-(2-methyl propylidene)cyclohexylamine was dried over magnesium sulfate and distilled at a vapor temperature of 61° to 67°C (pressure: 13 to 14 mm Hg).

(b) Reaction of Schiff Base with Grignard Reagent: Into a 3-liter flask purged with ni-trogen, 680 ml (2.02 mols) of methyl magnesium chloride in tetrahydrofuran was added. The contents of the flask were heated to 60°C. Over a period of 1 hour, 282 grams of the Schiff base produced in part (a) was added, maintaining the temperature in the range of 50° to 70°C. After addition, the contents were heated for 4 hours until the evolution of hydrogen ceased.

(c) Reaction of the Schiff Base—Grignard Reagent with Myrtenyl Chloride: Over a period of 2 hours 444 grams of 71.3% (wt) myrtenyl chloride were added to the reaction prod-uct produced in part (b), while maintaining the temperature in the range of 65° to 70°C. After addition was completed, the reaction mass was stirred for a period of 8 hours, main-

taining the temperature in the range of 60° to 72°C.

(d) Hydrolysis of Schiff Base Product Formed in (c): The pH of the reaction mass was brought to 4 by addition of 1,140 grams of 10% aqueous sulfuric acid. The mass was then heated for a period of 30 minutes at 65°C after which the aqueous phase was separated from the organic phase. The aqueous layer was extracted with 550 ml of toluene and the toluene extract was bulked with organic layer. The organic phase was then washed per the following sequence:

(1) One 550 ml volume of 5% aqueous hydrochloric acid;
(2) One equal volume of saturated sodium chloride solution;
(3) One equal volume of a 3% sodium bicarbonate solution (bringing the pH to 8.0);
(4) One equal volume of a saturated sodium chloride solution (bringing the pH to 7.0).

The solvent was then stripped off and the reaction product was distilled in a 12" Goodloe column at a vapor temperature of 91° to 94°C (pressure: 2.6 to 3.0 mm Hg; reflux ratio 9:1). 236 grams of the reaction product, α-pinyl isobutyraldehyde was recovered, the structure of which, confirmed by NMR, infrared and mass spectral analysis is

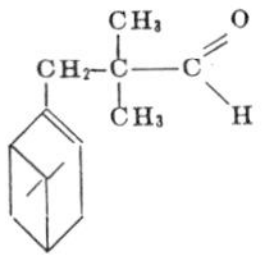

The α-pino-isobutyraldehyde had a highly persistent, fresh, soft floral, woodsy, ozone-like odor reminiscent of early morning dew-laden vegetation.

Example 3: The following mixture was prepared:

Ingredients	Parts by Weight	Ingredients	Parts by Weight
Coumarin	100	Hydroxycitronellal	20
Linalol	200	Sauge Sclaree	20
Benzylacetate	50	Neroli bigarade	20
Geranium absolute	30	Isobutylsalicyclate	10
Methylacetophenone	50	Ylang-Ylang Bourbon	10
Bergamot	40	Patchouli oil	10
Lavender, Barreme	120	Vetiver acetate	5
Pinoacetaldehyde		Mousse de Chene absolute	5
(Product of Ex 1)	80	Anis alcohol	10
Benzophenone	25	Basilicum absolute	5
Trichloromethylphenyl-			
carbinyl acetate	25		

A pleasing new fragrance results giving an interesting variation which can be described as a fresh-air quality to the basic classic Foin Coup cologne blend.

Additional studies with the pinane derivatives, α-alkyl and α, α-dialkyl-6,6 dimethyl bicyclo-[3.1.1] hept-2-ene-alkanals are described by *J.B. Hall; U.S. Patent 3,636;113; January 18, 1972; assigned to International Flavors & Fragrances, Inc.*

Myrcene Epoxide Diels-Alder Adducts

According to a process described by *J.O. Bledsoe, Jr.; U.S. Patent 3,671,551; June 20, 1972; assigned to SCM Corporation,* Diels-Alder adducts of myrcene epoxide have been found to exhibit excellent olfactory and perfumery properties. The adducts are made by reacting myrcene epoxide with an α,β-unsaturated carbonyl compound (dienophile), such as acrolein, in a Diels-Alder reaction. Additionally the adducts can be hydrogenated to form the saturated adduct which also possesses excellent olfactory properties.

Hydrolyzed Diels-Alder Adducts of Ocimenol

According to a process described by *J.O. Bledsoe, Jr. and J.M. Derfer; U.S. Patent 3,758,590; September 11, 1973; assigned to SCM Corporation,* hydrolyzed Diels-Alder adducts of ocimenol have been synthesized and found to have good olfactory and perfumery properties. The hydrolyzed adducts are made by reacting ocimenol and an α,β-unsaturated carbonyl compound, preferably acrolein, methacrolein or crotonaldehyde, in a Diels-Alder reaction, followed by hydrolysis.

Aldehydes from 1,2-Epoxides

A process described by *W.D. Niederhauser; U.S. Patent 3,130,233; April 21, 1964; assigned to Rohm & Haas Company* relates to β-hydroxyaldehydes and α,β-unsaturated aldehydes. The process comprises treating 1,2-epoxides with carbon monoxide and hydrogen gases under pressure and elevated temperatures in the presence of a hydroformylation catalyst, resulting in useful aldehydes.

The process is applicable to compounds containing one or a plurality of 1,2-epoxide groups. When there are employed as starting materials, polyepoxides, such as alkyl esters of epoxidized water-insoluble fatty acids or epoxidized glyceryl esters, there may be obtained products which are mixtures of poly-β-hydroxyaldehydes and of poly-α,β-unsaturated aldehydes. However, it is preferred to use somewhat simpler starting materials which may be classified within the following three groups:

Group A which may be represented by

(I)
$$ R-\underset{\diagdown O \diagup}{CH-CH}-R^1 $$

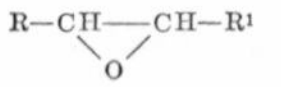

where R and R^1 are hydrogen atoms or alkyl groups containing from one to preferably twelve carbon atoms, R and R^1 being alike or different;

Group B which may be represented by

(II)
$$ R^2-\underset{\diagdown O \diagup}{CH-CH}-\left(CH_2\right)_{n-1}-\overset{O}{\overset{\|}{C}}-OR^3 $$

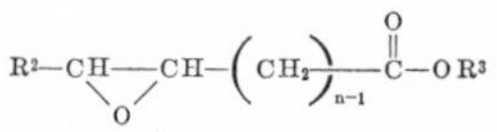

where R^2 represents an alkyl group containing from one to eleven carbon atoms, R^3 represents an alkyl group containing one to eighteen, preferably one to eight carbon atoms, and n is an integer from eight to eleven, the total number of carbon atoms of compounds of group B preferably ranging from twenty to thirty; and

Group C which may be represented by

(III)
$$ A-\underset{\diagdown O \diagup}{CH_2-CH-CH}-R^4 $$

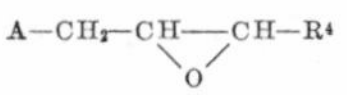

where A is an aryl group, preferably containing from six to eight carbon atoms, such as phenyl, tolyl, and xylyl, and R^4 is an alkyl group containing from one to six, preferably one, carbon atoms.

The process yields valuable compounds. The products resulting from the groups A, B, and C, respectively, may be represented by the following formulas, in which the alphabetical designation corresponds to that given to the starting epoxides and the even numbers designate the α,β-unsaturated aldehydes, whereas the uneven numbers specify the β-hydroxyaldehyde products,

(A IV)

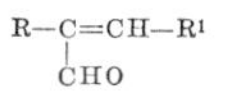

$$R-\underset{\underset{CHO}{|}}{C}=CH-R^1$$

(A V)

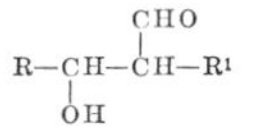

$$R-CH-\underset{\underset{OH}{|}}{\overset{\overset{CHO}{|}}{C}}H-R^1$$

(B VI)

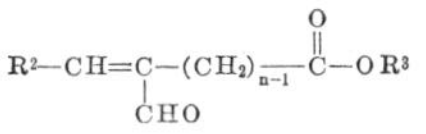

$$R^2-CH=\underset{\underset{CHO}{|}}{C}-(CH_2)_{n-1}-\overset{\overset{O}{\|}}{C}-OR^3$$

(B VII)

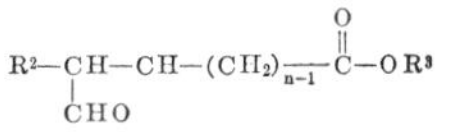

$$R^2-CH-\underset{\underset{CHO}{|}}{C}H-(CH_2)_{n-1}-\overset{\overset{O}{\|}}{C}-OR^3$$

(C VIII)

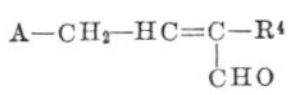

$$A-CH_2-HC=\underset{\underset{CHO}{|}}{C}-R^4$$

(C IX)

$$A-CH_2-CH-\underset{\underset{CHO}{|}}{\overset{\overset{OH}{|}}{C}}H-R^4$$

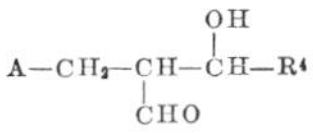

in which R, R¹, R², R³, R⁴, A and n have the definitions assigned above. In each case illustrated above, the α,β-unsaturated aldehyde products include the isomers in which the formyl group and the vicinal vinylene hydrogen atom are on either carbon of the vinylidene unsaturation. Likewise, in the β-hydroxyaldehyde products there are included the isomers in which the hydroxyl and formyl groups are interchangeably bonded onto either of the vicinal carbon atoms onto which originally the epoxy oxygen was bonded.

Typical β-hydroxyaldehydes prepared in accordance with the method include:

> 2-methyl-3-hydroxy-4-phenylbutanal;
> 2-benzyl-3-hydroxybutanal;
> 2-butyl-3-hydroxy-4-phenylbutanal;
> 2-methyl-3-hydroxy-4-xylylbutanal;
> 2-(2,4-dimethylbenzyl)-3-hydroxybutanal; and
> methyl 9,(10)-hydroxy-10,(9)-formylstearate.

Typical of α,β-unsaturated aldehydes prepared in accordance with this method include:

> 2-methyl-4-phenyl-2-butenal, and its isomer;
> 2-benzyl-2-butenal;
> 2-butyl-4-phenyl-2-butenal;
> 2-methyl-4-xylyl-2-butenal;
> methyl 9,(10)-formyloleate; and
> octyl 9,(10)-formyloleate.

The α,β-unsaturated aldehydes are valuable for preparing unsaturated dibasic acids by oxidation. Oxidation, such as with hydrogen peroxide, under mild conditions yields hydroxyacids. Another use for the α,β-unsaturated aldehydes is as adjuncts in odoriferous compositions. The more pungent α,β-unsaturated aldehydes may be useful in insect repellent preparations, the other aldehydes which have more pleasant fragrance may be used as bases or additives in cosmetic preparations. The following examples illustrate the process. Unless otherwise indicated, all parts are by weight.

Example 1: To a stainless steel autoclave of 300 cc capacity, there are charged 29 parts of propylene oxide, 40 parts of xylene, and 5 parts of a solution of cobalt carbonyl in benzene containing 3% cobalt. The vessel is closed and it is filled with a mixture of carbon monoxide and hydrogen in a 1 to 1 volume ratio until a pressure of 2,100 psi is recorded. The vessel is heated to within a temperature range of 130° to 140°C with rocking for one hour to insure mixing. The pressure drops smoothly during the reaction. When pressure dropped to 960 psi and no further drop is recorded, the autoclave is cooled to 20°C. The product is removed; it is distilled rapidly and the distillate is separated from the lower water layer. The product is redistilled through a packed column to give 5.5 parts of methacrolein and 9 parts of crotonaldehyde.

Example 2: To a hydrogenation bomb of 300 cc capacity, there are charged 87 parts of methyl 9,10-epoxystearate, 50 parts of benzene and 8 parts of cobalt carbonyl in benzene having a 3% cobalt content. Carbon monoxide and hydrogen are fed into the bomb to a pressure of 2,600 psi and heat is applied to and maintained at 120° to 150°C for one hour, with rocking. Upon a drop of pressure to 1,420 psi and when no further uptake of gas is recorded, the bomb is cooled to room temperature. Catalyst is separated and solvent is distilled from the product. There is obtained 91 parts of an oil, which is a mixture of the isomers of methyl 9,(10)-hydroxy-10,(9)-formylstearate and of methyl 9,(10)-formyloleate. These products are separated by fractional distillation under reduced pressure.

Example 3: Following the procedure of Example 2, octyl-9,10-epoxystearate is treated in the presence of cobalt carbonyl with a mixture of carbon monoxide and hydrogen under pressure to yield octyl-9,(10)-hydroxy-10,(9)-formylstearate and octyl-9,(10)-formyloleate. The products are separated by fractional distillation under reduced pressure. Methyl 13,(14)-epoxybehenate is treated in a similar manner to yield methyl 13,(14)-hydroxy-14,(13)-formyldocosanoate and methyl 15,(16)-formylerucate. The products are separated by fractional distillation under a reduced pressure of 1 mm of mercury.

KETONES

Silylorganoaryl Ketones

E.V. Wilkus and A. Berger; U.S. Patent 3,391,109; July 2, 1968; assigned to General Electric Company describe organosilicon materials having at least one aroylorgano radical attached to silicon by carbon-silicon linkages. The organosilicon materials or aryl ketone-containing organosilicon materials are selected from

(A) Silylorganoaryl ketones of the formula

$$(Q\overset{O}{\overset{\|}{C}}R'') R_2 SiO_{\frac{(1-a)}{2}}$$

with R'_a

(B) Polymers consisting essentially of chemically combined units of the formula

$$Q'\overset{O}{\overset{\|}{C}}R''SiO_{\frac{(3-b)}{2}}$$

with R_b

(C) Copolymers composed of 0.01 to 99.99 mol percent of organosiloxy units of the formula

$$SiO_{\frac{(4-c)}{2}}$$

with R_c

chemically combined with 99.99 mol percent to 0.01 mol percent of units of (B), and

(D) Curable compositions comprising a curing agent and a silanol chain-stopped polymer selected from

(a) Homopolymers consisting essentially of chemically combined units of the formula

$$Q'\overset{O}{\overset{\|}{C}}R'SiO$$

with R

(b) Copolymers of from 5 to 95 mol % of (a) units chemically combined with from 95 mol % to 5 mol % of R_2SiO units

where R is a member selected from monovalent radicals, halogenated monovalent hydrocarbon radicals, cyanoalkyl radicals, halogen radicals, alkoxy, R′ is selected from R radicals, R″ is a divalent hydrocarbon radical selected from arylene radicals and alkylene radicals, Q is a monovalent aromatic radical selected from aryloxyaryl radicals, arylthioaryl radicals, arylsulfonylaryl radicals and heteroaromatic radicals. Q′ includes all of the above Q radicals, aromatic hydrocarbon radicals and halogenated aromatic hydrocarbon radicals, a and b are whole numbers equal to 0 or 1, c is a whole number equal to 0 to 3, inclusive, and the sum of b and c in the copolymers of (C) can have a value between 1 to 2.01, inclusive.

Some of the aryl ketone containing organosilicon materials of the process can be made directly by acylating an aryl nucleus with a silyl acid halide of the formula

$$\underset{Y_{3-c}}{} \overset{R_c}{\underset{|}{Si}} R' \overset{O}{\overset{||}{C}} X$$

where R, R′ and c are as defined above, and X is a halogen radical, such as chloro.

Some of the silylorganoaryl ketones are for example, trimethylsilylbutyrylthiophene, 1,3-bis(4-phenoxybenzoylpropyl)tetramethyldisiloxane, 1,3-bis(furoylpropyl)tetramethyl-disiloxane, 2-trimethylsilylpropionylxanthene and furoylpropyldimethylsilanol. These materials can be used as perfumes, oil bases in cosmetics, etc. The following examples illustrate the process. All parts are by weight.

Example 1: There was added 130 parts of anhydrous stannic chloride to a mixture of 90 parts of trimethylsilylbutyryl chloride, 100 parts methylene chloride and 84 parts of thiophene under a nitrogen atmosphere. Hydrogen chloride was continually evolved as the mixture was stirred resulting in the production of a deep colored complex. The mixture was allowed to warm to room temperature and stirred for an additional 3 hours. It was then heated to reflux for 3 more hours.

The mixture was then stirred with a mixture of crushed ice and dilute hydrochloric acid. After the reaction product had been completely hydrolyzed, the organic layer was separated, dried and fractionated. There was obtained 70 parts of a product boiling at 134° to 137°C at 1.5 mm. Based on method of preparation and its infrared spectrum, the product was trimethylsilyl butyryl-2-thiophene having the formula

$$(CH_3)_3Si(CH_2)_3\overset{O}{\overset{||}{C}}(C_4H_3S)$$

Example 2: There was added uniformly over a 30-minute period, 4.2 parts of anhydrous aluminum chloride to a mixture of 15 parts of diphenyl ether, 5 parts of β-trimethylsilyl propionyl chloride, and 50 parts of methylene chloride while the mixture was stirred. During the addition hydrogen chloride was continuously evolved.

The mixture was then stirred for an additional hour and then refluxed for two more hours. The mixture was then hydrolyzed in accordance with the procedure described in Example 1, and the crude oily product was purified by chromatography on a column packed with Alco F-20 alumina in hexane. Elution with hexane removed the excess diphenyl ether; elution with ether gave 7 parts of a colorless oil whose infrared spectrum showed absorption for alkylaryl ketone at 6.0 microns, for methyl-to-silicon at 8.0 microns, and for the trimethylsilyl grouping at 11.6 microns.

In addition, absorption characterizing diphenyl ether was found at 6.3 microns, 6.8 microns, 8.3 microns, 7.5 microns, 13.3 microns and 14.4 microns. Based on its method of preparation and its infrared spectrum, the product was (β-trimethylsilylpropionyl)diphenyl ether having the formula

$$(CH_3)_3Si(CH_2)_2\overset{O}{\overset{||}{C}}C_6H_4OC_6H_5$$

2-Cyclohexylcyclohexanone

L.O. Winstrom, J.M. Becker and J.C. Park; U.S. Patent 3,246,036; April 12, 1966; assigned to Allied Chemical Corporation describe the production of 2-cyclohexylcyclohexanone. 2-cyclohexylcyclohexanone, although not a large tonnage commodity finds importance for use as a flavoring agent, an insect repellent and perfume fixative, and has previously been prepared by a variety of procedures. In one such procedure 2-cyclohexylcyclohexanone is prepared by passing cyclohexanol vapors over a catalyst consisting of a mixture of the chromites of zinc, copper and cadmium. In another procedure, 2-cyclohexylcyclohexanone is prepared by liquid-phase dehydrogenation of cyclohexylcyclohexanol in the presence of a copper chromite catalyst.

It has been found that 2-cyclohexylcyclohexanone can be produced in small but nevertheless commercially recoverable amounts by passing hydrogen in contact with phenol in the presence of palladium catalyst at a temperature within the range of from 150° to 250°C preferably 175° to 225°C for a sufficient length of time to convert the phenol to 2-cyclohexylcyclohexanone and concomitantly cyclohexanone and cyclohexanol, separating the cyclohexanone and cyclohexanol from the reaction mixture leaving as residue a mixture containing usually more than 50% by weight 2-cyclohexylcyclohexanone with the remainder substantially all high boiling constituents less volatile than cyclohexanone and cyclohexanol and separating and recovering substantially pure 2-cyclohexylcyclohexanone from the residue by fractional distillation under reduced pressure, e.g., from about 5 to 50 mm Hg absolute pressure.

The resultant light distillate, substantially pure cyclohexylcyclohexanone is recovered in good yields up to about 75% or more based on the weight of the 2-cyclohexylcyclohexanone in the residue. If an especially light color 2-cyclohexylcyclohexanone product is desired the 2-cyclohexylcyclohexanone product of the process may be contacted with absorbent charcoal for example, under agitation at ambient temperature for about 30 minutes and the mixture filtered to remove the charcoal.

2-Propenyl-2-Cyclohexanone

B. Thompson and T.E. Buckner; U.S. Patent 3,431,305; March 4, 1969; assigned to Eastman Kodak Company describe aliphatic 2-substituted carbocyclic ketones which are aliphatic 2-allylidene carbocyclic ketones of the formula:

$$\begin{array}{c} O \qquad\qquad R^3 \\ \| \qquad\qquad / \\ C-C=CH-CH=C \\ / \quad\quad\quad\quad\quad \backslash \\ R^1-CH \quad\ HC-R^2 \quad R^4 \\ \backslash \qquad / \\ (CH_2)_n \end{array}$$

and aliphatic 2-propenyl carbocyclic ketones of the formula:

$$\begin{array}{c} O \quad H \qquad\qquad R^3 \\ \| \quad \| \qquad\qquad / \\ C-C-CH=CH-CH \\ / \quad\quad\quad\quad\quad \backslash \\ R^1-CH \quad\ HC-R^2 \quad R^4 \\ \backslash \qquad / \\ (CH_2)_n \end{array}$$

where n is an integer from 0 to 8; each of R^1 and R^2, when taken singly, is hydrogen; R^1 and R^2, when taken collectively, represent an alkylene group having 1 to 2 carbon atoms, R^3 and R^4 when taken singly, are hydrogen or alkyl of 1 to 8 carbon atoms; and R^3 and R^4, when taken collectively with the carbon atom to which they are attached, represent a saturated carbocyclic ring having 4 to 8 ring carbon atoms.

The process is preferably carried out by heating a mixture containing the acetylenic alcohol and the aliphatic carbocyclic ketone in the presence of the acidic catalyst. The reaction can be carried out with equimolar amounts of the acetylenic alcohol and the aliphatic carbocyclic ketone or with a molar excess of either the acetylenic alcohol or the aliphatic carbocyclic ketone. However, it is preferred to use an excess of the aliphatic carbocyclic ketone. The reaction is catalyzed by virtually any type of acidic material. The following example illustrates the process.

Example: A solution containing 3,920 grams of cyclohexanone, 1,120 grams of propargyl alcohol, 10 grams of hydroquinone, 0.5 gram of methionic acid, and 510 grams of p-xylene was heated in a reaction still having means for removing water at the still-head. Enough benzene, 120 grams, was added to the reaction mixture to aid in the separation of water at the still-head. The mixture was heated for about 13½ hours during which time about 370 cm^3 of water containing some propargyl alcohol was removed at the still-head.

The crude product was removed from the reaction still and stripped in a flash still to remove unreacted feed materials. The ratio of ketone to alcohol in the unreacted feed materials was adjusted to 2 mols ketone to 1 mol of alcohol and the reaction was repeated with the unreacted feed materials. The higher boiling products from each of the reactions were fractionated to separate 2-(propenyl)-2-cyclohexenone, BP 63° to 65°C at 2.0 mm. Elemental analysis confirmed the formula $C_9H_{12}O$. Infrared and nuclear magnetic resonance analysis confirmed the structure of the major portion of the reaction product to be 2-(propenyl)-2-cyclohexenone. Another fraction having the same elemental analysis was shown to be 2-allylidenecyclohexanone. These compounds are useful as odor-imparting agents in the preparation of perfumes and other scented compositions. For example, they can be incorporated in milled soap in a concentration of from about 0.5 to about 2 weight percent to give the soap a pleasant scent.

Glyoxylylbenzophenone Derivatives

W.H. Edgerton; U.S. Patent 3,128,312; April 7, 1964; assigned to Smith Kline & French Laboratories describes glyoxylylbenzophenone derivatives which are represented by the following basic formula:

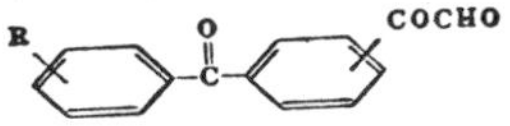

in which R represents hydrogen or glyoxylyl (—COCHO). The benzophenone derivatives are prepared from the dihaloacetyl analogs by their reaction with sodium or potassium ethylate to form the methyl or ethyl acetals which are then hydrolyzed to the glyloxal derivatives or, preferably, from the acetyl analogs by direct oxidation with selenium dioxide.

Example 1: A mixture of 3.9 grams of selenium dioxide, 1 ml of water and 15 ml of dioxane is heated on the steam bath while 5.6 grams of 4'-acetylbenzophenone in 60 ml of dioxane is added. After a reflux period of 6 hours, the hot reaction mixture is filtered and evaporated to give 4'-glyoxylylbenzophenone hydrate. The hydrate is heated under vacuum in a drying pistol at 78°C for 10 hours to yield the free glyoxal. This compound (500 mg) is heated at reflux in methanol. Evaporation gives the methylate addition products. The glyoxal (500 mg) heated on the steam bath in butanol gives upon evaporation in vacuo the butylate.

Example 2: A mixture of 10 grams of 2,2'-diethylbenzophenone, 15 grams of potassium permanganate, 15 grams of magnesium nitrate and 100 ml of water is heated for 30 hours at 80° to 85°C. An excess of oxalic acid solution is added to destroy the unused permanganate. The oxidation sludge is extracted several times with benzene. Drying and evaporating the organic solvent gives the desired 2,2'-diacetylbenzophenone. A mixture of 2.7 grams of the diacetyl derivative, 2.3 grams of selenium dioxide and 100 ml of anhydrous dioxane is heated at reflux for 10 hours, filtered hot and evaporated to give the desired 2,2'-bisglyoxylylbenzophenone. This compound (750 mg) is dissolved in anhydrous ethanol and evaporated on the steam bath to give the ethylate addition product. Another portion of the parent compound (500 mg) is heated in aqueous dioxane. The hydrate is isolated by evaporation.

The compounds have utility as fixatives for perfumes, such as in the manufacture of soaps.

Alkyl Cyclopentyl Ketones

A process described by *J.C. Leffingwell and R.E. Shackelford; U.S. Patent 3,689,562; September 5, 1972; assigned to R.J. Reynolds Tobacco Company* involves the pyrolysis of trans-1-hydroxy-2-acetoxycyclohexanes to produce alkyl cyclopentyl ketones. The synthesis can be illustrated generally by the following reaction:

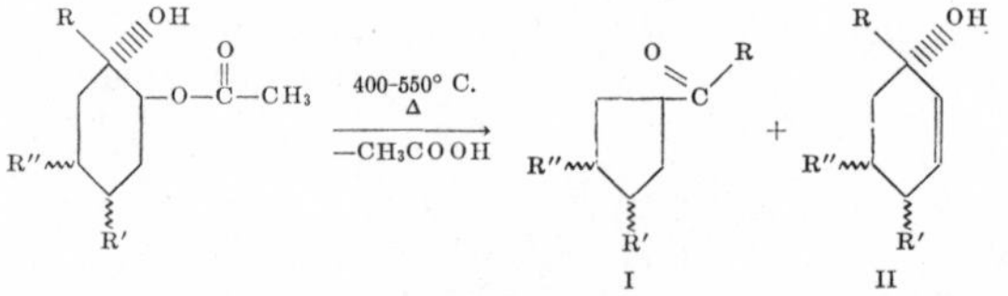

where R is methyl or isopropyl; R' is methyl, isopropyl or isopropenyl; R" is hydrogen; and R' + R" is dimethylmethylene; with the hydroxyl and acetate groups being in trans position with respect to one another and R' and R" being in trans or cis position with respect to one another. As seen in the above reaction, an allylic alcohol (II) is also formed by pyrolysis. The alkyl cyclopentyl ketone (I) can be separated from the allylic alcohol by fractional distillation, chromatography and the like.

In the following examples, the pyrolysis apparatus employed consisted of a vertical tube, 18 inches long and 1 inch in diameter filled with ¼ inch glass helices, mounted in a combustion furnace. The sample was directed through the apparatus by means of a pressure equalizing funnel mounted on the top of the pyrolysis tube. The sample was carried through the pyrolysis tube by gravity and the pressure due to vaporization. The effluent pyrolyzate was condensed by means of a cold water condenser and trapped in an ice cooled vessel. The samples used in pyrolysis were 20% hydroxyacetates by weight in acetone (a solvent being employed for convenience but not required). A drop of 0.5 to 2.0 drops/second was generally employed.

The reaction temperatures reported are external wall temperatures of the pyrolysis tube. After pyrolyses were complete, the samples were neutralized with a sodium bicarbonate solution and extracted with either hexane or ether. Multiple vapor phase chromatographic analyses were done on each sample using a 10 foot, 10% diethyleneglycolsuccinate column under several conditions. Product analyses were done by comparison of the retention times and spectra with known samples, when available.

Example 1: 4-hydroxyneomenthylacetate is prepared by treating 3-menthene with an organic peroxyacid such as peracetic acid to form (±) cis and trans-3-menthene epoxides. Reaction of the cis-3-menthene epoxide with acetic acid in a sodium acetate buffered solution produces 4-hydroxyneomenthylacetate. The 4-hydroxyneomenthylacetate when subjected to vapor phase pyrolysis afforded a product mixture of isopropyl 3-methylcyclopentyl ketone and trans-2-menthene-4-ol. In the following table are set forth the results of vapor phase pyrolysis of 4-hydroxyneomenthylacetate at different temperatures.

Pyrolysis Temperature	% Acetate Pyrolyzed	- - - - - - - - Product Ratio - - - - - - - -	
		% Ketone*	% Allylic Alcohol**
410°	27.6	81	19
430°	73	68	32
444°	86.2	65	35
475°	100	60	40

*Isopropyl 3-methylcyclopentyl ketone
**trans-2-menthene-4-ol

The isopropyl 3-methylcyclopentyl ketone was identified from its characteristic spectral data. Identification of trans-2-menthene-4-ol was made by spectral comparison with a known sample.

Example 2: 1-hydroxyneocarvomenthylacetate is prepared by acetylation of 1-hydroxy-neocarvomenthol. The results of pyrolysis at different temperatures are tabulated below.

Pyrolysis Temperature	% Acetate Pyrolyzed	- - - - - - - - Product Ratio - - - - - - - -	
		% Ketone*	% Allylic Alcohol**
417°	20	22	78
438°	79	22	78
449°	94	23	77

*3-Isopropylcyclopentyl methyl ketone
**trans-2-menthene-1-ol

Identification of the trans-2-methen-1-ol was made by comparison with a known sample. The 3-isopropylcyclopentyl methyl ketone was identified by its characteristic spectra and semicarbazone.

β-Disubstituted α-Indanones

H.A. Bruson and H.L. Plant; U.S. Patent 3,466,332; September 9, 1969; assigned to Olin Mathieson Chemical Corporation describe a process for preparing beta-disubstituted alpha-indanones by reacting carbon monoxide and an aryl-substitute aliphatic halide in the presence of an aluminum halide selected from the group consisting of aluminum chloride and aluminum bromide. The aryl-substituted aliphatic halides suitable for use in preparing beta-di-substituted alpha-indanones include aryl-substituted halogenated alkanes, such as 1-halogeno-2-methyl-2-phenylpropane, aryl-substituted halogenated alkenes, and halogenated aryl-substituted halogenated alkanes and mixtures thereof. All parts and percentages are by weight unless otherwise specified in the following examples which illustrate the process.

Example 1: In this example 2,2-dimethylindanone-1 is prepared from neophyl chloride. 67.5 grams (0.4 mol) of neophyl chloride was added dropwise over a period of three hours to a vigorously stirred mixture of 54 grams (0.4 mol) $AlCl_3$ in 188 grams (2.4 mol) benzene maintained at 21° to 22°C. Carbon monoxide was rapidly bubbled through the mixture during the entire 4½ hour reaction period. The solution was poured onto 400 grams crushed ice, stirred, the benzene layer separated, washed, dried, and distilled eventually under reduced pressure.

Fraction 1 BP 62° to 85°C/0.1 mm 8.0 grams (oil and solid). Fraction 2 BP 85° to 101°C at 0.1 mm 51.0 grams (solid). The two fractions were combined and dissolved in ligroin (BP 30° to 60°C) with warming. The solution was cooled to –40°C and the crystalline 2,2-dimethylindanone-1 filtered off. Yield = 52 grams (81% of theory), MP 42° to 43°C.

42 grams (0.25 mol) of neophyl chloride was added dropwise to a vigorously stirred mixture of 34 grams $AlCl_3$ in 200 grams of carbon disulfide during a period of 2⅓ hours, while rapidly bubbling carbon monoxide through the reaction mixture for a period of 5 hours at 20° to 25°C. The product was poured onto 500 cc of crushed ice and the organic layer was separated, washed, and distilled, to remove the CS_2. The 2,2-dimethylindanone-1 distilled under reduced pressure at 110° to 158°C/0.1 mm and crystallized on cooling. Yield = 17.4 grams. Upon recrystallization from cold ligroin it formed white crystals, MP 42°C.

Example 2: In this example 2,2-dimethylindanone-1 is prepared from 1-phenyl-2-chloro-2-methylpropane. 42 grams (0.25 mol) of 1-phenyl-2-chloro-2-methylpropane was added dropwise to a vigorously stirred mixture of 35 grams (0.25 mol) $AlCl_3$ in 156 grams (2.0 mol) benzene while a continuous stream (120 cc/min) of CO was being bubbled through the solution. The temperature was controlled at 23° to 25°C during the four hour reaction period. After working up by hydrolysis, washing, drying and distillation under reduced pressure as described in Example 1, 24.3 grams (60% of theory) of pure, recrystallized 2,2-dimethylindanone, MP 44°C, was obtained. The 1-phenyl-2-chloro-2-methylpropane used above was prepared by refluxing neophyl chloride for 17 hours under an 8-plate column and recovering by distillation, a mixture of 1-phenyl-2-methylpropene-1, 1-phenyl 2-methylpropene-2, and 1-phenyl-2-chloro-2-methylpropane. This mixture was then treated in toto with hydrogen chloride at 0°C which converted the 1-phenyl-2-methylpropene-1 and the 1-phenyl-2-methylpropene-2 into 1-phenyl-2-chloro-2-methylpropane. In this manner 65% of the original neophyl chloride was converted to 1-phenyl-2-chloro-2-methylpropane boiling at 88°/10 mm.

In related work *H.A. Bruson and H.L. Plant; U.S. Patent 3,466,333; September 9, 1969; assigned to Olin Mathieson Chemical Corporation* describe a process for preparing beta-disubstituted alpha-indanones by reacting carbon monoxide, an aromatic compound such as benzene, and certain aliphatic halides in the presence of an aluminum halide catalyst. Products of the process include 2-methyl-2-phenylindanone-1; 2,2-dimethylindanone-1; 2,2,3,3-tetramethylindanone-1; 2,3-dimethyl-2-phenylindanone-1; and 2-methyl-2-(o-chloro-phenyl)-4-chloroindanone-1.

Derivatives of 2-Acyl-3-Carenes

A process described by *D.C. Heckert; U.S. Patent 3,530,171; September 22, 1970; assigned to The Procter & Gamble Company* concerns the new compounds, 2α-acyl-3-carenes, the 2α-(1'-hydroxyalkyl)-3-carenes, the 2α-(1'-acyloxyalkyl)-3-carenes. These have the following generic formula:

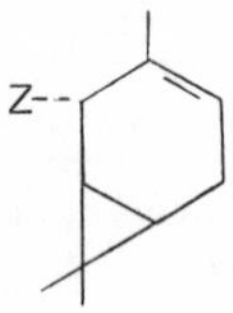

In this formula Z is

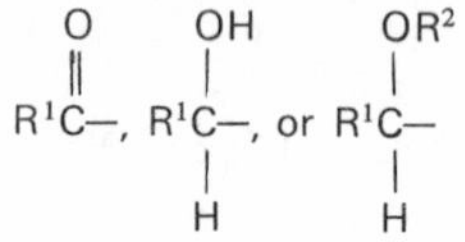

$$
\underset{H}{\overset{O}{\underset{\|}{R^1C-,}}} \quad \underset{H}{\overset{OH}{\underset{|}{R^1C-,}}} \quad or \quad \underset{H}{\overset{OR^2}{\underset{|}{R^1C-}}}
$$

where R^1 is an alkyl group having from 1 to about 5 carbon atoms and R^2 is an acyl group containing from 1 to about 6 carbon atoms. In addition, this process concerns a photo-chemical reaction for the preparation of the 2α-acyl-3-carenes by the irradiation with ultra-violet light of the 4α-acyl-2-carenes; a process for the preparation of the 2α-acyl-3-carenes by selective acylation of 2-carene with organic acid anhydrides or acid halides in the presence of a Friedel-Crafts catalyst, a process for the preparation of the 2α-(1'-hydroxyalkyl)-3-carenes by reduction of the 2α-acyl-3-carenes, and a process for the preparation of the 2α-(1'-acyloxyalkyl)-3-carenes. In the photochemical synthesis of the 2α-acyl-3-carenes, the 4α-acyl-2-carenes, either as neat samples or as a soluttion in an inert solvent, are irradiated with any source of ultraviolet irradiation. The irradiation process is schematically shown by the following:

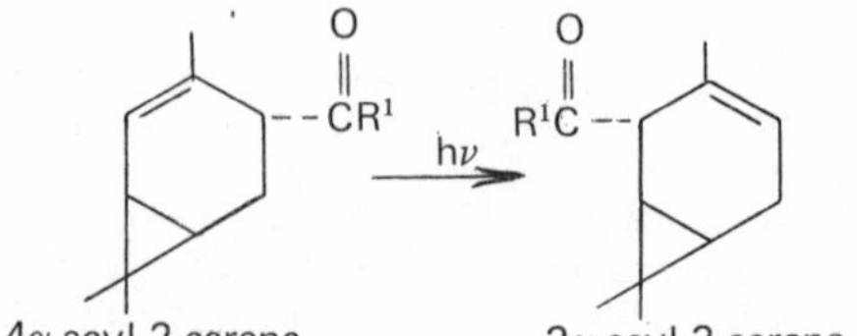

4α-acyl-2-carene   2α-acyl-3-carene

where R^1 in the above equation is an alkyl group having from 1 to 5 carbon atoms. In the nonphotochemical process for the preparation of the 2α-acyl-3-carenes, 2-carene is reacted with an organic acid anhydride or an acid halide in the presence of a Friedel-Crafts catalyst according to the following:

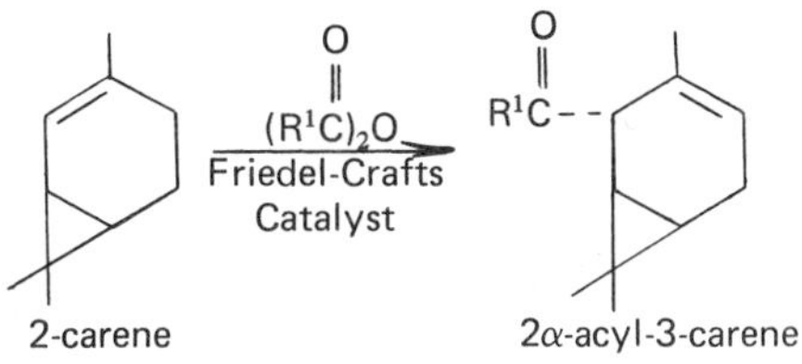

$$(R^1C)_2O \xrightarrow[\text{Catalyst}]{\text{Friedel-Crafts}}$$

2-carene   2α-acyl-3-carene

where R^1 in the above equation is an alkyl group having from 1 to 5 carbon atoms (the R^1's in the above two synthesis, e.g., the photochemical and nonphotochemical synthesis are identical). The above synthesis of the 2α-acyl-3-carenes is quite selective and occurs even in the presence of 3-carene mixtures to the exclusion of the acylation of 3-carene. The 2α-acyl-3-carenes produced by either the photochemical or the nonphotochemical synthesis shown above are useful as perfume components. The following examples in which all percentages and ratios are by weight, unless otherwise indicated, illustrate the process.

Example 1: A solution of 2 grams of 4α-acetyl-2-carene in 150 ml of benzene was placed in a Vycor irradiation vessel under nitrogen and irradiated for 1 hour. During the course of irradiation, with a 654A Hanovia 200-watt lamp, nitrogen was bubbled through the solution. The benzene was distilled off at atmospheric pressure leaving a slightly yellow oil. Gas chromatographic analysis of the oil indicated that it was composed of 34% of the 2α-acetyl-3-carene and 43% of the 4α-acetyl-2-carene. Distillation on an 18 inch spinning band column separated the mixture of 4α-acetyl-2-carene and 2α-acetyl-3-carene (BP 53° to 58°C, 0.65 mm Hg) from the minor products and impurities. Gas chromatographic separation of the two remaining components of the mixture yielded pure 2α-acetyl-3-carene as a colorless oil.

Example 2: The procedure of Example 1 was repeated except that 4α-propionyl-2-carene replaced the 4α-acetyl-2-carene. After irradiation, 2α-propionyl-3-carene was obtained in 30% yield. The 2α-propionyl-3-carene was isolated by preparative gas chromatography as a colorless oil.

Example 3: A 4.42 gram sample of 2α-acetyl-3-carene in 30 ml of diethyl ether was added dropwise to 0.51 gram of lithium aluminum hydride in 100 ml of ether. The mixture was stirred at room temperature for 3 hours, then a second 100 ml of ether was added. A total of 2 ml of water was added dropwise to the stirred solution, and the reaction mixture was stirred for an additional ½ hour. The inorganic solids were removed by filtration and washed with 250 ml portions of ether. The ether portions were combined and the ether was removed at atmospheric pressure. The remaining oil was distilled under vacuum to yield 4.04 grams (90%) of a 2α-(2'-hydroxyethyl)-3-carene in the form of a colorless liquid, BP 70° to 77°C (1.2 mm Hg).

The members of the class referred to as 2α-acyl-3-carenes each have a resinous, woody odor; the members of the class referred to as 2α-(1'-hydroxyalkyl)-3-carenes each have a light, fruity citrus odor; while each of the members of the third class, the 2α-(1'-acyloxyalkyl)-3-carenes, give off a light, sweet, fruity citrus odor.

Caranone Derivatives

D. Lamparsky and P. Schudel; U.S. Patent 3,660,489; May 2, 1972; assigned to Givaudan Corporation describe odorant compositions which are characterized in that they contain olfactorily-desirable compounds of the general formula whose structure is shown on the following page.

R_1, R_2 and R_3 represent hydrogen atoms or lower alkyl groups, X signifies a CO, CHOH, CHOAc, CH_2 or $=CH$ group (double bond directed toward C_9), Ac denotes the acyl residue of a lower alkanecarboxylic acid, and $---$ signifies a C—C single or double bond. Preferred compounds of the general formula are those in which at least one of the three R-symbols signifies hydrogen, i.e., compounds where (a) all three R-symbols signify hydrogen, or (b) those where two of the R-symbols signify hydrogen and the third represents lower alkyl or (c) those where one of the R-symbols is hydrogen and the other two stand for lower alkyl groups.

Example 1: 20 grams of 3-caranone dissolved in 25 ml of ethanol are added to a solution of 0.6 grams of sodium in 25 ml of absolute ethyl alcohol. The solution of 18.7 grams of methyl vinyl ketone in 25 ml of ethanol is subsequently added dropwise with stirring in the course of an hour at room temperature and under N_2-gassing. The stirring at about 25°C is continued overnight and the dark-colored solution is then heated to boiling for a further 2 hours. The reaction mixture is poured onto ice, extracted with ether, the ethereal solution washed neutral, dried and concentrated. The residue (35 g) is distilled at 138° to 140°C and 0.03 mm Hg. There are thus obtained 21.3 grams (79%) of 4,4,7-tri-methyl-tricyclo [5.4.0.0^{3,5}]-undec-11-en-10-one of MP 103° to 104°C (from pentane). UV: λ_{max} 240 mμ, ϵ 16,700. Odor: green, slightly woody.

Example 2: 20 grams of 3-caranone are added to a sodium ethylate solution freshly prepared from 0.61 grams of sodium and 25 ml of absolute ethanol. The solution of 12.25 grams of ethyl vinyl ketone in 25 ml of ethanol is added dropwise in the course of an hour with stirring, N_2-gassing and slight external cooling at 18° to 20°C and the reaction mixture is stirred overnight at room temperature. It is subsequently boiled at reflux for 2.5 hours and worked up as in Example 1. There is thus obtained 4,4,7,11-tetramethyl-tricyclo [5.4.0.0^{3,5}]-undec-11-en-10-one, MP 74° to 75°C. Yield 73%. UV: λ_{max} 249 mμ, ϵ 14,900. Odor: Interesting wood note, harmonizing well with cedar and sandalwood oils.

Example 3: A sodium ethylate solution is prepared from 0.305 gram of sodium and 12.5 ml of absolute ethanol. After the addition of 10 grams of 3-caranone, the solution of 10.9 grams of isopropenyl methyl ketone (3-methyl-3-buten-2-one) in 25 ml of ethanol is added dropwise in the course of 45 minutes with stirring, N_2-gassing and maintenance of a temperature of 10° to 15°C. The mixture is stirred overnight at room temperature and then boiled at reflux for a further 1 hour. The further working up is effected as described in Example 1. There is thus obtained 4,4,7,9-tetramethyl-tricyclo[5.4.0.0^{3,5}]-undec-11-en-10-one of BP 93°C/0.06mm; MP 63°C; UV: λ_{max} 241.5 mμ, ϵ 13,800; yield: 75%. Odor: woody, spicy.

Dehydration of 4-Acyloxy-3-Caranols to Produce Carenes

P.J. Kropp; U.S. Patent 3,510,510; May 5, 1970; assigned to The Procter & Gamble Company has found that reaction of a 4-acyloxy-3-caranol with certain dehydrating agents results in the formation of a 4-acyloxy-3(10)-carene and a new 2-acyloxy-4-isopropenyl-1-methylbicyclo[3.1.0]hexane. It has further been found that the relative proportion of the 4-acyloxy-3(10)-carene to the 2-acyloxy-4-isopropenyl-1-methylbicyclo[3.1.0]hexane is directly dependent upon the stereochemical configuration of the hydroxyl and acyloxyl groups in the 4-acyloxy-3-caranol starting material. The compounds prepared by the process have desirable and useful odors. The 4-acyloxy-3(10)-carane compounds have odors generally characterized as floral-camphoraceous. The 2-acyloxy-4-isopropenyl-1-methylbicyclo[3.1.0]hexane compounds have odors generally characterized as woody-camphoraceous. Mixtures comprising a 4-acyloxy-3(10)-carane compound and a 2-acyloxy-4-isopropenyl-1-methylbicyclo[3.1.0]-hexane compound have odors that are generally characterized as spicy-camphor with animal and/or hay side notes. The 2-hydroxy-4-isopropenyl-1-methylbicyclo-[3.1.0]hexane has a minty-camphoraceous odor. The 4-isopropenyl-1-methylbicyclo[3.1.0]hexan-2-one has strong sweet clove odor with a hay side note. The following examples illustrate the process. All percentages and ratios in the following examples are by weight unless otherwise indicated.

Example 1: A solution containing 9.70 grams of (–)-trans-3,4-caranediol 4-acetate (0.055 M) and 82.6 ml of phosphorous oxychloride (1.1 M) in 826 ml of pyridine was maintained at 100°C under an atmosphere of nitrogen for three hours. The resulting brown solution was poured over ice water and exhaustively extracted with ether. The ether extracts were combined and washed with 10% hydrochloric acid and dried over saturated sodium chloride solution followed by anhydrous sulfate. Removal of the solvent by distillation gave 6.88 grams of amber residue which was shown by gas chromatography to contain 3(10)-caren-4-ol acetate (34%) and 2-hydroxy-4-isopropenyl-1-methylbicyclo[3.1.0]hexane acetate (31%), which were purified by preparative gas chromatography.

Also observed were peaks corresponding to lower molecular weight material (13 to 17%) and additional unidentified olefinic acetates (6 to 7%). From among the former fractions, peaks were isolated having retention times and infrared and NMR spectra identical with p-cymene, α,p-dimethylstyrene and 1,1,4-trimethylcycloheptatriene. The 2-hydroxy-4-isopropenyl-1-methylbicyclo[3.1.0]-hexane acetate was obtained as a colorless oil having a woody-camphoraceous odor, BP 72° to 74°C (1.2 mm). The compound was formally characterized as (–)-2-endo-hydroxy-4-exo-sipropenyl-1-methylbicyclo[3.1.0]hexane. The 3(10)-caren-4-olacetate was obtained as a colorless oil having a floral-camphoraceous odor, BP 80° to 82°C (1.2 mm). This compound was formally identified as (–)-3(10)-caren-4α-ol acetate.

Example 2: A solution containing 865 mg of trans-3,4-caranediol 4-butyrate (0.229 M) and 1.7 ml of phosphorous oxychloride (1.1 M) in 17 ml of pyridine was stirred at 100°C for three hours under an atmosphere of nitrogen. Isolation of the product mixture in the same manner as in Example 1, supra, gave 820 mg of a dark amber liquid. Short-path distillation of this liquid at 100°C (0.2 mm) gave a 1:1 mixture of 3(10)-caren-4α-ol butyrate and 2-endo-hydroxy-4-exo-isopropenyl-1-methylbicyclo[3.1.0]hexane butyrate as a colorless liquid having a spicy-camphor, animal-hay odor, $[\alpha]_{5461}{}^{25}$ –16° (c 1.04); λ_{max} 5.76.

Synthesis of cis-β-Bergamotene

A process described by *T.W. Gibson and W.F. Erman; U.S. Patent 3,481,998; December 2, 1969; assigned to The Procter & Gamble Company* relates to the synthesis of cis-β-bergamotene and therefore represents the first total synthesis of a π-substituted pinene sesquiterpene. A multistep process starting with readily preparable 2-carboalkoxymethylnopinol, through the formation of several intermediate compounds, and resulting ultimately in the formation of cis-β-bergamotene has been found. A key step in this process and an important feature of this porcess is the cyclization of certain nopinol compounds to form oxatricyclo [5.2.0.0⁴,⁹] nonyl compounds.

β-Bergamotene is a known compound, having been isolated from Valerian root oil by Kulkarni et al as reported in *Tetrahedron Letters,* 8, 505 (1963). A comparison of the nuclear magnetic resonance spectrum of the β-bergamotene prepared by this process (Example 1) with that of naturally occurring β-bergamotene as reported by Kulkarni et al in *Tetrahedron,* 22, 1917 (1966) revealed the nonidentity of these compounds.

This nonidentity is believed to reside in the cis-trans stereo configuration of the compounds. It is also to be noted that the cis structure for β-bergamotene has been assigned to naturally occurring β-bergamotene in the above-cited *Tetrahedron* (1966) reference. However, due to the unambiguous nature of the synthesis of the process, it is concluded that the product obtained hereby is cis-β-bergamotene, and therefore the naturally occurring isomer is believed to be trans-β-bergamotene. In any event, cis-β-bergamotene prepared by the process has a unique and desirable odor and thus has utility as an odorant or as a component of perfume compositions. In addition, the oxatricyclo[5.2.0.0^{4,9}]nonyl compounds mentioned above also have utility based on their olfactory properties. Oxo derivatives of these oxatricyclo[5.2.0.0^{4,9}]nonyl compounds have also been prepared as a part of this process and these compounds likewise have useful olfactory characteristics. The synthesis of cis-β-bergamotene, comprises:

(a) cyclizing 2-carboalkoxymethylnopinol (preferably 2-carboethoxymethylnopinol) to form alkyl-1-methyl-3-oxatricyclo[5.2.0.0^{4,9}]nonyl-2-acetate (preferably alkyl is ethyl);

(b) hydrolyzing the acetate to form 1-methyl-3-oxatricyclo[5.2.0.0^{4,9}]nonyl-2-acetic acid;

(c) decarboxylating and halogenating the acetic acid to form 1-methyl-4-halomethyl-3-oxatricyclo[5.2.0.0^{4,9}]nonane (preferably halo is chloro);

(d) cleaving the nonane to form 9-hydroxy-β-pinene;

(e) tosylating the pinene to form 9-toluenesulfonyloxy-β-pinene;

(f) displacing the pinene with sodium iodide to form 9-iodo-β-pinene;

(g) displacing the pinene with lithium acetylide to form 9-ethynyl-β-pinene;

(h) hydroborating the pinene with disiamylborane to form 9-(β-pinyl)-acetaldehyde; and

(i) reacting the aldehyde with triphenylisopropylidene phosphorane to form cis-β-bergamotene.

The above-identified process for the synthesis of cis-β-bergamotene comprising steps (a) through (i) is described in more detail in Example 1. Respective steps (b) through (i) each involve individual reactions whose conditions are known in the art. References where these conditions are described are summarized in the following table. This table also shows preferred temperature conditions for each step.

	Preferred Temperature Conditions		
Step	Broad Range, °C.	Narrow Range (Highly Preferred), °C.	Reference
(b)	20–100	25–50	N. A. Abraham et al., Compt. rend., 248, 2880 (1959).
(c)	50–100	75–85	J. Kochi, J. Org. Chem. 30, 3265 (1965).
(d)	70–125	80–90	R. C. Blume et al., J. Org. Chem., 30, 1553 (1965).
(e)	−5–12	0–10	M. F. Ansell et al., J. Chem. Soc., 1788 (1957).
(f)	40–100	55–65	M. F. Ansell et al., J. Chem. Soc. 1788 (1957).
(g)	0–35	10–30	Copending U.S. Patent application of Erman et al., Ser. No. 549,812, filed May 13, 1966.
(h)	0–40	0–10	H. C. Brown et al., J. Am. Chem. Soc., 83, 3834 (1961).
(i)	50–100	60–70	U. H. M. Fagerlund et al., J. Amer. Chem. Soc., 79, 6473 (1961).

Example 1: cis-β-bergamotene is synthesized in this example. (a) To a mixture of 20.2 grams of 2-carboethoxymethylnopinol and 33 grams yellow HgO in 500 ml pentane was added 22 grams Br$_2$. During addition the pentane was kept at reflux (~36°C) and a stream of Ar was passed through the system to remove HBr. After addition, reflux was continued for 1 hour, the mixture cooled, filtered, and dried over MgSO$_4$. Removal of drying agent and solvent gave 20.4 grams dark oil, which was filtered through 150 grams of Al$_2$O$_3$ twice to give 16.0 grams of ethyl-1-methyl-3-oxatricyclo[5.2.0.0^{4,9}]nonyl-2-acetate (80%), which appeared to be pure by gas chromatography. Purification was carried out by gas chromatography followed by short-path distillation to give the acetate with BP 88°C (0.2 mm).

(b) and (c) Hydrolysis of 15.5 grams of the product of (a) with KOH in aqueous methanol at 25°C gave a quantitative yield of 1-methyl-3-oxatricyclo-[5.2.0.0^{4,9}]nonyl-2-acetic acid. To a solution of 12.43 grams of the acid at room temperature in 250 ml benzene was added 44 grams Pb(OAc)$_4$, and the mixture stirred until homogeneous, when 4.31 grams NaCl was added, the system evacuated repeatedly to afford an Ar atmosphere, and then heated at 80°C overnight. As the reaction proceeded, CO$_2$ was given off and the color became lighter as Pb^{+2} salts were precipitated. The solution was decanted from the gummy salts, washed with dilute HClO$_4$, saturated Na$_2$CO$_3$, saturated NaCl, dried over MgSO$_4$, filtered, the benzene removed in vacuum, and the residue chromatographed on 50 grams Al$_2$O$_3$. Elution with 10% ether in pentane gave 5.50 grams pure 1-methyl-4-chloromethyl-3-oxa-tricyclo[5.2.0.0^{4,9}]nonane. An additional 0.834 grams was obtained on rechromatography of the latter fractions. Purification by gas chromatography gave the nonane above with BP 65°C (1.3 mm).

(d) To a solution of 14.4 grams of 1-methyl-4-chloromethyl-3-oxatricyclo[5.2.0.0^{4,9}]nonane in 150 ml dry monoglyme was added 4.6 grams sodium, and the solution refluxed over-night (85°C). After cooling, the excess sodium was decomposed by the addition of meth-anol, the solution diluted with water and extracted thoroughly with ether. The ether solu-tion was washed with water, dried over MgSO$_4$, filtered and stripped. Distillation of the residue gave 5.6 grams (48%) pure 9-hydroxy-β-pinene BP 55°C (0.5 mm).

(e) To a solution of 5.20 grams of 9-hydroxy-β-pinene in 90 ml dry pyridine at 0°C was added 6.55 grams toluene-sulfonyl chloride (tosylate), and the solution put in a 0°C refrig-erator overnight. The mixture was poured onto ice, extracted with ether, the ether washed with dilute HCl, saturated NaHCO$_3$, dried over MgSO$_4$, filtered and stripped. Crystallization of the residue from ether-pentane gave 7.4237 grams pure 9-toluene-sulfonyloxy-β-pinene (71%) MP 115°C.

(f) A solution of 4.20 grams of the compound of (e) and 5.60 grams of NaI in 50 ml of purified acetone was refluxed for 18 hours (55°C). After cooling in an ice bath to ~10°C and filtration of the sodium tosylate, the acetone was removed in vacuum and the oily residue taken up in ether. The ether solution was washed with a dilute Na$_2$S$_2$O$_3$ solution and dried over MgSO$_4$. Distillation of the residue after filtration and removal of ether gave 3.20 grams (89%) of 9-iodo-β-pinene, BP 66°C (0.4 mm).

(g) A solution of 2.4748 grams of product of (f) and 1.72 grams of the ethylene-diamine complex of lithium acetylide in 50 ml DMSO was stirred at room temperature under Ar for 20 hours. The solution was poured into water, neutralized with NH$_4$Cl solution, and extracted with pentane. The pentane solution was washed with saturated NaCl solution, dried over Na$_2$SO$_4$, filtered and stripped. Short-path distillation of the residue gave 1.0673 grams (71%), BP ~50°C (0.5 mm), which showed two peaks on gas chromatography in the ratio of 4:1 (planimeter). Spectral data for material giving the minor peak suggested an internal isomer while the major product was shown to be the desired product, 9-ethynyl-β-pinene.

(h) To a solution of 0.303 gram of the mixture of products obtained in step (g) in 20 ml THF, cooled in an ice bath (10°C), was added 2.0 ml of 1 M diisamylborane by syringe. The solution was then stirred four hours at room temperature, decomposed with 2 ml of 3 N NaOH and 2 ml of 30% H$_2$O$_2$, poured into water, and the water solution extracted with pentane. The pentane extract was dissolved with water, dried over Na$_2$SO$_4$, filtered and stripped to give 0.320 gram crude product. Gas chromatography analysis indicated the presence of a number of compounds, the major peak of which (~30%) was shown to be the desired product, 9-(β-pinyl)-acetaldehyde. Material collected by gas chromatography showed BP 90° to 95°C (0.6 mm).

(i) Triphenylisopropylidenephosphorane was generated from 1.93 grams of triphenyliso-propylphosphonium bromide in 50 ml THF by the addition of one equivalent of butyl lithium. After two hours at room temperature, 0.305 grams of the product of step (h), as the crude product, was added and the mixture heated to 60°C overnight. After cooling, the mixture was poured into water, extracted with pentane, and the pentane washed with water, dried over MgSO$_4$, filtered and stripped to give 0.235 gram crude product. This material was filtered through 6 grams Al$_2$O$_3$ to give 0.099 gram hydrocarbons, consisting of 90% (+)-cis-β-bergamotene and 10% acetylenes. Purification gave (+)-cis-β-bergamotene with BP ~105°C (0.5 mm), having odor characterized as lemon-lime with a woody, slightly camphoraceous background with a touch of minty sweetness. As is evident from this example, each of the products of steps (a) through (h) has utility as an intermediate in the synthesis of cis-β-bergamotene.

Example 2: In this example, cyclization of alkylnopinol to form 1-methyl-4-alkyl-3-oxatricyclo[5.2.0.0^{4,9}]nonane is shown. To a solution of 100.8 grams of methylnopinol in 1 liter distilled pentane was added 200 grams yellow mercuric oxide. The mixture was heated to reflux (~36°C) under N$_2$ and 20.0 ml bromine added dropwise over about two hours. After an additional two hours reflux at ~36°C, the mixture was cooled, filtered and dried over MgSO$_4$ and Na$_2$CO$_3$. Filtration through 450 grams Al$_2$O$_3$ followed by vacuum distillation gave 69.0 grams of 1,4-dimethyl-3-oxatricyclo-[5.2.0.0^{4,9}]nonane, BP 64°C (10.5 mm), and 15 grams nopinone, for an 82% yield of pure product. The material purified by gas chromatography had an odor characterized as fenchone-eucalyptol.

Hydrogenation of Allene-Ketones

G.Saucy; U.S. Patent 3,330,867; July 11, 1967; assigned to Hoffmann-La Roche Inc. describes a process for the manufacture of olefinic ketones from allene-ketones. The process is carried out by treating an allene-ketone of the formula

$$R_1H_2C$$
$$\diagdown$$
$$C=C=CH-CH-CO-CH_2R_3$$
$$\diagup \qquad\qquad |$$
$$R_4 \qquad\qquad R_2$$

where R$_1$, R$_2$ and R$_3$ are hydrogen or lower alkyl groups and R$_4$ is a hydrocarbon residue (preferably containing 1 to 12 carbon atoms) which may be substituted by oxygen-containing groups (e.g., hydroxy, lower-alkoxy, or lower-acyloxy) and may, together with the neighbouring C-atom and the —CH$_2$R$_1$ group, form a carbocyclic radical, preferably a 5 to 7 membered carbocyclic radical (e.g., the cyclohexylidene group) with hydrogen in the presence of a hydrogenation catalyst until approximately one mol of hydrogen is reacted per mol of allene-ketone. The following examples illustrate the process.

Example 1: 31.1 grams of 6-methyl-4,5-heptadien-2-one are dissolved in 200 ml of petroleum ether, and, after the addition of 0.3 gram of Lindlar catalyst and 0.3 gram of quinoline, the mixture is hydrogenated at room temperature and normal pressure in a shaking apparatus. The hydrogenation almost comes to a standstill after the uptake of 5.6 liters of hydrogen (=1 mol equivalent H$_2$). (Time taken: 6 hours, wherein 5 liters of hydrogen are taken up in 2.5 hours). The catalyst is filtered off and the filtrate evaporated under vacuum. There is thus obtained a product (n$_D^{24}$ = 1.4405) which, according to a gas chromatogram, contains the following components: 87.9% 6-methyl-5-hepten-2-one; 11.9% 6-methyl-4-hepten-2-one; and 1% 6-methyl-2-heptanone. The 6-methyl-4-hepten-2-one can be isolated by preparative gas chromatography in the form of a mixture (about 1:1) of the cis and trans isomers, BP 54° to 55°C/11 mm.

The 6-methyl-4,5-heptadien-2-one used as the starting material can be obtained as follows: 172 grams of 2-methyl-3-butyn-2-ol, 800 ml of petroleum ether, 0.4 gram of hydroquinone and 432 grams of isopropenyl methyl ether are added to a flask. While stirring, the mixture is treated with 0.2 gram of p-toluene-sulfonic acid. The reaction solution is boiled under reflux for 15 to 24 hours. After cooling, a solution of 0.2 gram of sodium acetate in 20 ml of methanol is added to the reaction solution and the mixture is stirred for 10 minutes at room temperature. Thereafter, the entire mixture is evaporated in a water-jet vacuum at 40°C. The evaporation residue is distilled under high vacuum. 230 grams of 6-methyl-4,5-heptadien-2-one are obtained as the main fraction, BP of the pure product 70°C/19 mm.

Example 2: 9.6 grams of 6,10-dimethyl-4,5,9-undecatrien-2-one are diluted in 100 ml of petroleum ether and, after the addition of 1 gram of Lindlar catalyst and 0.2 ml of quinoline, the mixture is hydrogenated under normal conditions up to the cessation of hydrogen uptake (1.08 liters). The usual working up yields 9.7 grams of hydrogenation product (n_D^{20} = 1.4702) which, on the basis of gas chromatographical analysis, contains 64.7% cis geranyl-acetone and 31.3% trans geranyl-acetone. The hydrogenation product is almost free from the isomeric β,γ-unsaturated ketone 6,10-dimethyl-4,9-undecadien-2-one. The allene-ketone introduced as the starting material was prepared by the condensation of 3,7-dimethyl-6-octen-1-yn-3-ol(dehydro-linalool) with isopropenyl ether and was subjected to hydrogenation as a crude product.

ALCOHOLS

1-(α-Furyl)-2,2-Dialkyl-1,3-Dihydroxypropane Derivatives

A process described by *K. Kulka; U.S. Patent 3,227,731; January 4, 1966; assigned to Fritzsche Brothers, Inc.* relates to 1-(α-furyl)-2,2-dialkyl-1,3-dihydroxypropanes; the mono and di lower alkyl and the mono and di phenyl carbonates and the mono and di lower alkyl and mono and di phenyl carbamates thereof; 1-(α-tetrahydrofuryl)-2,2-dialkyl-1,3-dihydroxypropanes; and the mono and di lower alkyl and the mono and di phenyl and the cyclic carbonates, the mono and di carbamates and the mono and di lower alkyl and the mono and di phenyl carbamates of 1-(α-tetrahydrofuryl)-2,2-dialkyl-1,3-dihydroxypropanes.

The mono and di lower alkyl and the mono and di phenyl carbonates of 1-(α-furyl)-2,2-dialkyl-1,3-dihydroxypropanes and the mono and di lower alkyl, the mono and di phenyl and the cyclic carbonates of 1-(α-tetrahydrofuryl)-2,2-dialkyl-1,3-dihydroxypropanes are useful in producing the corresponding carbamates, while the carbonates of both types of glycols are useful in perfume compounding. The 1-(α-furyl)-2,2-dialkyl-1,3-dihydroxypropanes have the formula:

$$
\begin{array}{c}
\text{CH}\!\!-\!\!\text{CH} \quad \text{H} \quad \ \ \text{R} \quad \text{H} \\
\|\qquad\ \| \qquad | \qquad\ | \qquad | \\
\text{CH} \quad\ \ \text{C}\!-\!\text{C}\!-\!\text{C}\!-\!\text{CH} \\
\diagdown\ \diagup \qquad\quad |\ \quad |\ \ \ | \\
\text{O} \qquad\quad \text{OH}\ \ \text{R}_1\ \ \text{OH}
\end{array}
$$

in which R is an alkyl group, R_1 is an alkyl group and the total number of carbon atoms in both alkyl groups is less than eight. The 1-(α-tetrahydrofuryl)-2,2-dialkyl-1,3-dihydroxypropanes have the formula.

$$
\begin{array}{c}
\text{CH}_2\!\!-\!\!\text{CH}_2 \quad \text{H} \quad \ \ \text{R} \quad \text{H} \\
|\qquad\ \ | \qquad | \qquad\ | \qquad | \\
\text{CH}_2 \quad \text{CH}\!-\!\text{C}\!-\!\text{C}\!-\!\text{CH} \\
\diagdown\ \diagup \qquad\quad |\ \quad |\ \ \ | \\
\text{O} \qquad\quad \text{OH}\ \ \text{R}_1\ \ \text{OH}
\end{array}
$$

in which R is an alkyl group, R_1 is an alkyl group and the total number of carbon atoms in both alkyl groups is less than eight. The 1-(α-furyl)-2,2-dialkyl-1,3-dihydroxypropanes are produced by reacting furfural in the presence of a methanolic solution of an alkali metal hydroxide with an aldehyde having the formula:

$$
\begin{array}{c}
\text{R} \\
| \\
\text{CH}\!-\!\text{CHO} \\
| \\
\text{R}_1
\end{array}
$$

The desired glycol is recovered. The 1-(α-tetrahydrofuryl)-2,2-dialkyl-1,3-dihydroxypropanes are prepared by the hydrogenation of the required 1-(α-furyl)-2,2-dialkyl-1,3-dihydroxypropanes in the presence of metallic hydrogenation catalysts. The lower alkyl carbonates of the resulting 1-(α-tetrahydrofuryl)-2,2-dialkyl-1,3-dihydroxypropanes are obtained by reacting a solution of the required glycol, desirably containing a tertiary amine, such as a trialkyl amine or pyridine, with an alkyl chloroformate in which the alkyl group preferably contains less than six carbon atoms. The carbamates of the 1-(α-tetrahydrofuryl)-2,2-dialkyl-1,3-dihydroxypropanes are produced from a lower alkyl carbonate of the glycol by ammonia treatment desirably with agitation of a solution of the corresponding lower alkyl carbonate. The mono lower alkyl or phenyl carbamates of the 1-(α-tetrahydrofuryl)-2,2-dialkyl-1,3-dihydroxypropanes are obtained by reacting one mol of the desired lower alkyl or phenyl isocyanate with the glycol. If the corresponding di lower alkyl or diphenyl dicarbamate is desired, two mols of the lower alkyl or phenyl isocyanate are reacted. The following examples illustrate the process.

Example 1: Preparation of 1-(α-Furyl)-2,2-Dimethyl-1,3-Dihydroxypropane — To a solution of 180 grams of sodium hydroxide in 1,000 ml of methanol was added over a period of 3 hours, under agitation, a mixture of 288 grams of freshly distilled furfural and 540 grams of isobutyraldehyde. During the addition, the temperature is kept between 48° to 52°C. After the addition, agitation was continued, for 3¼ hours whereby the reaction temperature decreased to 29°C. The reaction mixture was acidified with glacial acetic acid, 500 ml of water were added and the reaction mixture was permitted to stand overnight. The next day 800 ml, consisting mostly of methanol, were distilled off from a steam bath, under agitation, using a 1½ ft Vigreux column. The remaining organic part was diluted with 800 ml of benzene and this solution was washed twice with 300 ml portions of warm water. The solvent was distilled off in a slight vacuum from a steam bath. The residue crystallized to a yellow compound. It was fractionated through a 2 ft Vigreux column, as follows:

| | Temperature, ° C. | | Vac., mm. | Ml. | Wt., g. |
	Vapor	Flask			
Front Section	99–118	128–132	4	60	56
Main Section	125–133	136–158	4	340	358
Residue					23
Total					437

The main section which crystallized had a melting point of 60° to 61°C and a purity by a wet analysis (acetylation) of 99%. It was recrystallized from a benzene-hexane mixture, had a melting point of 61° to 62°C and was represented by the following formula:

$$
\begin{array}{c}
\text{CH—CH} \quad \text{H} \quad \text{CH}_3 \quad \text{H} \\
\text{CH} \quad \text{C—C—C—C—CH} \\
\backslash_{\text{O}}\diagup \quad \text{OH} \quad \text{CH}_3 \quad \text{OH}
\end{array}
$$

An IR curve indicated that the desired compound was obtained.

Example 2: Preparation of 1-(α-Tetrahydrofuryl)-2,2-Dimethyl-1,3-Dihydroxypropane — Using 5 grams of Raney nickel catalyst, a solution containing 250 ml of isopropanol and 255 grams of 1-(α-furyl)-2,2-dimethyl-1,3-dihydroxypropane, prepared as described in Example 1, were hydrogenated at an initial pressure of 100 psi and a reaction temperature of 50°C. The theoretical amount of hydrogen was consumed in 7 hours. The reaction mixture was filtered off from the catalyst and the solvent was removed by distillation in a slight vacuum from a steam bath. The residue was examined by IR spectroscopy and the IR curve was found to be in correlation with that of the expected product. The product was fractionated without a column, as follows:

| | R.I. 20° | Temperature, ° C. | | Vac., mm. | Ml. | Wt. |
		Vapor	Flask			
Front Section	1.4750	124–126	129–130	4	5	4.6
Main Section	1.4785	126–136	130–140	4	222	235.5
Residue						5.7
Total						245.8

The wet analysis (acetylation) was 98.5%. IR spectrum indicated the correct structure.

Example 3: Preparation of Monomethyl Carbonate of 1-(α-Tetrahydrofuryl)-2,2-Dimethyl-1,3-Dihydroxypropane — To a well agitated mixture of 44 grams of 1-(α-tetrahydrofuryl)-2,2-dimethyl-1,3-dihydroxypropane, 70 ml of benzene and 24 grams of pyridine was added over a period of 30 minutes, a solution of 27 grams of methylchloroformate dissolved in

30 ml of benzene. During the addition, the reaction mixture was cooled and maintained between 7° and 12°C. The reaction mixture was then agitated at 22° to 23°C for one hour. It was then heated to 51° to 58°C under agitation for a period of about 4½ hours thereafter. The reaction mixture stood overnight at room temperature. The following day, the reaction mixture was washed successively once with 150 ml of water, twice with 100 ml of a 2% aqueous hydrochloric acid solution, once with 100 ml of an aqueous saturated sodium bicarbonate solution, and twice with 100 ml of water. The solvent was then distilled off at a light vacuum on a steam bath. A viscous amber liquid remained consisting of 44 grams of crude reaction product. The actual yield was 75.2%. IR curves indicated the desired reaction product was obtained.

Example 4: Preparation of Monocarbamate of 1-(α-Tetrahydrofuryl)-2,2-Dimethyl-1,3-Dihydroxypropane — A stream of ammonia gas was passed for a period of 17 hours through a solution containing 40 grams of ammonia water, 80 ml of isopropanol and 40 grams of the mono methyl carbonate of 1-(α-tetrahydrofuryl)-2,2-dimethyl-1,3-dihydroxypropane, prepared as described in Example 3. During the introduction of the ammonia gas, the solution was agitated and maintained at room temperature. After the 17 hour period, the ammonia water and solvent were distilled off. A viscous yellow oil of 36.4 grams resulted.

On standing, it partially crystallized. It was treated with 100 ml of isopropanol and 3 grams of activated carbon under reflux and filtered hot. On standing crystals formed which were collected on a Buchner funnel. 15 grams of crystals representing a 40% yield of the theoretical were obtained. The melting point was 136° to 141°C. The nitrogen determination by Kjeldahl was 6.81% compared with a theoretical of 6.45%. A molecular weight determination by the Rast method was 219 as contrasted with a theoretical value of 217. An IR curve indicated that the desired compound was obtained.

Cyclopropyl-Substituted Cyclohexanols

According to a process described by *R.A. Comes; U.S. Patent 3,770,836; November 6, 1973; assigned to Philip Morris Incorporated* cyclohexanes and cyclohexanols having a cyclopropane substituent which are useful as fragrances or flavors are prepared from terpenes. The compounds of the process fall within the scope of the following illustrative chemical structure:

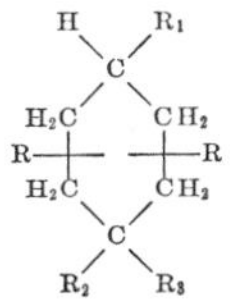

In the structural formula shown, R is intended to represent hydrogen or a hydroxy radical, R_1 stands for 2-hydroxyisopropyl or an alkyl radical of 1 to 4 carbon atoms but preferably methyl, with R_2 standing for hydrogen and R_3 representing an alkyl substituted cyclopropyl radical, or when R_2 and R_3 are taken together with a carbon of the cyclohexane ring, they represent a cyclopropyl or a dimethylcyclopropyl ring of a spiro[2.5]octane or spiro[2.5]-octanol. The compounds are synthesized from corresponding unsaturated compounds, which may be represented by the three cyclohexane derivatives shown below:

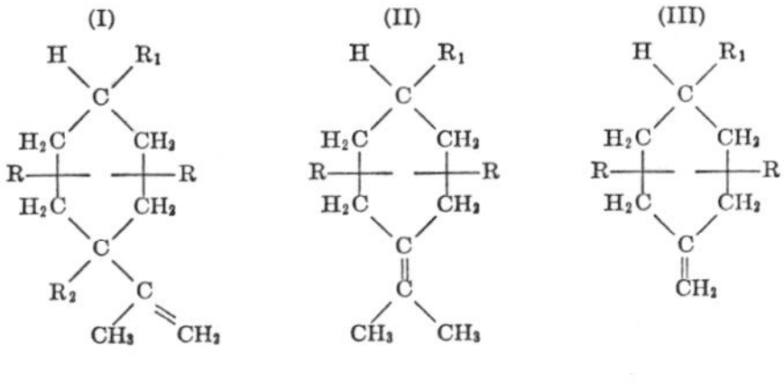

in which R, R_1 and R_2 have the previously indicated meanings. The starting materials represented by Formulae I, II and III are known compounds described in the text *The Terpenes,* by J.L. Simonsen, vol 1, Cambridge University Press, New York (1953).

Reaction of the unsaturated starting compounds with methylene iodide using a zinc-copper couple in an anhydrous ether solvent, following a procedure for the preparation of nor-carane described by R.D. Smith and H.E. Simmons in *Organic Syntheses,* vol 41, pages 72 to 75, John Wiley, New York (1961) will give rise to the corresponding cyclopropyl compounds. In the process described by the authors, the reaction is carried out with cyclohexane whereas the starting compounds utilized here are of the type in which the double bond is in a radical attached to a cyclohexane nucleus.

Preferred starting materials for preparing the compounds are p-menth-8-en-2-ol (dihydro-carveol), p-menth-8-en-1-ol (β-terpineol), p-menth-8-en-1,2-diol, p-menth-4(8)-en-1-ol (γ-terpineol), p-menth-4(8)-en-3-ol (pulegol), p-menth-8-en-3-ol (isopulegol), and 7-methylene-4-(2-hydroxyisopropyl) cyclohexane.

Branched Chain Alkenols

According to a process described by *G.J. Brendel; U.S. Patent 3,493,623; February 3, 1970; assigned to Ethyl Corporation* branched chain alkenols are prepared by hydrolyzing an intermediate formed by reaction among aluminum, tetrahydrofuran or an alkyl substituted tetrahydrofuran, a hydrocarbyl aluminum hydride (e.g., diisobutyl aluminum hydride), and a conjugated diene (e.g., isoprene). The resultant alkenols have utility as perfumes, monomers, chemical intermediates, and surface active agents. The following examples illustrate the process.

Example 1: Into a 250 ml autoclave equipped with stirring means were placed approximately 16 grams of aluminum, 50 ml of tetrahydrofuran, 50 ml of isoprene and 10 ml of diiso-butylaluminum hydride. The autoclave was sealed and the mixture heated for 1 hour at 140° to 150°C. On opening the autoclave, it was found to be filled with a solid reaction product. This procedure was thereupon repeated three more times under virtually identical conditions and the products from each of the four runs were combined for further handling. A sample of this solid reaction product was subjected to deuterolysis which resulted in the formation of a carbon-deuterium bond showing that an aluminum-carbon bond was present in the product.

The remaining combined solid product was hydrolyzed with dilute hydrochloric acid. Thereupon, 1,000 ml of toluene was added to the product and the phases were separated. The toluene was then removed from the organic phase leaving approximately 80 grams of an organic product, 90% of which was a C_9 saturated alcohol. Analysis of this C_9 alcohol showed it to contain approximately 80 weight percent of 5,6-dimethyl-6-hepten-1-ol and 20 weight percent of 5,5-dimethyl-6-hepten-1-ol.

Example 2: Approximately 10 grams of aluminum, 15 ml of isoprene, 10 ml of diisobutyl aluminum hydride and 100 ml of tetrahydrofuran were charge into the autoclave and the contents of the sealed reactor were stirred for one hour at 140° to 150°C. On opening the autoclave the system was found to be a slurry of unreacted aluminum in an homo-genous organic phase. The aluminum was separated by filtration, the organic phase subjected to hydrolysis conditions (dilute HCl) and thereupon hexane was added as an extractive solvent. The hexane solution was isolated and the hexane removed therefrom by vacuum distillation leaving 8.2 grams of 90% pure C_9 unsaturated alcohol corresponding in makeup to the alcohol product of Example 1. The yield of alcohol was approximately 90% based on the hydride atom of the diisobutyl aluminum hydride reactant, and 39% based on the quantity of isoprene charged into the autoclave.

Example 3: The procedure of Example 2 was repeated with the exception that the quantity of diisobutyl aluminum hydride reactant was 20 ml. In this instance the yield of the alcohol product was 77% based on the hydride atom of the diisobutyl aluminum hydride reactant, and 58% based on the isoprene reactant.

In related work *G.J. Brendel and L.H. Shepherd; U.S. Patent 3,692,847; September 19, 1972; assigned to Ethyl Corporation* prepared nonionic compounds in which an aluminum atom is part of an olefinically unsaturated ring system by causing interaction among aluminum, a conjugated diene and a hydrocarbon aluminum hydride in the presence of a suitable Lewis base such as 1,4-dioxane or N-methyl pyrrolidine. The resulting cyclic organoaluminum compound is useful in the synthesis of olefins and branched chain alkenols.

Thus by subjecting the cyclic organoaluminum compound to hydrolysis, one or more olefins may be produced. To prepare branched chain alkenols, the cyclic organoaluminum compound is reacted with a cleavable cycloparaffinic monoether having a 3, 4 or 5 membered ring. The reaction mixture is then subjected to hydrolysis. The following compounds were prepared by this procedure:

1-chloromethyl-3,4-dimethyl-4-penten-1-ol
1-chloromethyl-3,3-dimethyl-4-penten-1-ol
2,2-bis(chloromethyl)-4,5-dimethyl-5-hexen-1-ol
2,2-bis(chloromethyl)-4,4-dimethyl-5-hexen-1-ol
1,5,5-trimethyl-6-hepten-1-ol
1,5,6-trimethyl-6-hepten-1-ol
4,5,6-trimethyl-6-hepten-1-ol
2,2,3-trimethyl-5,5-bis(chloromethyl)tetrahydropyran

Example 1: Reaction of 1-Isobutyl-3-Methyl-Aluminacyclopent-3-ene with Epichlorohydrin — 1-Isobutyl-3-methyl-aluminacyclopent-3-ene was prepared by reacting activated aluminum powder with isoprene and diisobutyl aluminum hydride in excess 1,1-dioxane at 150°C for two hours. The unreacted aluminum metal was removed by filtration of the liquid reaction mixture. To 43 millimols of the 1-isobutyl-3-methyl-aluminacyclopent-3-ene contained in 30 ml 1,4-dioxane was slowly added 6 ml (78 millimols) of epichlorohydrin.

An exothermic reaction occurred. Then the reaction mixture was diluted with diethyl ether and the mixture hydrolyzed with dilute aqueous HCl. Excess reaction solvent was removed under vacuum and the product was distilled. The main fraction boiled at 65° to 66°C at 1.8 mm Hg. Analysis of this fraction by nuclear magnetic resonance and vapor phase chromatography showed this product to be a mixture of 1-chloromethyl-3,4-dimethyl-4-penten-1-ol, the former isomer predominating by about 9:1.

Example 2: Reaction of 1-Isobutyl-3-Methyl-Aluminacyclopent-3-ene with Bis(Chloromethyl)-Oxetane — Another portion of the dioxane solution of 1-isobutyl-3-methyl-aluminacyclopent-3-ene of Example 1 (21 millimols) was reacted with 4.1 grams (26.5 millimols) of bis(chloromethyl)-oxetane for three hours at 150°C. After hydrolysis of the reaction product, distillation resulted in the isolation of 4.8 grams of a liquid boiling over a wide range, 60°C at 1.5 mm Hg to 134°C at 7 mm Hg. Redistillation resulted in the isolation of 128° to 144°C and 9 mm Hg of 2,2-bis(chloromethyl)-4,5-dimethyl-5-hexen-1-ol, 2,2,3-trimethyl-5,5-bis-(chloromethyl)tetrahydropyran, and 2,2-bis(chloromethyl)-4,4-dimethyl-5-hexen-1-ol.

According to another process described by *G.J. Brendel; U.S. Patent 3,674,846; July 4, 1972; assigned to Ethyl Corporation* 7-octen-1-ols having one or two methyl groups in the 6 position are prepared by hydrolyzing an intermediate formed by reaction among aluminum, tetrahydropyran or an alkyl substituted tetrahydropyran, a hydrocarbyl aluminum hydride and butadiene or butadiene substituted on either or both of the internal carbon atoms. During at least a portion of the reaction period the reaction temperature must be in the range of from about 185° to about 210°C so that there is formed an intermediate condensation product via cleavage of the ring of the tetrahydropyran reactant. The 7-octen-1-ols are useful as perfumes, monomers, chemical intermediates and surface active agents.

Example 1: A mixture of 500 millimols of isoprene, 15 grams of activated aluminum powder, 1.03 mols of tetrahydropyran and 85 millimols diisobutylaluminum hydride was heated in a closed reaction vessel for 1 hour at 150°C and then for 2 hours at 185°C. After cooling to room temperature, a portion of the reaction product was hydrolyzed at 0° to 5°C using dilute hydrochloric acid. This resulted in the liberation of 6,7-dimethyl-7-octen-1-ol along with a lesser quantity of 6,6-dimethyl-7-octen-1-ol. These alkenols possess very desirable fragrance characteristics.

Example 2: Repetition of the procedure of Example 1 using a reaction temperature of 200°C for 1.5 hours followed by hydrolysis results in a higher yield of the same alkenols.

Example 3: On heating 500 millimols of butadiene, 15 grams of activated aluminum, one mol of tetrahydropyran, and 85 millimols of diisobutylaluminum hydride in a sealed autoclave for 3 hours at 200°C and then hydrolyzing the reaction mixture with water, 6-methyl-7-octen-1-ol is produced.

Example 4: By substituting 2,3-dimethyl butadiene-1,3 for the butadiene of Example 3, the hydrolysis reaction results in the formation of 6,6,7-trimethyl-7-octen-1-ol.

Example 5: Example 1 is repeated using 2-ethyl butadiene in place of isoprene. Upon hydrolysis, a mixture of 6-methyl-7-ethyl-7-octen-1-ol and 6-methyl-6-ethyl-7-octen-1-ol is formed.

Hydroxy Ethers of 1-Octene and 1-Octyne

W. Kimel; U.S. Patent 3,248,430; April 26, 1966; assigned to Hoffmann-La Roche Inc. describes ethers of 3,7-dihydroxy-3,7-dimethyl-1-octyne and ethers of 3,7-dihydroxy-3,7-dimethyl-1-octene. The compounds are selected from the group consisting of ethers having the formula:

$$
(1) \quad R_1-CH_2-\underset{\underset{OH}{|}}{\overset{\overset{CH_3}{|}}{C}}-\underset{}{\overset{\overset{R_2}{|}}{C}}H-CH_2-CH_2-\underset{\underset{OR_3}{|}}{\overset{\overset{CH_3}{|}}{C}}-C\equiv CH
$$

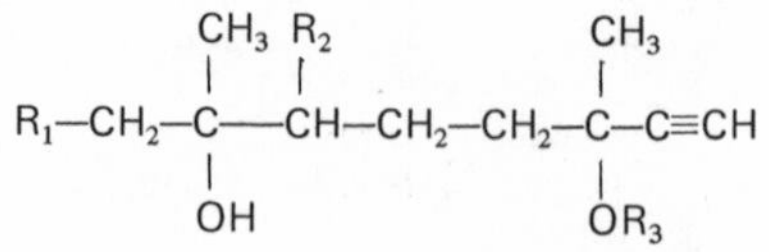

and ethers having the formula:

$$
(2) \quad R_1-CH_2-\underset{\underset{OH}{|}}{\overset{\overset{CH_3}{|}}{C}}-\underset{}{\overset{\overset{R_2}{|}}{C}}H-CH_2-CH_2-\underset{\underset{OR_3}{|}}{\overset{\overset{CH_3}{|}}{C}}-CH=CH_2
$$

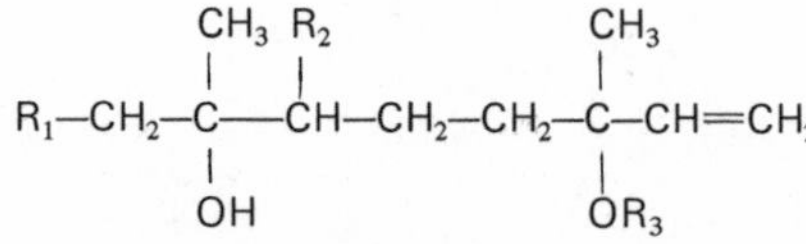

where, in each of Formulas 1 and 2, R_1 represents hydrogen or a lower alkyl group, preferably, an alkyl group having 1 to 3 carbon atoms; R_2 represents hydrogen or a lower alkyl group, preferably, an alkyl group having from 1 to 3 carbon atoms; and R_3 represents a lower alkyl group, preferably, an alkyl group having from 1 to 3 carbon atoms. Two or all three of the alkyl groups represented by the symbols R_1, R_2 and R_3 can be the same group or all three groups can be different. The products of this process are prepared by the hydration of a compound having the formula.

$$
(3) \quad R_1-CH_2-\overset{\overset{CH_3}{|}}{C}=\overset{\overset{R_2}{|}}{C}-CH_2-CH_2-\underset{\underset{OR_3}{|}}{\overset{\overset{CH_3}{|}}{C}}-C\equiv CH
$$

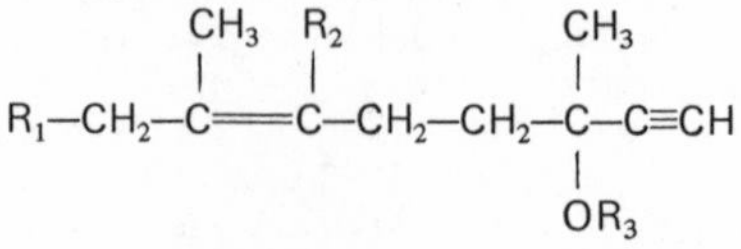

where R_1, R_2 and R_3 have the same meanings as in Formulas 1 and 2. The hydroxy ethers of Formula 2 are obtained by hydrogenating the ethers of Formula 1. The following examples illustrate the process. All parts given in the examples are parts by weight unless otherwise indicated.

Example 1: In this example 200.0 grams of 3,7-dimethyl-3-methoxy-6-octen-1-yne (Formula 3 where $R_1 = R_2 = H$ and $R_3 = CH_3$) were added to a mixture of 400 grams of sulfuric acid (98%), 800 cc of acetic acid and 800 cc of water. The mixture was warmed to, and maintained for a period of about 3 hours at, a temperature within the range of from about 45° to 50°C. Thereafter, the mixture was diluted with 2.0 liters of water, and then extracted with ether. The ether layer was next washed with sodium bicarbonate and then with water until neutral in reaction. The solution was dried over calcium sulfate and distilled at diminished pressure. There was obtained 3,7-dimethyl-3-methoxy-1-octyn-7-ol (Formula 1 where $R_1 = R_2 = H$ and $R_3 = CH_3$), having a boiling point of 104° to 106°C (6 mm).

Example 2: A mixture of 100.0 grams of 3,7dimethyl-3-methoxy-6-octen-1-yne, 100.0 grams of concentrated sulfuric acid (98%), 400 cc of acetic acid, and 400 cc of water was heated to, and maintained for a period of about 3 hours at a temperature of 60° to 65°C, with vigorous stirring. The reaction mixture was allowed to stand overnight, following which it was diluted with about 2.0 liters of water. The mixture was then extracted with ether and it was washed first with sodium bicarbonate and then with water until neutral in reaction. Vacuum distillation yielded 3,7-dimethyl-3-methoxy-1-octyn-7-ol, having a boiling point of 106° to 108°C (7 mm).

Example 3: 3,7-dimethyl-3-methoxy-1-octyn-7-ol produced by the method described in Example 1, was converted by hydrogenation into 3,7-dimethyl-3-methoxy-1-octen-7-ol (Formula 2: $R_1 = R_2 = H$; $R_3 = CH_3$). The procedure employed was as follows: a solution was prepared by dissolving 388.4 grams of 3,7-dimethyl-3-methoxy-1-octyn-7-ol in 400.0 grams of hexane. To this solution, 11.6 grams of Lindlar catalyst [5% palladium-on-calcium carbonate, modified by deposition of lead thereon, as specifically disclosed by Lindlar, *Helvetica Chimica Acta* 35, 450, (1952)] were added. The ether was then reacted with an equimolar quantity of hydrogen at room temperature and atmospheric pressure. Approximately, 95% of the theoretical amount of hydrogen had been consumed when uptake ceased. The reaction mixture was, thereafter, distilled and 3,7-dimethyl-3-methoxy-1-octen-7-ol, having a boiling point at 78°C (0.5 mm), was obtained in quantitative yield.

Example 4: In this example, a mixture of 169 grams of 3-methoxy-3,6,7-trimethyl-6-octen-1-yne (Formula 3 where $R_1 = H$ and $R_2 = R_3 = CH_3$), 338 grams of sulfuric acid (98%), 676 grams of acetic acid and 676 grams of water was stirred vigorously at a temperature of from about 45° to 50°C for a period of about six hours. The mixture was thereafter diluted with about 3.0 liters of water, following which it was extracted with ether. The ether layer was washed with sodium bicarbonate and water until neutral in reaction. The ether solution was subsequently subjected to fractional distillation. After recovery of some unreacted starting material at 82° to 84°C (7 to 8 mm), there was obtained 3-methoxy-3,6,7-trimethyl-1-octyn-7-ol, boiling point of 113° to 116°C (7.5 mm).

Example 5: In this example, a mixture of 159.7 grams of 3,7-dimethyl-3-methoxy-6-nonen-1-yne (Formula 3 where $R_1 = R_3 = CH_3$ and $R_2 = H$) 319.4 grams of sulfuric acid (98%), 639 cc of acetic acid and 639 cc of water was heated at a temperature of about 50°C for about 6 hours. The reaction mixture was continuously and vigorously stirred during the heating step. Thereafter, the reaction was allowed to continue overnight at room temperature with continuous stirring. The reaction mixture was then diluted with 3.5 liters of water, extracted with ether and worked up in the manner described in Example 1. 3,7-dimethyl-3-methoxy-1-nonyn-7-ol (Formula 1 where $R_1 = R_3 = CH_3$ and $R_2 = H$) was obtained at boiling point 114° to 116°C (7 mm).

Example 6: In this example, 23.0 grams of the ether produced in Example 5, that is, 3,7-dimethyl-3-methoxy-1-nonyn-7-ol (Formula 1 where $R_1 = R_3 = CH_3$ and $R_2 = H$) were dissolved in 46 cc of hexane. To this solution, 1.2 grams of Lindlar catalyst (same catalyst as described in Example 3) was added. The ether was then reacted with an equimolar quantity of hydrogen at room temperature and atmospheric pressure. The consumption of 99% of the hydrogen theoretically required was noted. By distillation, 3,7-dimethyl-3-methoxy-1-nonen-7-ol, boiling point 127° to 129°C (14 mm), was isolated in quantitative yield.

Example 7: In this example, 101.5 grams of 3,7-dimethyl-3-ethoxy-6-nonen-1-yne (Formula 3 where R_1 = CH_3, R_2 = H, and R_3 = C_2H_5) were added to a mixture of 406 cc of acetic acid and 609 grams of 33% aqueous solution of sulfuric acid (98%). The reaction mixture was stirred for a period of about 8 hours at a temperature of from about 45° to 50°C. Thereafter, the reaction mixture was diluted with 2,200 cc of water, and worked up in the manner described in Example 1. After isolation of the unreacted starting material by distillation, there was obtained 3,7-dimethyl-3-ethoxy-1-nonyn-7-ol, boiling point 125° to 126°C (10 mm).

8-Mercapto-p-Menthan-3-ol

D. Lamparsky and P. Schudel; U.S. Patent 3,769,328; October 30, 1973; assigned to Givaudan Corporation describe p-menthane derivatives which have the following formula

where R represents a hydrogen atom or a C_1 to C_5 acyl group. The p-menthane derivatives of the above general formula are distinguished by particular fragrance and flavor properties. According to the process, the p-menthane derivatives are manufactured by reducing p-menthane-8-thiol-3-one with a complex metal hydride and, if desired, acylating the hydroxyl group of the resulting 8-mercapto-p-menthan-3-ol.

8-mercapto-p-menthan-3-ol has, for example, fragrance and flavor properties which may be termed fruity, flat-camphoraceous tending towards buccu camphor, reminiscent of bread-crust, with a slight indole note and a warm-woody side-note reminiscent of oak-moss. 8-mercapto-p-menthan-3-yl acetate, which is particularly interesting for use in aromas, has fragrance and flavor properties which can be paraphrased as follows: fruity, green, floral, minty with marked cassis and buccu oil note. The following examples illustrate the process.

Example 1: A solution of 9.3 grams of p-menthane-8-thiol-3-one in 30 ml of absolute ether is slowly added dropwise with cooling, stirring and exclusion of moisture to 1.0 gram of lithium aluminum hydride in 30 ml of absolute diethyl ether in such a way that the solution boils quite weakly. After completion of the addition, the mixture is stirred for a further 1 hour at the boiling temperature of the ether and subsequently cooled to about 0°C.

The excess reducing agent is then decomposed by the cautious addition of water. The mixture is thereupon made weakly acidic with a dilute mineral acid (or an organic acid such as tartaric acid), the ether layer is separated off and the aqueous phase is exhaustively extracted with ether. The combined ether solutions are washed neutral, dried and the ether is removed. There are thus obtained 7.6 grams (about 80% of theory) of 8-mercapto-p-menthan-3-ol in the form of a stereoisomer mixture in the ratio 60:36:4. The mixture boils at 67° to 69°C/0.06 mm Hg. In this case, the main component is enriched in the most volatile fractions, while the content of the two other isomers lies markedly higher in the end fraction than at the beginning of the distillation.

The p-menthane-8-thiol-3-one used as the starting material can be prepared as follows: 114.0 grams of technical pulegone with a pulegone content of about 93% are dissolved in 150 ml of technical absolute ethanol and treated with a solution of 7.5 grams of potassium hydroxide in 50 ml of ethanol. Hydrogen sulfide is conducted into the solution, cooled to −75°C, until the increase in volume amounts to 40 ml. The cold solution is immediately transferred into a suitable previously cooled pressure vessel and allowed to stand for 16 hours, the temperature gradually rising to room temperature. The autoclave is subsequently heated at an internal temperature of 50°C for 2 hours; the pressure thereby rising to at most 7.4 atmospheres. After completion of the reaction, the mixture is cooled to room temperature. 140 ml of ethanol are distilled off from the reaction mixture in vacuo on a rotary evaporator. The residue (153 grams) is taken up in 250 ml of ether, washed twice with 100 ml of saturated sodium chloride solution each time and subsequently twice with 100 ml of water each time to neutrality. The ether solution is dried and the ether is subsequently removed. The residue (122.4 grams) is fractionally distilled. The p-menthane-8-thiol-3-one (102 grams, 73%) obtained boils at 74° to 75°C/0.1 mm Hg; n_D^{20} = 1.4951; ratio of the stereoisomers about 4:1.

Example 2: 1.15 grams of sodium borohydride and 2 grams of calcium chloride are dissolved in 10 ml of absolute ethanol. 10 grams of p-menthane-8-thiol-3-one are added to this mixture and the resulting mixture is left to stand overnight at room temperature with exclusion of moisture. On the next morning, 5 ml of 10 N sodium hydroxide are added. After heating for a short time, the mixture is allowed to cool, 10 ml of water are added and insolubles are filtered off. The filtrate is acidified with 7.5 ml of glacial acetic acid and subsequently concentrated. The residue is made alkaline and extracted twice with 75 ml of chloroform each time. The combined chloroform solutions are washed with saturated sodium chloride solution and dried and the solvent is removed. The residue (8.7 grams) contains about 70% of 8-mercapto-p-mentan-3-ol and is fractionally distilled in the manner described in Example 1, the pulegone occurring as a byproduct and the 10% of starting material still present being separated off with the head fractions.

Example 3: A mixture of 4.5 grams of acetic acid anhydride and 4.3 grams of pyridine is added with external cooling to 8.2 grams of 8-mercapto-p-menthan-3-ol. The mixture is allowed to stand overnight at a temperature of about 0°C, then poured onto crushed ice and dilute hydrochloric acid and exhaustively extracted with ether. The ethereal solution is washed neutral and dried, and the ether is removed. The residue (10 grams) is fractionally distilled in the vacuum of an oil-pump and yields a stereoisomer mixture of 8-mercapto-p-menthan-3-yl acetate of boiling point 72°C/0.8 mm Hg; n_D^{20} = 1.4887 to 1.4893.

OTHER COMPOUNDS

Benzylthioindoles

A process described by *A. Hofmann and F. Troxler; U.S. Patent 3,143,551; August 4, 1964; assigned to Sandoz Ltd., Switzerland* is concerned with compounds having the formula

(1)

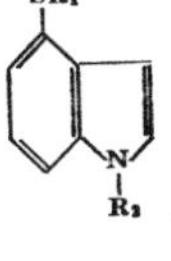

in which R signifies a lower alkyl radical or an aralkyl radical, and R_2 signifies a hydrogen atom, or a lower alkyl or alkenyl radical, or an aralkyl radical. The process for the production of the compounds 1, is characterized in that a substituted nitrotoluene of Formula 2,

(2)

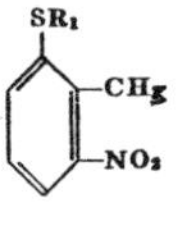

in which R_1 has the above significance, is condensed in the presence of an alkali metal alcoholate with an oxalic acid diester. The resulting phenyl-pyruvic acid ester of Formula 3 in which R signifies the radical of any alcohol, preferably a lower alkyl radical, is saponified to the corresponding acid of Formula 4.

(3) 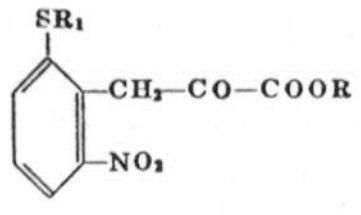   [structure: benzene ring with SR₁ at top, —CH₂—CO—COOR substituent, and —NO₂]

(4) 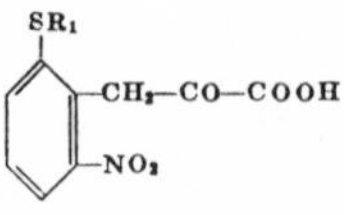   [structure: benzene ring with SR₁ at top, —CH₂—CO—COOH substituent, and —NO₂]

This is cyclized in the presence of sodium dithionite of ferrous hydroxide to an indole-2-carboxylic acid of Formula 5:

(5) 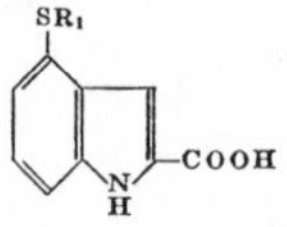   [indole structure with SR₁ substituent and —COOH at 2-position, N-H]

Alternatively, the compound (5) may also be prepared by cyclizing the ester (3) in the above manner, and saponifying the resulting indole-2-carboxylic acid ester of Formula 6:

(6) 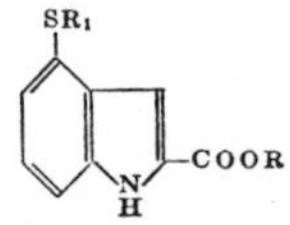   [indole structure with SR₁ substituent and —COOR at 2-position, N-H]

The acid (5) is then decarboxylated and, if desired, the resulting indole, substituted in the 4 position, treated in the presence of an alkaline condensing agent with a lower alkyl or alkenyl halide, or an aralkyl halide.

At room temperature, these compounds are oils or crystalline substances having a low melting point; they have an intense characteristic smell. With Keller's color reagent (ferric chloride containing glacial acetic acid and concentrated sulfuric acid) and Van Urk's reagent (p-dimethylaminobenzaldehyde and dilute sulfuric acid) they give characteristic color reactions. Compounds 1 may be used as scents or in the perfumery. Due to their odor, they may further be used in agriculture for attracting bee swarms or for attracting or repelling other insects.

Example 1: 4-Methylthioindole — 2-Nitro-6-methylthiotoluene is prepared as follows: a mixture of 425 grams of 2-nitro-6-amino-toluene, 189 cc of concentrated sulfuric acid, 4 liters of water and 2.5 kg of ice are diazotized at 0°C by adding a solution of 210 grams of sodium nitrite in 350 cc of water dropwise. After 30 minutes the mixture is brought to a pH value of 6 by the addition of sodium acetate and the solution added at 0°C to a mixture of 200 grams of sodium hydroxide, 2 liters of water, 200 cc of liquid methyl-mercaptan and 200 grams of copper bronze, while stirring.

Gaseous methylmercaptan is passed through for a further 15 minutes, 1.5 kg of common salt added and the mixture left to be stirred in an ice bath overnight. The mixture is acidified with concentrated hydrochloric acid, extracted 7 times with 2.5 liters of chloroform, the chloroform extract dried over magnesium sulfate and potash (1:1) and then evaporated. The residue is distilled in a high vacuum. Boiling point 130°C/0.2 mm of Hg. For analysis the mixture is sublimed in a high vacuum at 40° to 45°C. Melting point 56° to 58°C.

(2-Nitro-6-methylthiophenyl)-pyruvic acid is prepared as follows: a solution of 9.5 grams of 2-nitro-6-methylthiotoluene and 15.3 grams of oxalic acid diethyl ester in 50 cc of ether are added dropwise to a solution of potassium ethylate, prepared from 3.53 grams of potassium and 16 cc of absolute ethanol in 150 cc of ether, at 0°C. After standing for 10 days at room temperature the precipitate is filtered off with suction, washed with ether and then shaken with 100 cc of ether, 150 cc of water and 30 cc of a 2 N sodium hydroxide solution for one hour at room temperature. The ethereal phase is separated, shaken again in 100 cc of water, the aqueous solution filtered through highly purified fuller's earth until clear and slowly acidified with concentrated hydrochloric acid at 0°C. The oily (2-nitro-6-methylthiophenyl)pyruvic acid precipitating is extracted with chloroform and crystallizes from benzene in druses having a melting point of 107° to 109°C.

4-Methylthioindole-2-carboxylic acid is prepared as follows: 10 grams of sodium dithionite are added portionwise to a solution of 6.651 grams of (2-nitro-6-methylthiophenyl)pyruvic acid in 50 cc of water containing 26 cc of 1 N sodium hydroxide solution while stirring and cooling with ice. A further 20 cc of 1 N sodium hydroxide solution are added, the mixture is filtered through highly purified fuller's earth after 30 minutes and the filtrate slowly acidified with 2 N hydrochloric acid. The precipitated carboxylic acid is filtered off with suction and recrystallized from ethanol (needles), methanol/benzene (needles) and from ethanol/glacial acetic acid (needles). Melting point 244° to 246°C. Keller's color reaction: negative. Van Urk's color reaction: negative.

4-Methylmercaptoindole is prepared as follows: 1.2 grams of 4-methylthioindole-2-carboxylic acid are decarboxylated in a distillation column at a pressure of 15 mm of Hg and 260° to 270°C. The mixture is subsequently distilled in a high vacuum at 0.02 mm of Hg and 180°C. The distillate is taken up in ether, shaken twice with a 10% soda solution and the ethereal solution dried over potash. The evaporation residue of the solution is again distilled at 0.05 mm of Hg and 145° to 155°C. Melting point of the solidified distillate 44° to 47°C. Keller's color reaction: brown-violet. Van Urk's color reaction: blue tinged with violet.

Example 2: 4-Benzylthioindole — 2-Nitro-6-benzylthiotoluene is prepared as follows: 369 grams of 2-nitro-6-aminotoluene are diazotized in a manner analogous to that described in Example 1. After 30 minutes the solution is brought to a pH value of 6 by the addition of sodium acetate and the solution added portionwise to a mixture of 300 grams of benzylmercaptan, 282.2 grams of sodium hydroxide, 172.5 grams of copper bronze and 1.5 liters of water, while stirring. After working up in a manner analogous to that described in Example 1 the resulting, dried chloroform extract is concentrated until the 2-nitro-6-benzylthiotoluene crystallizes. The crystallate is filtered with suction and dried. Melting point 106° to 108°C.

(2-Nitro-6-benzylthiophenyl)pyruvic acid is prepared as follows: a solution of 725 grams of oxalic acid diethyl ester and 442.5 grams of 2-nitro-6-benzylthiotoluene in 3 liters of tetrahydrofuran are added dropwise to a potassium ethylate solution, prepared from 189 grams of potassium and 850 cc of ethanol in 2 liters of absolute tetrahydrofuran, cooled to 0°C. After the mixture has stood for 12 days at room temperature, the tetrahydrofuran is distilled off, 3 liters of ether are added to the residue and after a short while the mixture decanted. The residue remaining in the flask is dissolved in the required quantity of water (about 6 to 7 liters) with the addition of 40% solution of sodium hydroxide, the mixture filtered and then strongly acidified with concentrated hydrochloric acid. The oily (2-nitro-6-benzylthiophenyl)pyruvic acid is extracted with chloroform and the chloroform extract dried over magnesium sulfate/potash (1:1) and evaporated.

4-Benzylthioindole-2-carboxylic acid is prepared as follows: 400 grams of raw oily (2-nitro-6-benzylthiophenyl)pyruvic acid are dissolved in 1 liter of benzene and diluted with 475 cc of a 2 N sodium hydroxide solution and quickly shaken with 2 liters of water. The combined red colored aqueous extracts are filtered through highly purified fuller's earth and 624 grams of sodium dithionite and 475 cc of a 2 N sodium hydroxide solution added portionwise at 0° to 5°C.

The mixture is made alkaline with a 40% sodium hydroxide solution, filtered through highly purified fuller's earth and acidified with concentrated hydrochloric acid whilst cooling with ice. The precipitated 4-benzylthioindole-2-carboxylic acid is filtered off with suction and recrystallized from ethanol and ethanol/glacial acetic acid. Melting point 191° to 192°C.

Keller's color reaction: chrome green like. Van Urk's color reaction: negative.

4-Benzylthioindole is prepared as follows: 2.11 grams of 4-benzylthioindole-2-carboxylic acid are decarboxylated in a distillation column at 15 mm of Hg and 210°C. The temperature is increased to 240°C and the mixture then distilled in a high vacuum. The distillate is taken up in ether, shaken twice with a 10% soda solution and the ethereal solution dried over potash. The evaporation residue of the solution is again distilled at 0.02 mm of Hg and 155°C. Melting point of the solidified distillate 32° to 35°C. Keller's color reaction: before shaking, violet, then brown. Van Urk's color reaction: turbid violet. It is to be noted that the cyclization may also be effected with ferrous hydroxide instead of sodium dithionite.

Cyclic Sulfides

According to a process described by *R.W. Campbell; U.S. Patent 3,345,381; October 3, 1967; assigned to Chevron Research Company* thiophane and thiophane-like cyclic sulfides are produced by the cobalt sulfide catalyzed reduction of cyclic carboxylic acid anhydrides using hydrogen sulfide.

Cyclic sulfides, for example thiophane and the like, are useful as odorants in natural gas while the less volatile higher molecular weight sulfides are useful as oxidation inhibitors, in rubber chemistry, as modifiers of perfume fragrances and the like. It has been found that cyclic sulfides can be produced by reacting cyclic organic acid anhydrides with hydrogen sulfide in the presence of cobalt sulfide at a temperature in the range of about 180° to 325°C. The anhydride compounds useful in the process may be represented by the general formula

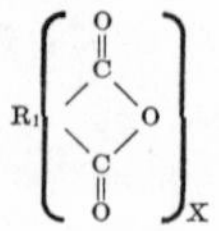

$$R_1 \left[\begin{array}{c} O \\ \| \\ C \\ \diagdown \\ \diagup O \\ C \\ \| \\ O \end{array} \right]_X$$

In which R_1 is a hydrocarbon radical having from 2 to about 18 carbon atoms and X is a whole number less than three. The resulting cyclic sulfides are also representable by a general formula,

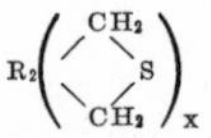

$$R_2 \left(\begin{array}{c} CH_2 \\ \diagdown \\ S \\ \diagup \\ CH_2 \end{array} \right)_x$$

and in this case R_2 is a saturated hydrocarbon radical having from 2 to about 18 carbon atoms and X is one or two. The acid anhydrides contemplated contain the anhydride functionality in a 5- or 6-membered carbon-oxygen heterocyclic ring containing at least 4 but less than 6 carbon atoms. The net chemical transformation occurring in the process may be represented by the representative equation:

$$(CH_2CO)_2O + 5H_2S \longrightarrow \underline{SCH_2CH_2CH_2CH_2} + 3H_2O + 4S$$

Under the process conditions, sulfur reacts readily with hydrogen gas to form hydrogen sulfide. Hydrogen is therefore desirably added to the reaction system since the conversion of sulfur to hydrogen sulfide tends to drive the reaction more fully towards completion. A further advantage found in the use of added hydrogen is that the substantial absence of elemental sulfur in the product mixture facilitates work-ups. The following examples illustrate the process.

Example 1: A 4.5-liter shaker bomb was charged with 200 grams (2 mols) of succinic anhydride, 10 grams of cobalt chloride, and 545 grams (16 mols) of H_2S. After this, it was pressured to 950 lb with hydrogen. The reaction mixture was agitated for 18 hours at 230° to 260°C during which time the maximum pressure observed was 3,400 psi. After cooling down, the liquid contents were removed from the bomb and the small amount of aqueous material discarded.

The organic layer, after drying, was analyzed by vapor-phase chromatography using appropriate standards and found to contain 27% thiophane, 11% thiophene, and 5% γ-butyrothiolactone. These yields are mol percent based on the succinic anhydride starting material. When the intermediates, thiophene and γ-butyrothiolactone, are recycled to the process, the yield of saturated cyclic sulfide is correspondingly increased.

Example 2: A 4-liter autoclave was charged with 150 grams (1.32 mols) of methyl succinic anhydride, 5 grams of cobalt acetate, and 540 grams (15.9 mols) of H_2S. The bomb was then pressured to 950 psi with hydrogen and agitated for 2 hours at 260°C. The products were worked up as previously described. In this case, the yields were based upon nuclear magnetic resonance spectra. The product contained 20% 2-methyl thiophane and 29% methyl-γ-thiobutyrolactone.

Example 3: As in Example 2 except that no cobalt catalyst was added, the conversion of methyl succinic anhydride to methyl thiophane was attempted. None was detectable in the reaction mixture.

Example 4: The 4-liter shaker bomb was charged with 154 grams (1 mol) of 1,2,3,6-tetrahydrophthalic anhydride, 5 grams of cobalt chloride, and 340 grams (10 mols) of H_2S. The bomb was pressured to 1,000 psi with hydrogen and heated at 280° to 300°C for 18 hours. The work-up of the products gave 53% of 8-thiabicyclo[4.3.0]nonane (I) and a small amount of 8-thiabicyclo[4.3.0]nonadiene-6,9 (II).

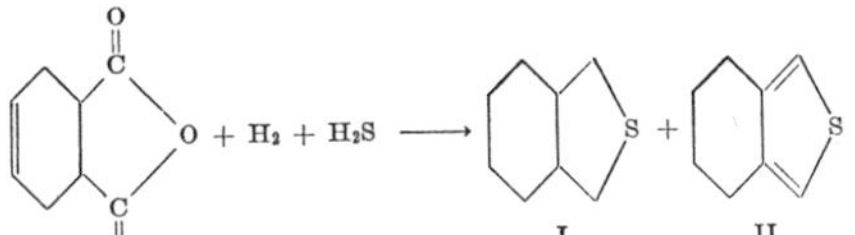

This latter compound (II) was identified by the NMR spectra.

Example 5: This was carried out as in Example 4 except that the feed was hexahydrophthalic anhydride. An experiment was carried out and found to result in a 69% yield of 8-thiabicyclo[4.3.0]nonane (I) obtained as a mixture of the cis- and trans-isomers. These isomers were separated by the vapor-phase chromatograph and identified by comparing the IR spectras with those of the known isomers.

Example 6: In the same manner as in Example 1, a 2.5-liter shaker bomb was charged with 86 grams (1.0 mol) of γ-butyrolactone, 2 grams of cobalt chloride, 360 grams (10.5 mols) of H_2S and then pressured to 850 psi with hydrogen. Reaction was carried out for 2 hours at 260°C, and then the product was worked up as in Example 1. In this case, conversion of lactone was in excess of 99%. The product contained 35% thiophane and 45% γ-butyrothiolactone. This example demonstrates that lactones corresponding to partially hydrogenated acid anhydrides of the general formula:

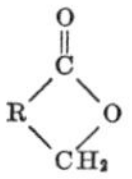

wherein R is a hydrocarbon radical having from 2 to 18 carbon atoms and in which the lactone ring is a 5- or 6-membered heterocyclic ring, are readily converted to the cyclic sulfides of the aforedescribed general formula.

10-Undecenyl Alkylene Glycol Borates

I.S. Bengelsdorf; U.S. Patent 3,189,638; June 15, 1965; assigned to United States Borax & Chemical Corporation describes the preparation of 10-undecenyl alkylene glycol borates having the formula

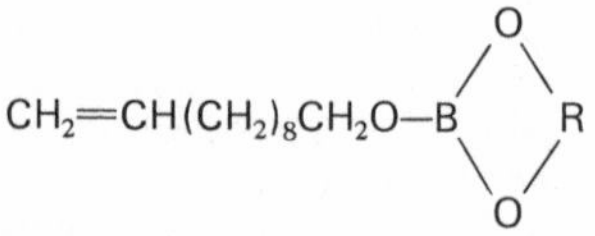

$$CH_2=CH(CH_2)_8CH_2O-B \begin{array}{c} O \\ \diagup \diagdown \\ \diagdown \diagup \\ O \end{array} R$$

where R is an alkylene radical of 2 to 3 carbon atoms in length and containing a total of 2 to about 20 carbon atoms. When R is an alkylene radical of 2 carbon atoms in length, the compounds contain a 1,3-dioxa-2-borolane ring. When R is an alkylene radical of 3 carbon atoms in length, the boron-containing ring is that of a 1,3-dioxa-2-borinane. The carbon atoms of the rings can be unsubstituted or they can be substituted with lower alkyl groups. The preferred compounds are those that have one or more lower alkyl groups, for example, methyl, as substituents on the carbon atoms of the ring. The borates are readily prepared by reaction of 10-undecenyl alcohol with the appropriate alkylene glycol monoborate or a lower alkyl ester of the appropriate glycol monoborate.

Example 1: A solution of 95.0 grams (0.557 mol) of 10-undecenyl alcohol and 80.3 grams (0.557 mol) of 2-hydroxy-4,4,6-trimethyl-1,3-dioxa-2-borinane in 150 ml of cyclohexane was stirred in a 500 ml flask at reflux temperature. The by-product water was removed by means of a Dean-Stark trap as it was formed. Refluxing was continued until the theoretical amount of water had been taken off (about 2.5 hours). The cyclohexane was removed by distillation under reduced pressure to give the crude product as an oily residue. The crude product was distilled under reduced pressure and 2-(10-undecenoxy)-4,4,6-trimethyl-1,3-dioxa-2-borinane collected at 125° to 127°C/0.4 mm. The product is a colorless, mobile liquid.

Example 2: A mixture of 10-undecenyl alcohol (170.1 grams, 1.0 mol), 2,2,4-trimethyl-1,3-pentanediol (146.6 grams, 1.0 mol) and boric acid (62.1 grams, 1.0 mol) was stirred and heated in the presence of 300 ml toluene. The by-product water was removed with the use of a Dean-Stark trap. Refluxing was continued until the theoretical amount of water (54 ml) had been liberated (10 hours). The toluene was removed at reduced pressure and the crude oily residue was distilled. The 2-(10-undecenoxy)-4-isopropyl-5,5-dimethyl-1,3-dioxa-2-borinane was collected at 165° to 167°C/0.3 mm as a colorless, mobile liquid.

Methallyl Methoxyphenyl Ethers

W.J. Houlihan; U.S. Patent 3,328,260; June 27, 1967; assigned to Universal Oil Products Company has found that allyl and methallyl methoxyphenyl ethers have unusual and useful odors which make them of specific value to the perfume and related industries. These compounds have the following structural formula:

where R is $-CH_2CH=CH_2$ (allyl) or $-CH_2\overset{\overset{\displaystyle CH_3}{|}}{C}=CH_2$ (methallyl).

Beta-methallyl-p-methoxyphenyl ether has an odor resembling that of bergamot oil. Bergamot oil is a relatively expensive oil which differs somewhat in composition and quality depending upon its source and method of production. Beta-methallyl p-methoxyphenyl ether, however, can be economically produced and is constant in its odor and composition. Naturally occurrring bergamot oil often possesses certain overtones or perfume notes which are desirable in many perfumed compositions and, therefore, beta-methallyl p-methoxyphenyl ether can also be used as an additive or extender with natural bergamot oil. The other compounds of the process in direct contrast to the beta-methallyl p-methoxyphenyl ether have fruity or phenolic type odors which make them useful in compounding a wide range of perfume compositions. The following examples illustrate the process:

Example 1: A stirred mixture of 2 mols (248 grams) of p-hydroxyanisole, 2 mols (181 grams) of beta-methallyl chloride, 2.2 mols (304 grams) of potassium carbonate and 300 grams of acetone is refluxed for 12 hours. Water is added to the reaction mixture to dissolve the salts. The organic layer is separated from the water layer and the latter is extracted with benzene. The combined organic layers are washed with a 10% sodium hydroxide solution until phenol-free. The mixture is then distilled through a column to yield beta-methallyl p-methoxyphenyl ether, BP 104° to 106°C. at 1 mm.

The compound thus obtained has a strong bergamot odor and may be used by itself in perfumes or perfumed products. However, it will ordinarily be used in combination with other agents in a compounded perfume composition where the product replaces part or all of the bergamot oil which would otherwise be employed.

Example 2: A stirred mixture of 248 grams of p-hydroxyanisole (2.0 mols), 242 grams of allyl bromide (2.0 mols), 304 grams of potassium carbonate (2.2 mols), and 300 grams of acetone is refluxed for eight hours. The reaction mixture is cooled to 25°C and sufficient water is added to dissolve the salts and the aqueous layer is separated. The aqueous layer is extracted with 200 ml of benzene and the organic phases are combined and washed twice with 100 ml portions of an aqueous 10% solution of sodium hydroxide. The mixture is then distilled through a column to yield p-methoxyphenyl allyl ether. The compound has a fruity odor.

Example 3: A stirred mixture of 248 grams of guaiacol (2.0 mols), 181 grams of methallyl chloride (2.0 mols), 304 grams of potassium carbonate (2.2 mols) and 200 grams of acetone is refluxed for eight hours. The resulting viscous, light brown solution is allowed to cool to 25°C and sufficient water is added to the cooled solution to dissolve the salts. The organic layer is separated and the aqueous layer extracted with 200 ml of benzene. The combined organic layers are washed three times with an aqueous 10% solution of sodium hydroxide. The mixture is then distilled through a column to yield o-methoxyphenyl methallyl ether. The yield was 41%. The compound has a phenolic type odor useful in producing perfumes and perfumed products.

Example 4: A stirred mixture of 248 grams of guaiacol (2.0 mols) 242 grams of allyl bromide (2.0 mols), 304 grams of potassium carbonate (2.2 mols) and 400 grams of acetone is refluxed for 2.25 hours. The reaction mixture is allowed to cool to 25°C and sufficient water is added to dissolve the salts. The organic layer is separated and the aqueous layer extracted with 200 ml of benzene. The organic layers are combined and washed twice with 100 ml solution of 10% sodium hydroxide. The mixture is then distilled through a column to yield o-methoxyphenyl allyl ether in about 56% yield. The compound has a pungent phenolic odor useful in the perfume industry.

Butyrolactones

L.V. Phillips; U.S. Patent 3,299,100; January 17, 1967; assigned to Gulf Oil Corporation describes a method of manufacturing α-substituted γ-butyrolactones. The process may be represented by the following sequence of reactions:

The improvement which has been effected in the synthesis of α-substituted γ-butyrolactones resides primarily in the use of sodium alkoxide in both the reaction of the substituted malonic ester with ethylene oxide and in the subsequent reaction in only quantities large enough to be considered catalytic. The second or de-carbethoxylation step performed by refluxing in the presence of ethanol and a catalytic quantity of sodium ethoxide finds no correspondingly similar procedure in the prior art with which it can be compared, de-carbethoxylation being usually accomplished under acid conditions. The following examples illustrate the process.

Example 1: Preparation of α-Carbethoxy-α-Methyl-γ-Butyrolactone — A solution of 1.7 grams (0.0316 mol) of sodium methoxide in 5 ml of absolute ethanol was added to 137.3 grams of commercial diethyl methylmalonate which gas chromatographic analyses indicated to contain about 33% diethyl dimethylmalonate. While the solution was stirred and maintained at 30° to 35°C, 38.3 grams (0.87 mol) of ethylene oxide in 65 ml of absolute ethanol was added during the course of 3.5 hours. The reaction continued to be exothermic for about 2.5 hours and occasional cooling was required to maintain the temperature below 35°C.

After the reaction mixture had stood overnight at room temperature, it was acidified with sulfuric acid and distilled to give 39.4 grams of diethyl dimethyl malonate, BP 63° to 73°C (4 mm); and 89.1 grams of ethyl α-carbethoxy-α-methyl-γ-butyrolactone, BP 110° to 115°C (4 mm). Based upon the amount of received diethyl dimethylmalonate, this represents a 92% yield of carbethoxylactone.

Example 2: (A) Preparation of α-Methyl-γ-Butyrolactone — A solution of 500 grams (2.86 mols) of diethyl methylmalonate, 6.2 grams (0.114 mol) of sodium methoxide and 40 ml of absolute ethanol was maintained at 35°C while a solution of 140 grams (3.18 mols) of ethylene oxide and 140 ml of absolute ethanol was added over a 1¼ hours period. The reaction became exothermic after approximately ½ of the ethylene oxide solution had been added and a cold finger condenser was employed to keep the temperature below 38°C.

After stirring for 7 hours, the reaction ceased to be exothermic and it was allowed to stand overnight at room temperature. An additional 6.2 grams of sodium methoxide and 330 ml of absolute ethanol were added then the solution was refluxed for 17 hours. After the addition of 5.7 ml (0.09 mol) of sulfuric acid, the solution was distilled to give 232 grams of diethyl carbonate, 239.8 grams of α-methyl-γ-butyrolactone, BP 66° to 69°C (1 mm); and 60.9 grams of α-carbethoxy-α-methyl-γ-butyrolactone, BP 83° to 91°C (1 mm).

Diethyl ethylmalonate and diethyl isobutylmalonate were also reacted with ethylene oxide then decarbethoxylated under similar conditions to give an 80% yield of α-ethyl-γ-butyro-lactone and 92% yield of α-isobutyl-γ-butyrolactone. The conversion of α-methyl-γ-butyro-lactone to other useful products is demonstrated in parts B and C below.

(B) Preparation of Methyl α-Methyl-γ-Chlorobutyrate — A mixture of 268 grams (2.65 mols) of α-methyl-γ-chlorobutyrolactone, 5 grams of freshly fused zinc chloride and 250 ml of methylene chloride was placed in a glass lined autoclave. The autoclave was pressured to 200 psi with anhydrous hydrogen chloride then stirred and heated at 100° to 110°C for 5 hours. After removal of methylene chloride under reduced pressure, the residue was re-fluxed overnight with 1,070 ml of methanol and 3.5 grams of p-toluenesulfonic acid. The product was distilled to give 264.1 grams, BP 74° to 76°C (22 mm), of mixture which con-tained 90% methyl α-methyl-γ-chlorobutyrate and 10% α-methyl butyrolactone. A higher boiling fraction, 36.7 grams, BP 77° to 85°C (22 mm), consisted largely of α-methylbutyro-lactone with a small amount of methyl α-methyl-γ-chlorobutyrate.

(C) Preparation of Methyl α-Methylcyclopropanecarboxylate — A slurry of 133 grams (2.46 mols) of sodium methoxide, 800 ml of benzene and 369.9 grams of a mixture which contained 90% methyl α-methyl-γ-chlorobutyrate and 10% α-methyl-γ-butyrolactone was refluxed for 2 hours then 450 ml of the methanol-benzene azeotrope was removed over an 8 hr period. After the mixture had cooled, 21 ml of concentrated hydrochloric acid in 350 ml of water was added. The organic phase was dried and distilled through an

efficient column to give 247.7 grams of methyl α-methylcyclopropanecarboxylate, BP 121° to 123°C. There remained 36 grams of α-methyl-γ-butyrolactone as a distillation residue.

Example 3: Preparation of α-Phenoxy-γ-Butyrolactone — A mixture of 40 grams (0.159 mol) of diethyl phenoxymalonate, 1 gram (0.018 mol) of sodium methoxide and 10 ml of absolute ethanol was heated to 40°C then 18.4 grams (0.42 mol) of ethylene oxide in 20 ml of absolute ethanol was added. The reaction mixture maintained its temperature at 36° to 39°C for 3 hours. After standing at room temperature overnight, the solution was refluxed for 1 hour then distilled to give 22 grams of α-phenoxy-γ-butyrolactone, BP 140° to 143°C (1 mm). The product solidified upon standing.

PRODUCT APPLICATION

DETERGENTS AND CLEANING PRODUCTS

Titanate Esters of Alcohols

B.G. Jaggers, K.F. Ufton and H.R. Wagner; U.S. Patent 3,779,932; December 18, 1973 describe solid washing compositions comprising one or more monomeric titanium or zirconium compounds containing at least one group of the formula M—O—R, where M is titanium or zirconium and R is the residue of a perfumery alcohol or phenol. Such compounds have the general formula MA_4 where M is titanium or zirconium and the groups A are the same or different organic groups at least one of which is a group of the formula [—O—R].

The perfumery alcohol or phenol may be any odoriferous mono- or polyhydric alcohol or phenol used or suggested for use in perfumery compositions, for example, such as described in the books *Synthetic Perfumes* by West, Strausz and Barton, published by Arnold & Co. (London) 1969, *Soap, Perfumery and Cosmetics,* 7th edition by W.A. Poucher, published by Chapman & Hall (London), 1959 and *Perfume and Flavour Chemicals* by Steffen Arctander, published by the author (Montclair) 1969.

Particularly preferred esters are tetra-eugenyl orthotitanate tetra-α-terpinyl orthotitanate, tetra-linalyl orthotitanate, tetra-β-phenyl ethyl orthotitanate, tetra-citronellyl orthotitanate, tetra-geranyl orthotitanate, tetra-neryl orthotitanate, tetra-benzyl orthotitanate, tetra-cinnamyl orthotitanate and tetra-2-amyl-cinnamyl orthotitanate. The following examples illustrate the process. All parts are by weight.

Example 1: The preparation of tetra-eugenyl orthotitanate is as follows: To 74 grams of tetra-n-butyl orthotitanate in a dry 250 ml flask, 144 grams of eugenol were added. The pressure in the distillation system was 20 mm Hg; the contents of the flask were heated and n-butanol was given off and collected as distillate. When the pot temperature reached 120°C the pressure in the system was cautiously reduced to 5 mm Hg and more butanol was collected. The temperature fell and rose again to 120°C. A pressure of 0.1 mm Hg was applied until no more butanol was distilled. The theoretical amount of butanol was collected, (65 grams). 153 grams of tetra-eugenyl orthotitanate was obtained as a dark red extremely viscous liquid.

Example 2: The preparation of tetra-α-terpineyl orthotitanate is as follows: The method used was that of Example 1 except that 136 grams α-terpineol (0.88 mol) was used in place of the eugenol. The theoretical amount of butanol was collected leaving 145 grams tetra-α-terpineyl orthotitanate as a very viscous liquid.

264

Example 3: A lilac perfume incorporating orthotitanates was prepared from the following ingredients:

	Parts
Coumarin	5
Lauryl aldehyde	5
Citronellyl acetate	10
Heliotropin	10
Rose base	10
Anisaldehyde	20
Cyclamen aldehyde phenyl acetaldehyde	20
Dimethyl acetal	20
Terpineyl acetate	20
Benzyl acetate	30
Phenyl ethyl alcohol	30
Linalool	50
Musk xylene	50
Terpineol	400
Tetra-α-phenyl ethyl titanate	30
Tetralinalyl titanate	40
Tetraterpineyl titanate	250
Total	1,000

Quantities of this perfume were thoroughly mixed into a standard solid domestic spray dried detergent powder comprising approximately 35% sodium tripolyphosphate, 22% sodium perborate, 18% sodium dodecyl benzene sulfonate, 12% sodium sulfate together with small quantities various other additives such as coconut monoethanolamide, ethylenediamine tetraacetic acid, sodium carboxymethylcellulose and optical brighteners. The thus perfumed detergents comprised from 0.05 to 0.25% of the above perfumery formulation. The alcohols present as titanate esters were retained during storage and hydrolyzed rapidly on addition of the perfumed detergent to water, giving off their characteristic perfumery notes.

5-Alkoxy-2-Pentanones

A. Cahn and A.H. Gilbert; U.S. Patent 3,479,301; November 18, 1969 and U.S. Patent 3,316,305; April 25, 1967; both assigned to Lever Brothers Company describe the production of compounds with desirable odor characteristics which retain their fragrances in the presence of bleaching ingredients and which are stable in alkaline media. It has been found that this can be attained by a compound of the formula:

$$R-O-(CR^1R^2)_n-(CR^3R^4)_m-(CR^5R^6)_p-CO-R^7$$

where R is a straight or branched-chain alkyl group having at least 4 carbon atoms; R^1, R^2, R^3, R^4, R^5, and R^6 each are radicals selected from the group consisting of hydrogen and straight or branched-chain alkyl groups having from 1 to 3 carbon atoms with not more than two of the radicals being alkyl; R^7 is a straight-chain or branched-chain alkyl group having from 1 to 4 carbon atoms; m, n and p are integers whose sum is greater than 2; the total number of carbon atoms in the molecule being no more than about 20.

Preferred compounds are those in which R ranges from 4 to 12 carbon atoms and the sum of m, n and p is less than 6. Examples of compounds coming within the above formula are the following: 5-isobutoxypentanone-2, 5-(2,4-dimethylpentoxy)pentanone-2, 5-(n-pentoxy)pentanone-2, 2-methyl-6-isobutoxyhexanone-3, 4-methyl-5-isobutoxypentanone-2, 6-isobutoxyhexanone-2, etc.

In the preparation of 5-alkoxy-2-pentanones, a suitable method has been developed which involves the use of α-acetyl-γ-butyrolactone as a starting material. The reaction equation is shown on the following page.

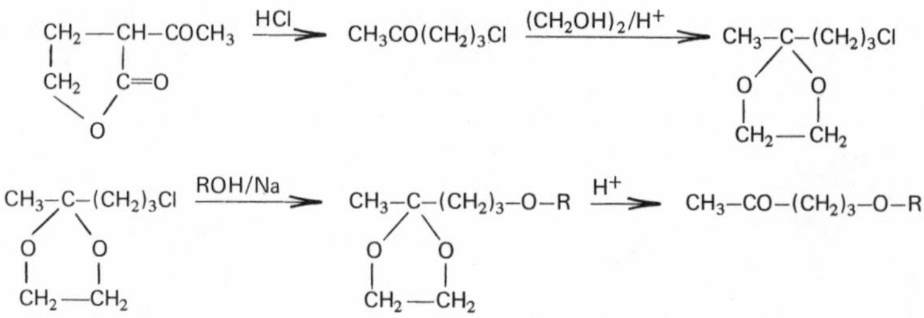

$$CH_2-CH-COCH_3 \xrightarrow{HCl} CH_3CO(CH_2)_3Cl \xrightarrow{(CH_2OH)_2/H^+} CH_3-\underset{\substack{O \quad O \\ | \quad | \\ CH_2-CH_2}}{C}-(CH_2)_3Cl$$

(where the first structure has CH_2 and $C=O$ joined through O forming the lactone ring)

$$CH_3-\underset{\substack{O \quad O \\ | \quad | \\ CH_2-CH_2}}{C}-(CH_2)_3Cl \xrightarrow{ROH/Na} CH_3-\underset{\substack{O \quad O \\ | \quad | \\ CH_2-CH_2}}{C}-(CH_2)_3-O-R \xrightarrow{H^+} CH_3-CO-(CH_2)_3-O-R$$

Example 1: 15.6 grams of 2,4-dimethylpentylallyl ether (0.1 mol), 1.5 grams of ditertiary-butyl peroxide (0.01 mol) and 13.2 grams of acetaldehyde (0.3 mol) were placed in a glass-lined pressure reactor and heated at 115° to 125°C for 24 hours. Excess pressure was vented and the contents of the reactor removed and distilled to yield 9.3 grams of 5-(2,4-dimethylpentoxy)-2-pentanone, BP 107° to 112°C/10 mm. This material retained its fragrance when subjected to Cl₂ and alkali for two weeks at 105°F. The scent characteristics are: odor, lavender, fruity, jasmine; intensity, strong; and retention, good.

Effect of Temperature — The following table shows the effect of temperature on the yield of 5-(2,4-dimethylpentoxy)-2-pentanone. Different catalysts were used in these experiments to obtain approximately equal half-lives at the temperatures employed.

Molar Ratios of Reactants

2,4-Dimethylpentylallyl Ether	Acetaldehyde	Catalyst	Temperature, °C	Time, hr	Yield, %
1	3	0.1*	60 – 70	24	0
1	3	0.1*	85 – 90	24	0
1	3	0.1**	85 – 95	24	0
1	3	0.1***	115 – 125	24	45
1	3	0.1***	125 – 135	24	36

*α,α'-Azodi-isobutyronitrile.
**Benzoyl peroxide.
***Ditertiarybutyl peroxide.

Effect of Glass-Lining in the Pressure Vessel — The following table shows a comparison of two runs carried out in a reactor with and without a glass lining, respectively.

Molar Ratios of Reactants

2,4-Dimethylpentylallyl Ether	Acetaldehyde	Ditertiarybutyl Peroxide	Temperature, °C	Time, hr	Lining	Yield, %
1	3	0.1	115 – 125	24	None	<5
1	3	0.1	115 – 125	24	Glass	45

Example 2: 5-Chloro-2-pentanone was prepared in 76% yield from α-acetyl-γ-butyrolactone and hydrochloric acid. 90.5 grams of this ketone (0.75 mol) and 62 grams of ethylene glycol (1 mol) were refluxed in 600 ml of benzene containing 1 gram of p-toluenesulfonic acid using a Dean-Stark trap to remove the water formed in the reaction. After 6 hours, the benzene solution was washed with sodium bicarbonate solution and water, and then distilled to yield 106.4 grams of 5-chloro-2-pentanone dioxolane as a colorless oil, BP 66° to 68°C/0.4 mm.

75 grams of the dioxolane (0.46 mol) was added to a solution of 10.6 grams (0.46 mol) of sodium in 296 grams (4 mols) of isobutyl alcohol and the mixture refluxed for 16 hours, 500 ml of water was added followed by enough concentrated hydrochloric acid to make the solution distinctly acid to litmus paper. The solution was then refluxed for 1 hour after which the product was isolated by ether extraction. Distillation gave 57.6 grams of 5-isobutoxy-2-pentanone, a colorless pleasant smelling oil, BP 94° to 95°C/0.2 mm.

This compound displayed a fragrance resembling rose and lavender. It is chemically stable in soap and detergent formulations and is well retained by such media. Its manner of use in perfumery is illustrated by the following formula:

Rose Lavender

	Parts by Weight
Lavandin oil	400
5-Isobutoxy-pentanone-2	400
Coumarin	80
Eugenol	40
Diphenyl ether	50
Patchouli oil	20
Musk ambrette	10
Total	1,000

This perfume mixture displayed an adequate fragrance level when used at 0.8 to 1.0%.

Ethers and Esters of Tetrahydrofuran and Tetrahydropyran

V. Lamberti and R.R. Winnegrad; U.S. Patent 3,668,134; June 6, 1972; assigned to Lever Brothers Company describe perfumery compounds for use in the detergent compositions which are the ethers and esters of tetrahydrofuran and tetrahydropyran having the structural formula:

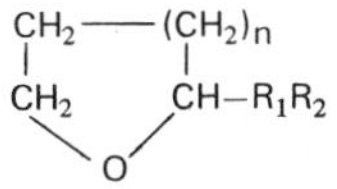

$$CH_2 \text{------} (CH_2)_n$$
$$CH_2 \qquad CH-R_1R_2$$
$$\diagdown O \diagup$$

where n is 1 or 2, R_1 is either —O— or CH_2O— and R_2 may be one of the following radicals:

(1) C_2 to C_{11} alkyl

(2) 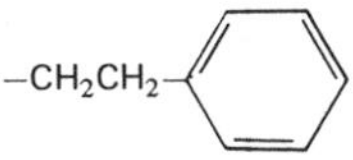 $-CH_2CH_2-$⟨benzene ring⟩

(3) 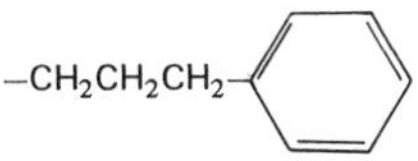 $-CH_2CH_2CH_2-$⟨benzene ring⟩

(4) 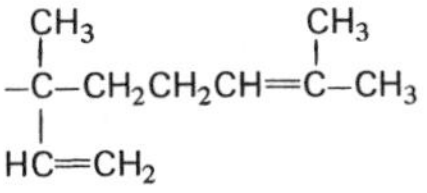
$$\begin{array}{cc} CH_3 & CH_3 \\ | & | \\ -C-CH_2CH_2CH=C-CH_3 \\ | \\ HC=CH_2 \end{array}$$

(5) 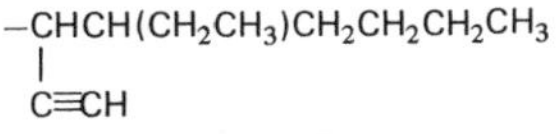
$$-CHCH(CH_2CH_3)CH_2CH_2CH_2CH_3$$
$$|$$
$$C\equiv CH$$

The alkali stability and chlorine stability of the perfumed detergent compositions of the process are illustrated by the following examples.

Example 1: Eight dishwasher products are provided with 0.1% by weight of each of the respective tetrahydropyran ethers R_1 = —O— having Formulas (1) (R_2 is hexyl), (2), (4), (5) above and tetrahydrofuran ethers R_1 = —O— (R_2 is hexyl), (2), (4), (5) above and the ingredients shown in the table on the following page.

Ingredients	Parts by Weight
Pentasodium tripolyphosphate*	44.00
Chlorinated trisodium phosphate*	9.60
N-silicate*	7.414
RU-silicate*	5.878
Nonionic detergent (Pluronic L62)	2.25
Nonionic detergent (Pluronic L61)	0.75
Colorants	0.004
Water	30.104
Total	100.00

*Expressed on dry basis.

After storage for 6 days at 95°F in both closed jars and commercial packages, these eight formulations lost none of their perfume odor.

Example 2: Eight liquid detergent formulations were perfumed with 0.1% by weight of each of the respective tetrahydropyran ethers $R_1 = -O-$ having Formulas (1) (R_2 is hexyl), (2), (4), (5) and tetrahydrofuran ethers R_1 is $-CH_2O-$ having Formulas (1) (R_2 is hexyl), (2), (4) and (5).

Ingredients	Parts by Weight
Potassium dodecylbenzene sulfonate	10
Sodium xylene sulfonate	8
Lauric/myristic diethanolamide	2.7
Lauric/myristic isopropanolamide	3.0
Potassium pyrophosphate	18.0
Sodium silicate	2.5
Sodium carboxymethylcellulose	0.15
Methylcellulose	0.57
Water	(to 100%)

The perfume odors of these eight formulations were unaffected after being stored in accordance with the procedure described in Example 1.

All the tetrahydropyran and tetrahydrofuran ethers and esters also passed the following soap bar stability test. The perfumery material is incorporated at the 1% level (or the 0.5% level if the odor is very intense as is the case for some of the acetylenic tetrahydropyran ethers) in an 80 to 20% tallow-coconut soap base. The perfumed soap chips are extruded and cut into minirectangular bars (about 45 grams each). The bars are enclosed in foil-laminated white cartons and aged at room temperature for 2 to 4 weeks. The bars are then rated for odor intensity, odor quality and any discoloration that may have taken place. Perfumery materials which satisfactorily cover the normal soapy base odor without causing significant discoloration of the bars are judged useful for incorporation in soap bar perfumes as well as in perfumes for use in alkaline detergent products.

2,4-Dialkyl-1,3-Dioxanes

A. Cahn and A.H. Gilbert; U.S. Patent 3,423,430; January 21, 1969 and U.S. Patent 3,326,746; June 20, 1967; both assigned to Lever Brothers Company have found that a synthetic perfume may be prepared which has a satisfactory geranium-rose note. Furthermore, this perfume may be advantageously employed in cleaning products including those products having chlorine-releasing agents. Such a perfume has the following generic structure:

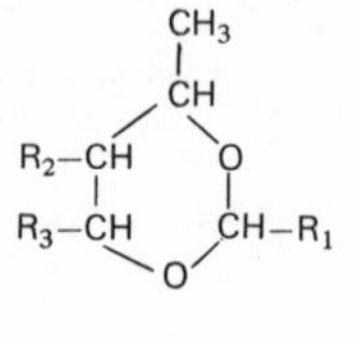

where R_1 is an alkyl group having 4 to 9 carbon atoms; R_2 is selected from the group consisting of hydrogen and a C_1 to C_4 alkyl group; and R_3 is selected from the group consisting of hydrogen and methyl.

The 2,4-dialkyl-1,3-dioxanes may be prepared in accordance with similar procedures known in the art for forming other 1,3-dioxanes. Generally about 1 to 1.5 equivalents of a 1,3-diol are reacted with about 1 equivalent of an aldehyde in the presence of, firstly, a solvent which azeotropes with water, e.g., chloroform, ethylene dichloride and benzene, and secondly, about 0.01 to 10% of an acid catalyst, e.g., sulfuric acid, hydrochloric acid, p-toluenesulfonic acid and an insoluble resin acid of the sulfonic acid type.

The temperature of the reaction is not critical but it is generally maintained between 40° and 150°C, preferably between 60° and 100°C; time varies inversely from 1 to 6 hours. Water is removed until the reaction is complete with subsequent cooling; neutralization with aqueous alkali, dry alkali, sodium carbonate or the like; washing; and distillation to provide the desired dioxane.

The 2,4-dialkyl-1,3-dioxanes having the geranium-rose note may be incorporated into a cleaning product, e.g., a dishwasher formulation, to overcome the strong odor resulting from the chlorine-releasing compounds. The other ingredients usually included in the cleaning products besides the dioxanes and chlorine-releasing agents are soaps or nonsoap detergents and phosphates.

Example: A dishwasher product was provided with 0.1% 2-isobutyl-4,5,6-trimethyl-1,3-dioxane and the ingredients shown below.

Ingredient	Parts
Sodium tripolyphosphate*	44.00
Chlorinated trisodium phosphate*	9.60
N-silicate*	7.414
RU-silicate*	5.878
Pluronic L62	2.25
Pluronic L61	0.75
Colorants	0.004
Water	30.104

*Expressed on dry basis.

After storage for six days at 95°F in both closed jars and commercial packages, this formulation lost none of its perfume odor.

α-Alkoxyisobutyrates

A.H. Gilbert and R.R. Winnegrad; U.S. Patent 3,368,943; February 13, 1968 have found that certain alkoxy-substituted isoalkanoates have perfumy properties and are suitable for use in cleaning products including products having chlorine-releasing agents. The compounds have the following generic structure:

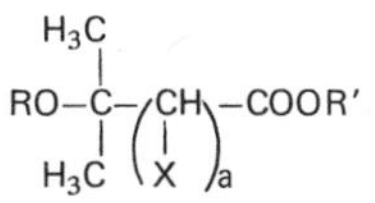

$$\underset{\underset{H_3C}{|}}{\overset{\overset{H_3C}{|}}{RO-C}}-\left(\underset{X}{\overset{CH}{|}}\right)_a-COOR'$$

where a is 0 or 1; X is chlorine or bromine; R is methyl or ethyl; and R' is a saturated C_4 to C_{12} aliphatic chain linear or branched, benzyl, phenylethyl or phenylpropyl. The compounds of the process, therefore, include α-alkoxyisobutyrates, i.e., when a is 0, and α-halo-β-alkoxyisovalerates, i.e., when a is 1. Preferred compounds are as follows: isobutyl α-methoxyisobutyrate; n-amyl α-methoxyisobutyrate; n-hexyl α-methoxyisobutyrate; phenylethyl α-methoxyisobutyrate; n-butyl α-ethoxyisobutyrate and n-amyl α-ethoxyisobutyrate.

Generally, the perfume is provided by reacting the appropriate α-alkoxyisobutyric acid or α-halo-β-alkoxyisovaleric acid with the appropriate alcohol under known conditions of esterification. An alternate method is the transesterification of an α-alkoxyisobutyrate or α-halo-β-alkoxyisovalerate with a suitable alcohol. The following examples illustrate the process. Unless otherwise indicated, all parts and percentages in the specification are based on weight.

Example 1: The compound, n-hexyl α-ethoxyisobutyrate, was prepared by adding chloroform (167.5 grams, 1.4 mol) dropwise over a 4 hour period to a cooled, stirred slurry of sodium hydroxide (233 grams, 5.8 mol), acetone (750 grams, 12.9 mol) and ethanol (46 grams, 1 mol). The mixture therefrom was refluxed for 2 hours and most of the acetone was removed subsequently by distillation. The residue was dissolved in hot water, filtered and evaporated to near dryness. The resulting residue was acidified with 25% sulfuric acid and ether extracted twice. The combined ether extracts were washed with brine, dried over anhydrous magnesium sulfate and distilled to form 34.2 grams (18.4%) α-ethoxyisobutyric acid (BP 90° to 112°C/18 mm).

The α-ethoxyisobutyric acid reactant was then esterified with excess n-hexanol by refluxing in xylene containing p-toluene-sulfonic acid. After distilling through the spinning band column, 29.7 grams (10%) pure n-hexyl α-ethoxyisobutyrate (BP 111° to 115°C/12 mm) was provided. The n-hexyl α-ethoxyisobutyrate was a perfume with a lavender-like note.

Example 2: The compound, n-hexyl α-chloro-β-methoxyisovalerate, was prepared by adding chlorine to a solution of methanol and dimethylacrylic acid at a temperature of 10°C. After 2.5 hours, the mixture was acidified with HCl and stirred overnight. The methanol was vacuum distilled until two layers appeared. The two layers were then ether extracted and the ethereal layer was washed with $KHCO_3$ solution.

The water layer was acidified with HCl and then concentrated under vacuum until the neutral salt began to appear. The aqueous layer was ether extracted, washed with salt solution, dried and concentrated to form α-chloro-β-methoxyisovaleric acid. The α-chloro-β-methoxyisovaleric acid reactant was esterified subsequently as described in Example 1. The resulting n-hexyl α-chloro-β-methoxyisovalerate was a perfume with a lavender-like note.

Example 3: Dry chlorinated bleaches in which the perfume odor during storage is not affected by the chlorine-releasing agents may be formed with the following ingredients therein.

| | - - - - - - - - - - - Parts - - - - - - - - - - - | | |
Ingredient	A	B	C
Isobutyl α-methoxyisobutyrate	0.10	–	–
Phenylethyl α-methoxyisobutyrate	–	0.10	–
n-Hexyl α-chloro-β-methoxyisovalerate	–	–	0.10
Sodium fatty alcohol sulfate	2.1	–	2.1
Potassium dichlorotriazinetrione	16.7	16.7	–
Sodium tripolyphosphate	36.2	36.2	36.2
Sodium silicate	0.4	0.4	0.4
Sodium sulfate	44.4	44.4	44.4
Sodium alkylbenzenesulfonate*	–	2.1	–
Halane**	–	–	16.7

    *Primarily a 1:1 mixture of alkylbenzene sulfonates in which the alkyl portion
        is a polypropylene group and has an average of 12 and 15 carbon atoms re-
        spectively.
    **Dichlorodimethylhydantoin.

Laundering Composition

According to a process described by *R.H. Blair; U.S. Patent 3,790,484; February 5, 1974* residual fragrance is imparted to laundered fabric articles by adding to such articles in course of laundering and during or at the inception of final rinse an aqueous composition comprising a fragrant oil, a cationic agent such as a dialkyl fatty quaternary ammonium halide, an organic amine base, and a nonionic detergent. A preferred cationic agent for inclusion in the composition is a dialkyldi(hydrogenated tallow) ammonium halide such as the dimethyldi(hydrogenated tallow) ammonium chloride available from Armour Chemical Corporation (Arquad 2HT-75). The quaternary ammonium halides exhibit an innate affinity for cellulosic fabrics and are believed to so condition the surface of the fabric as to transiently bind the fragrant oils thereto.

Preferably, from 8 to 12 parts by weight dialkyldi(hydrogenated tallow) ammonium chloride (75% active) is employed for from 2 to 4 parts by weight fragrant oil in 100 parts deionized water. Increased proportions of the fragrant oil, of course, call for additional increments of the cationic agent if fragrance retention through the drying cycle is to be maximized. In any case, the foregoing relative proportions have been found to serve admirably in imparting a useful, albeit not overpowering, degree of fragrance to laundered fabric when the preferred oils are employed, i.e., Alpine Aromatics, Inc., Jasmine 24-711, Orange Blossom 44-931, J.E. Type 42-431, Baby Powder 5606 and Ginger Spice 62-701.

Also employed in the fragrance-imparting composition is an organic amine base, preferably a tertiary amine base such as polyoxyethylene cocoamine available from Armour Chemical Corporation (Ethomeen C-25). The base is used in proportion sufficient to provide pH between 5 and 8, preferably from pH 6 to 7. In the case of the composition proportioned above, about 2.5 parts by weight polyoxyethylene cocoamine is preferably employed.

Finally, the composition desirably contains a substantial proportion of nonionic detergent, e.g., alkylphenoxy polyethoxyethanol (Rohm & Haas' Triton X-100), sufficient in amount as to solubilize the fragrant oil in the composition. Where the foregoing fragrances are employed in the proportions referred to above, about 25 to 50 parts by weight nonionic detergent may be employed, about 25 parts being the preferred proportion.

Sanitizing Concentrate with Lemon-Lime Fragrance

R.P. Wooden and W.G. Page; U.S. Patent 3,733,277; May 15, 1973; assigned to The Pillsbury Company have found that a subliminal quantity of a lemon-lime fragrance can be employed effectively without degradation in a liquid, low pH, sanitizing and cleaning solution containing quaternary ammonium halides to produce a fresh, clean fragrance sensation without producing an awareness of the specific lemon-lime odor. A cleaning and sanitizing concentrate is disclosed consisting essentially of (a) phosphoric or hydroxyacetic acid, (b) a nonionic synthetic detergent, (c) a quaternary ammonium halide, (d) water, and (e) lemon-lime fragrance.

Example: A cleaning and sanitizing concentrate was prepared from 40 parts phosphoric acid, 20 parts of a mixture of quaternary ammonium chlorides comprising 50% n-alkyl (60% C_{14}, 30% C_{16}, 5% C_{12}, 5% C_{18}) dimethylbenzyl ammonium chloride and 50 n-alkyl (50% C_{12}, 30% C_{14}, 17% C_{16}, 3% C_{18}) dimethylethylbenzyl ammonium chloride, 10 parts octyl phenoxy polyethoxy ethanol and 29.7 parts water. The concentrate was divided into 9 aliquots and to each aliquot was added 0.033 part of the fragrances listed below (0.033 parts fragrance divided by 2.22 parts quaternary equals 1.5 parts fragrance per 100 parts quaternary):

>   Aliquot 1 Fritzsche D&O Inc. No. 42149 (Lemon-Lime)
>   Aliquot 2 Fritzsche D&O Inc. No. 41994 (Pine)
>   Aliquot 3 Fritzsche D&O Inc. No. 42249 (Pine)
>   Aliquot 4 Fritzsche D&O Inc. No. 47314 (Woody Amber)
>   Aliquot 5 Fritzsche D&O Inc. No. 41985 (Musk)
>   Aliquot 6 Fritzsche D&O Inc. No. 54566 (Woody Amber)
>   Aliquot 7 Fritzsche D&O Inc. No. 43798 (Musk)
>   Aliquot 8 Fritzsche D&O Inc. No. 49745 (Orange)
>   Aliquot 9 Fritzsche D&O Inc. No. 42193 (Orange)

Bathroom testing was simulated by diluting each concentrate with 250 parts water per part of concentrate. One milliliter of the diluted concentrate was placed in a 500 ml jar. After about 15 minutes, fragrance experts odor tested these fragrances and found no degradation in the fragrance of aliquots 1, 8 and 9 and significant degradation in aliquots 2 through 7. After 12 hours, the fragrance of aliquots 2 through 7 and 9 had significantly degraded and were not desirable odors for this product. Concentrate 8 had a sweet, heavy orange odor which was unpleasant in the context of a bathroom.

The lemon-lime fragrance in aliquot 1 above did not degrade over a 30-day period. When used in the manner described above, a clean, fresh odor sensation was recognizable with no noticeable lemon-lime fragrance. This product, diluted as stated above, was used to clean a bathroom and left a clean, fresh odor sensation in the bathroom with no noticeable lemon-lime fragrance.

ODOR PROLONGATION

Trimethylnorbornyl-Alkylcyclohexanones

According to a process described by *H.C. Saunders; U.S. Patent 3,317,397; May 2, 1967; assigned to Universal Oil Products Company* the odor of perfumed materials is prolonged by incorporating into such materials a cyclohexanone compound of the following formula:

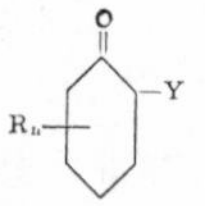

where n is an integer of from 0 to 2, Y is an alkyl group and R is a member selected from the group consisting of alkyl, cycloalkyl, aryl and a trimethylnorbornyl radical of the formula:

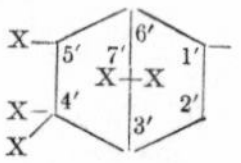

where X is selected from the group consisting of hydrogen and methyl radicals, provided at least three X's are methyl. Examples of the compounds which may be used either individually or as a mixture, according to this process, to prolong the odor of perfumed materials, and having the above general formula, include:

> 2-Dodecylcyclohexanone
> 2,6-Didodecylcyclohexanone
> 2-Cyclopentyl-6-methylcyclohexanone
> 2-(6',7',7'-trimethylnorborn-1'-yl)-6-methylcyclohexanone
> 2-(4',4',5',6'-tetramethylnorborn-1'-yl)-6-ethylcyclohexanone
> 2-(4',4',5'-trimethylnorborn-1'-yl)-6-ethylcyclohexanone, and
> 4-(4',4',5'-trimethylnorborn-1'-yl)-6-methylcyclohexanone

Example 1: A stabilizing compound was prepared for use according to the method to prolong the odor of perfumed material as follows. About 1,300 grams (12 mols) of orthocresol, about 560 grams of heptane and about 865 grams of polyphosphoric acid were added with mixing to a reaction flask over a period of about 15 minutes with the temperature maintained by cooling at 25° to 30°C. Then about 681 grams (5 mols) of camphene mixed with about 190 grams of heptane were added to the flask. After mixing for about 7 hours at a temperature maintained at about 25° to 30°C, the mixing was stopped and the mixture allowed to stand until it separated into organic and inorganic layers. The inorganic layer was extracted with about 500 grams of heptane and the heptane extract combined with the organic layer and the combined organic mixture was then washed with about a liter of water. Sodium carbonate was added to neutralize any remaining acid and the organic mixture thereafter dried by azeotropic distillation. The remaining mixture was then fractionated to recover about 953 grams of trimethylnorbornyl substituted ortho-cresol boiling at 168°C at about 1 mm Hg and having a refractive index of N_D^{20} 1.5465.

About 871 grams of this product were then changed to an autoclave containing about 87 grams of a nickel catalyst. The product was then hydrogenated at about 160°C and 600 pounds per square inch hydrogen pressure for about 4 hours. The hydrogenation product was removed and washed with isopropanol. After flashing off the isopropanol, the hydrogenation product was fractionally distilled to recover about 775 grams of trimethylnorbornyl substituted 2-methylcyclohexanol boiling at about 125° to 138°C and having a refractive index of N_D^{20} 1.4975 to 1.5072. About 670 grams of this product were then changed to a reaction flask containing about 1,820 grams of water.

With mixing, the mixture was heated to about 60°C and then over a period of about one-half hour were added about 570 grams of a 70 weight percent aqueous sodium dichromate solution and about 1,050 grams of a 50% sulfuric acid solution. The temperature of the exothermic reaction was maintained at about 60°C for about 1 hour and then the mixing was stopped and the mixture allowed to stand.

The resulting aqueous layer was separated, extracted with heptane and the heptane extract combined with the organic layer which was then neutralized with carbonate. After removal of the heptane, the remaining mixture was subjected to fractional distillation to recover about 414 grams of trimethylnorbornyl substituted 2-methylcyclohexanone boiling at about 136°C at 1 to 2 mm Hg pressure and having a refractive index of N_D^{20} 1.4980 to 1.5000.

Example 2: The following test was conducted to demonstrate the odor prolongation of perfumed materials. The following perfumes were prepared:

Perfume A—Rose

Component	Parts by Weight
Citronellol	45
Citronellyl acetate	6
Benzophenone	5
Nerol	10
Linalool	5
Hydroxy citronellal	10
Phenylethyl alcohol	3
Phenylethyl dimethyl acrylate	3
Oil bois de rose	8
Isoeugenol	½
Oil caraway	½
Aldehyde C-9, 10% alc	½
Isomenthol	1½
	98

Perfume B—Lavender

Component	Parts by Weight
Camphene 97%	3
Alpha-pinene	1
Linalool oxide	½
Ethyl amyl ketone	1
Alcohol C-6	½
Amyl alcohol	½
Methylheptenone	½

(continued)

Component	Parts by Weight
Isoborneol	2
Alpha-terpineol	3
Nerol	3
Linalool	40
Eucalyptol	½
Isobornyl acetate	2
Coumarin	½
Terpinyl acetate	2
Terpinyl isobutyrate	½
Dimethylacrylic acid	½
Vinyloctahydromethanoindinyl acetate	35
Ocimene	3
Oil lemon California	½
Oil clove	½
	100

Perfume C—Rose Geranium

Component	Parts by Weight
Isomenthone	6
Citronellyl formate	7
Geranyl formate	3
Citronellol	40
Geraniol	5
Linalool synthetic	3
Rose crystals	½
Benzophenone	3
Guaiacwood acetate	½
Isobornyl formate	1
Isoeugenol	½
Alpha-terpeniol	2
Isomenthol	1
Phenylethyl alcohol	5
Styralyl acetate	½
Isoamyl formate	½
Phenylethyl dimethyl acrylate	1
Ethyl salicylate	1
Methyl hexyl ketone	½
Oil cedarwood	5
Phenylacetaldehyde dimethyl acetal	6
	92

Perfume D—Eau de Cologne

Component	Parts by Weight
Oil petitgrain	10
Oil bergamot	6
Linalyl acetate	20
Terpinyl acetate	25
Oil mandarin	1
Oil marjoram	1
Cedryl acetate	8
Cinnamyl alcohol	11
Isobornyl formate	5
Citronellol	5
Coumarin	½
Oil lavandin	½

(continued)

Component	Parts by Weight
Benzoin 50% diethylphthalate	1
Yara-yara	½
Heptyl formate	½
Oil limes distilled	3½
Phenylpropyl alcohol	1½
	100

Each of the above perfumes, A, B, C and D, was divided into two parts and to one part was added a two weight percent proportion of a stabilizing compound comprising a trimethylnorbornyl substituent 2-methylcyclohexanone boiling from 119° to 124°C at 0.5 mm Hg and having a refractive index of N_D^{20} 1.4983 to 1.5003.

Soap cakes were prepared by first mixing about 50 grams of standard toilet soap pellets and about 0.5 gram of perfume. This mixture was then milled and finally plodded by extrusion until it became a plastic mass. The soap mass was then placed in a die and pressed into a cake. Two groups of soap cakes were prepared for each of the above perfumes. The first group contained the perfume without the stabilizing compound and the second group contained the perfume to which the stabilizing compound had been added.

The odors of the stabilized and unstabilized cakes were identical as prepared. The cakes were then exposed to daylight and air indoors over a period of about one month and were examined twice weekly for odor changes. It was observed that the odors of the unstabilized cakes began to fade rapidly and, in all cases, disappeared completely in from 1 to 2 weeks time. The odors of the stabilized soap cakes, however, even at the end of the test, were still very strong and unaltered as compared to their original odors.

Retention of Fragrance Using Chelate Coated Talc

L.L. Augsburger and J.R. Marvel; U.S. Patent 3,801,709; April 2, 1974; assigned to Johnson & Johnson have found that when chelating agents are addded to powdered substrates in an aqueous environment and the treated substrates are dried in situ, long-term fragrance stabilization is accomplished. Finely divided, solid materials such as talc can be suitably treated with an aqueous medium, containing small quantities of a chelating agent, in order to prevent the active components in the solid materials from causing degradation of odor imparting materials.

In general, the aqueous solution of chelating agent is applied to the finely divided solid materials by wetting the divided materials in any convenient conventional manner, such as by forming a slurry of the solid materials in a solution containing chelating agent, filtering and drying the resultant filter cake. It is also possible to apply the chelating agent by any other means resulting in the wetting of the powder, i.e., spraying the powder in a fluid bed process with a solution containing small amounts of chelating agent.

The resulting finely divided material, i.e., talc will usually contain from 0.05 to 3, preferably 0.1 to 2 and most preferably 0.1 to 1 weight percent chelating agent dispersed on the outer surfaces of each particle. It is important that the chelating agent be dried on the product since this step apparently provides a means to deactivate the active metal sites in the crystal lattice. This eliminates the possibility of their reaction with the perfume. The following examples illustrate the process.

Example 1: A finely-divided talc containing approximately 2.5% iron was acid treated in order to extract metals present therein: a solution of 236 ml of concentrated HCl was mixed with 764 ml of distilled water and added to 500 grams of the talc. After about 15 minutes of mixing, the slurry was kept at 50°C for 1 hour and a half on a steam bath.

The slurry was filtered and washed under vacuum until neutral. Approximately 700 ml of the first filtrate was saved for further analysis. The filtered talc was dried at 90°C in a forced draft oven for 21.5 hours. Analytical tests run on the filtrate showed the following concentrations of metals in miligram/milliliter of solution: Fe 0.462, Ni 0.048, Cu 0.00061. The resultant talc was washed free of acid, dried, and 0.2% by weight of perfume was added. The powder was thoroughly mixed in a V blender. Organoleptic evaluation indicated the same possessed a very chalky odor after aging for 4 weeks at 120°F. Thus, it is plain that extraction with acid to remove metal was not successful indicating some metal ions are very tightly bound. Analysis showed a considerable amount of metal remained in the talc.

Example 2: A portion of the untreated talc of Example 1 was treated with a warm aqueous solution of EDTA (ethylenediaminetetraacetate, tetrasodium salt) as follows. 40 grams of EDTA was mixed with 400 ml of distilled water. The mixture was stirred with a stirring rod until the EDTA had dissolved. The solution was added to the talc, which was then slurried to a paste. The resultant slurry was heated to 180°F and held there for an hour, after which it was filtered through a Buchner filter funnel and the original liquid was saved for metal analysis.

The remaining talc in the filter funnel was then washed thoroughly with distilled water and dried at 70°C. The first filtrate which was analyzed contained 0.318 mg/ml of Fe and 0.0033 mg/ml of Ni. 0.2% perfume was added to the dried powder. By organoleptic testing methods, the sample had a chalky odor after aging according to 75% of the panel members. From the above samples it is seen that the metals in the talc are tenaciously held in the crystal lattice and cannot be washed out with acids and therefore improved talc products insofar as fragrance stability is concerned cannot be made with these chemically obvious treatments.

Example 3: A series of five samples were prepared from the untreated talc (which contained approximately 2.5% total naturally present iron and nickel) of Example 1.

    (A) Untreated talc.
    (B) 0.5% Na$_2$ EDTA was added dry to talc of A.
    (C) 1.0% Na$_2$ EDTA was added dry to talc of A.
    (D) 0.5% Na$_4$ EDTA was added dry to talc of A.
    (E) 1.0% Na$_4$ EDTA was added dry to talc of A.

Each sample was mixed with 0.2% perfume and aged at 120°F. Organoleptic evaluation of the samples showed the following results given as percent of panel members sensing the characteristic undesired chalky odor. Dry addition of the chelating agents leaves the particle surfaces of talc intact causing no change in activities of the metal present thereon.

However, when talc samples are treated with chelating agent, the resulting powders are quite satisfactory. In each of the examples (F) through (I), the specified chelating agent is added at the indicated percentage by the following procedure. A solution containing the calculated amount of chelate to be deposited on 5,000 grams of talc is dissolved in 250 ml of water. The solution was sprayed onto the talc with mixing so that the solution uniformly coats the talc. The wet mixture was dried overnight in an oven at 60°C.

    (F) 0.5% of Na$_4$ EDTA is coated onto 99.3% of talc according to the procedure above, then 0.2% of perfume for 4, 8 and 12 weeks and subjected to organoleptic evaluation which showed respectively 5, 30 and 5% of response for chalkiness.

    (G) 1.0% of Na$_4$ EDTA was coated onto 98.8% of talc according to the procedure above, then 0.2% of perfume was mixed therewith. The sample was aged at 120°F for 4, 8 and 12 weeks and subjected to organoleptic evaluation. The results respectively were 20, 25 and 10% response for chalkiness.

    (H) 0.5% of Na$_2$ EDTA was coated onto 99.3% of talc according to the procedure above, then 0.2% of perfume was mixed therewith. The sample was aged at 120°F for 4, 8 and 12 weeks and subjected to organoleptic evaluation. The response for chalkiness were 30, 35 and 35 respectively.

(I) 1.0% Na₂ of EDTA was coated onto 98.8% of talc according to the proceduce above, then 0.2% of perfume was mixed therewith. The sample was aged at 120°F for 4, 8 and 12 weeks and subjected to organoleptic evaluation. Results were respectively 30, 35 and 15% chalkiness. The results obtained from Samples (A) through (I) are summarized below in the table. The use of chelates decreases the chalkiness odor.

Sample	4 Weeks	8 Weeks	12 Weeks	Average Response
A (control)	60	45	60	55
B	45	60	60	55
C	45	55	35	45
D	75	80	85	80
E	85	95	75	85
F	5	30	5	13
G	20	25	10	18
H	30	35	35	33
I	30	35	15	27

Perfume Adsorbed on Metallic Particles

D.E. Cashman and H.E. Remler; U.S. Patent 3,449,266; June 10, 1969; assigned to The Drackett Company describe a method for packaging a product scented with perfume in a polyethylene container to prolong the odor life of the perfume which otherwise is completely exhausted in a few days due to its migration through the walls of the polyethylene container. To accomplish this the perfume is adsorbed on metallic particles having a high internal pore volume and a large surface area which are contained in the package.

Specific examples of carrier materials are the synthetic or semisynthetic petroleum cracking catalysts of high surface area and high pore volume. Illustrative materials of the above type include mixtures of alumina and silica, in substantially any ratio. Other catalytic materials can be employed. Specific materials found particularly advantageous are (1) a microspheroidal material comprising about 13% alumina, 86.8% silica with the remaining 0.2% comprising salts and traces of heavy metals as impurities; (2) a silica gel having a pore volume of 1.10 ml/g and a surface area of 750 to 850 m²/g; (3) a gelled alumina having a pore volume of 0.20 ml/g and a high surface area; and (4) synthetic zeolites, often referred to as molecular sieves, described in U.S. Patents 2,818,137 and 2,818,455, which are highly porous alkali metal alumina silicates having pores of molecular dimensions and uniform size.

Example: A microspheroidal catalytic material composed of 13% alumina, 86.8% silica, and the remaining 0.2% being salts and heavy mineral impurities, having a pore volume of 0.88 ml/g and a surface area of 500 m²/g, was mixed with methyl salicylate in a ribbon mixer at a ratio of 1.0 part catalyst to 0.9 part perfume. During mixing, there was a heat rise of 20° to 25°F for a 10,000 gram or 22 lb mix. The resultant stabilized perfume was dry and free-flowing.

1.2 parts of the stabilized perfume was added to 100 parts of toilet bowl cleaner composed of 75% sodium bisulfate, 11% sodium carbonate, 11% sodium chloride, and 3% inert materials. The total granular composition was poured into a polyethylene container having a wall thickness of 0.030 to 0.045 inch and the container sealed. The product retained its pleasant scent for more than 30 days in an accelerated test, where the package was placed in an air-circulating oven at 125°F; equivalent to approximately 6 months of normal shelf life. An identical product merely scented with an equivalent amount of liquid perfume showed no trace of the perfume odor after only 3 days under the same test conditions.

Encapsulation Using Dextrinized Starch Acid-Esters

N.G. Marotta, R.M. Boettger, B.H. Nappen and C.D. Szymanski; U.S. Patent 3,455;838;

July 15, 1969; assigned to National Starch and Chemical Corporation describe a method for encapsulating water-insoluble substances which comprises the spray drying of an aqueous dispersion of a dextrinized starch acid-ester of a substituted dicarboxylic acid in which the water-insoluble substance has been emulsified. The resulting encapsulated particles are useful in a variety of applications, such, for example, as in the preparation of foods, pharmaceuticals and cosmetics.

It has been found that the use of a particular type of dextrin as an encapsulating agent provides spray dried products which are free from the characteristic color, aroma, and taste which have previously been associated with the use of ordinary dextrins. Moreover, the encapsulating dextrins have, surprisingly, been found to be superior in their encapsulating ability to these conventional dextrins as well as to various other encapsulating colloids such as gum arabic and gelatin. This superior encapsulating ability is believed to result from the finer particle size of the emulsions which are prepared from the encapsulating dextrins; this factor, in turn, resulting in spray dried products which exhibit a volatile oil loss substantially lower than that which is noted in the case of spray dried products made with ordinary dextrins and other encapsulating colloids.

The encapsulating agents comprise dextrins derived from ungelatinized starch acid-esters of substituted dicarboxylic acids. Such starch acid-esters may be represented diagrammatically by the following formula:

$$\text{starch-O-O-C-}\overset{\displaystyle R_1}{\underset{\displaystyle |}{R}}\text{-COOH}$$

where R is a radical selected from the class consisting of R_1-substituted dimethylene and R_1-substituted trimethylene radicals, and R_1 is a hydrocarbon constituent selected from the class consisting of alkyl, alkenyl, aralkyl, or aralkenyl groups. These ungelatinized starch acid-esters are prepared by reacting an ungelatinized starch, in an alkaline medium, with a substituted cyclic dicarboxylic acid anhydride having the following formula:

$$\begin{array}{c} \text{O} \\ \| \\ \text{C} \\ \diagup \quad \diagdown \\ \text{O} \qquad \text{R-R}_1 \\ \diagdown \quad \diagup \\ \text{C} \\ \| \\ \text{O} \end{array}$$

where R and R_1 represent the same substituent groups referred to above for these symbols. Substituted cyclic dicarboxylic anhydrides falling within this formula are the substituted succinic and glutaric acid anhydrides. Further details for the preparation of these starch derivatives may be found in U.S. Patent 2,661,349.

In using these acid-ester dextrins as encapsulating agents for the entrapment of volatile oils and other water-insoluble substances, it is first necessary to disperse or dissolve them in water; the resulting solution having a pH level preferably in the range of from 2 to 8. This is usually accomplished by adding the acid-ester dextrin, under agitation, to water which has previously been heated to a temperature of from 100° to 210°F. After solution of the dextrin is complete, the water-insoluble substance which is to be entrapped (e.g., oil, perfume or the like) is slowly added and the mixture is rapidly agitated until such time as emulsification is complete.

The resulting emulsion may then be dried by any suitable means, preferably by spray drying, although as noted earlier, drying may also be effected by passage of the emulsion over heated drums, by spreading it on belts which are then passed through a heating tunnel or by freeze-drying. The preferred spray drying technique may be accomplished using any commercially available spray drying equipment capable of providing an inlet temperature in the range of approximately 212° to 520°F.

Encapsulation

L.L. Balassa; U.S. Patent 3,495,988; February 17, 1970 describes the encapsulation and stabilization of a variety of organic chemical substances. The process comprises dispersing the material to be encapsulated in an aqueous hydrophilic colloid solution to form an emulsion, adding the colloid solution to a spinning liquid which under the process conditions forms a slurry with the emulsion and thereafter dehydrating the resulting slurry to form stabilized capsules which protect the encapsulated material against changes in its chemical and physical properties upon storage and exposure to oxygen. Included among the class of materials that may be encapsulated are aromas, flavors, vitamins, aroma bearing materials, flavor bearing materials, etc.

Water-Soluble Acrylate Polymers as Entrapping Agents

According to a process described by *F.E. Gould and T.H. Shepherd; U.S. Patent 3,772,215; November 13, 1973, U.S. Patent 3,681,248; August 1, 1972 and U.S. Patent 3,567,118; March 2, 1971; all assigned to National Patent Development Corporation* fragrant materials are entrapped in water-soluble hydroxyalkyl acrylate or methacrylate polymers to provide ready sources of the material by the deletion of water.

Thus there are employed copolymers of hydroxyethyl acrylate, hydroxypropyl acrylate, hydroxyethyl methacrylate or hydroxypropyl methacrylate with 0.5 to 20% of a water-solubilizing copolymerizable monomer. The copolymerizable monomer should be present in amount sufficient to be sure that the polymer is completely soluble in water. The following examples illustrate the process.

Example 1: Into a 30-gallon reactor was charged 40 lb of hydroxyethyl methacrylate, 4 lb of methacrylic acid, 120 lb of methanol and 0.05 lb of t-butyl peroctoate. The reactor was heated to 80°C and allowed to stir 6 hr to effect polymerization. To the polymer solution thus obtained was added 2.5 lb of sodium methoxide dissolved in 25 lb of methanol. The resulting solution was added slowly to a 10-fold excess of acetone to precipitate the polymer. After drying, a yield of 36 lb of water-soluble polymer was obtained.

Example 2: The polymer of Example 1 was dissolved in methanol to provide a 10 weight percent solution. To the solution was added orange oil at a level of 20% of the polymer content of the solution. The solution was then cast as a 20 mil film (wet) on a polyethylene sheet and dried. The resulting brittle film was ground to –60 mesh to yield a powder which exhibited only a slight odor of orange oil, but which released orange oil readily on contact with water.

Example 3: The orange oil-containing powder of Example 2 was blended with a commercial detergent (sodium dodecylbenzene sulfonate) at a level of 5% of the detergent. When the detergent was added to hot water, the orange oil odor was immediately apparent.

Example 4: Example 2 was repeated using citral in place of orange oil. A detergent composition prepared with citral-containing polymer in accordance with Example 3, immediately gave off a citrus-like odor when added to hot water.

Example 5: The citral-containing polymer of Example 4 (without detergents) was pulverized to –325 mesh in a hammermill. The micropulverized powder was milled with a saponified coconut oil soap base at a level of 1 lb of powder to 9 lb of the soap. The soap was extruded and stamped into cakes. On use of the soap cake for hand washing, the citral odor was evident on the hands. This effect persisted through the life of the soap cake.

In U.S. Patent 3,567,118 composite fiber materials which are adapted for odorizing, deodorizing, sanitizing and cleansing purposes by treating the fibrous material with a coating of a hydrophilic acrylate or methacrylate containing an appropriate essence, bactericide, cleansing agent or the like are described. Both natural and synthetic fibers can be treated with a solution of the hydrophilic polymer. Entrapment of the chemical agent can be prolonged by using a copolymer of the hydrophilic monomer with a minor amount of a hydrophobic monomer.

Diffusion of Odor Vapor from Polymers

G. Wilbert and T. Brown; U.S. Patent 3,567,119; March 2, 1971 describe improved methods for the incorporating of fragrance compounds or oil bouquets and/or topical antifungal or antibacterial agents, insect repellent compounds and certain odoriferous medicaments into polymeric or natural materials so that the fabricated product possesses the properties imparted by the additive or additives for a long period of time. The efficiency of incorporating these additives in the materials mentioned above is improved by the use of surfactants and the effectiveness and duration of the additive or additives in the fabricated product is enhanced by employing antioxidants and/or ultraviolet radiation absorbers.

The incorporation of a small quantity of additive into polymer, copolymer or polymer coated natural materials such as a quaternary ammonium compound, not only functions as a surfactant but also imparts to the surface of the manufactured product aseptic properties or establishes conditions for reducing the number of microbial organisms, some of which can be pathogenic. The following example illustrates the process.

Example: To 6.7 grams rose perfume oil was added 0.3 gram of an anionic surfactant. These two components were mixed and then thoroughly blended with 215.7 grams of intermediate density polyethylene beads and 11.35 grams of a red color concentrate. The entire mixture was then charged, in two portions, to the hopper of a Van Dorn Plastic Molder. With the average cylinder temperature of the molder, both front and rear, at about 300°F and a molding pressure of 450 to 500 psi, the material was processed in 16 minutes to give 24 retained molded pieces of irregular shape and thickness weighing about 8 grams each, run A. The initial molded pieces that were processed were discarded to insure that the machine's cylinder, piston and mold were adequately purged.

After processing it was readily apparent that no significant quantity of perfume oil had drained off the polyethylene beads since the oil was not observed at the bottom of the hopper adjacent to the retracted piston. A similar control, run B, without the addition of the surfactant showed distinct evidence of a portion of the perfume oil at the bottom of the hopper after processing. The same number of pieces weighing 5.0 grams were cut from similar parts of the molded objects from runs A and B, respectively, and placed in two 250-ml beakers marked A and B. These two beakers containing the pieces were retained for olfactory testing.

Panel olfactory testing by six individuals demonstrated that initially the odor from run A was significantly stronger than run B. After 8 weeks olfactory testing showed that the rose perfume oil odor was distinctly detectable from both run A and run B. However, run A had the more readily detectable and more pronounced odor.

Impregnated Plastic Article

W.H. Engel; U.S. Patent 3,688,985; September 5, 1972 describes a preformed synthetic resin which is dry to the touch containing a volatile matter which is gradually yielded in a chemically unchanged and dry state to the surrounding atmosphere over a considerable period of time.

The process involves forming a stable aqueous emulsion of a preferred essential oil with the help of a surfactant. Preferably the emulsion is contained within a closed vessel and a supply of a preformed synthetic resin in the form of a thin sheet, web, fiber or the like, is brought into intimate contact with the emulsion. The preformed synthetic resin is maintained in intimate contact with the emulsion for a predetermined period of time. It has been discovered that once the synthetic resin has become saturated it can be maintained in contact with the emulsion for an indefinite period of time without disintegrating. During the period of intimate contact between the preformed resin article and the emulsion, the temperature of the emulsion is maintained at a temperature below the boiling point thereof, and preferably at ambient temperatures and pressures.

Upon removing the impregnated resin from contact with the emulsion upon the lapse of a predetermined period the resin article is dried so that it feels dry to the touch. The dried preformed resin article is thus impregnated with volatile matter which will gradually be released or yielded to the surrounding atmosphere in a chemically unchanged, dry state over a considerable period of time.

Extrudable Polyvinyl Chloride Compositions

L.M. Grubb; U.S. Patent 3,725,311; April 3, 1973; assigned to Thuron Industries, Inc. describes an extrudable composition and the process of producing it comprising a polymer of 80 to 98% PVC, 2 to 20% PVAc, and 0 to 20% PVA, a plasticizer, a filler to maintain a dry mixture and a volatile odor-neutralizing or modifying agent, the composition being extrudable at a temperature of below 250°F in order to avoid loss of the volatile odor-neutralizing agent through degradation or evaporation. The following examples illustrate the process.

Example 1:

Union Carbide VAGH (copolymer of PVC, PVA, and PV acetate)	51.0%
Mineral oil (Nujoy)	0.3%
Diatomaceous earth	19.0%
Perfume (mint)	21.0%
Santicizer 213 (phthalate plasticizer blend)	8.7%

Material is mixed at 125°F in a Henschel mixer and extruded at temperatures between 100° and 150°F. The extrudate is cut into bars 2¼" x 10" x ¼" and weighing 110 grams.

Example 2:

Firestone resin 4301 (copolymer of PVC, and PV acetate)	46.95%
Diatomaceous earth	17.80%
Perfume (lemon oil)	27.00%
Mineral oil (Nujoy)	0.10%
Dyes and pigments	3.15%
Santicizer 213 (phthalate plasticizer blend)	5.00%

Mixed, extruded, as in Example 1, bars cut to 65 grams.

Example 3:

Firestone resin 4301 (copolymer of PVC, and PV acetate)	46.45%
Diatomaceous earth	19.00%
Perfume (floral)	20.00%
Mineral oil (Nujoy)	0.30%
Santicizer 213 (phthalate plasticizer blend)	13.00%
Dyes and pigments	3.15%

The products of the examples were tested and were found to continuously release the volatile perfume for a period greater than 30 days into the atmosphere where it overcame and neutralized any unpleasant odors that would arise in the environment of the composition. Bars of such composition may therefore be utilized by having a single bar of the approximate size of Example 1, and placed in a home-size room or office will be found to give continuous odor neutralization for a period in excess of 30 days and up to 3 months.

Polyolefin Composition

According to a process described by *B.L. Gaeckel; U.S. Patent 3,553,296; January 5, 1971* a polyolefin composition having improved odor retaining properties is prepared by blending polyethylene particles of a size of from 150 to 350 mesh with an odoriferous oil and then mixing the blend with the polyolefin in an amount of from 0.2 to 2.0% by weight.

Scented polyolefin such as low density polyethylene containing a perfume has become increasingly useful in recent years as applications are found for polyolefins as replacement for other materials. For example low density polyethylene is used to a great extent in the manufacture of artificial flowers. Such flowers were previously made of paper but polyethylene flowers are usually more life-like, have greater color retention and have a longer life span. It is desirable that a perfume imitative of the odor of the natural flower be manufactured into the polyethylene flower so that the odor could be retained over prolonged periods. The following example illustrates the process.

Example: The ease of incorporating five different perfumes in high density polyethylene powders of different particle size distributions was determined. The five perfumes which were used comprised the following essential oils in a volatile solvent containing a perfume-fixative: (1) oil of lilac, (2) oil of honeysuckle, (3) attar of roses, (4) oil of pepperpink, and (5) oil of carnation.

The perfumes which were used are those commercially available from Descollonges Inc., known as: (1) Lilas, (2) Honeysuckle Florafix, (3) Rose Cramoisie PY15, (4) Oeillet Poivre, PY15, and (5) Carnation Florafix. These perfumes were mixed with a high density grade of polyethylene powder (density 0.9600 g/cc) in a tumble blender using steel balls to prevent the formation of lumps during the blending.

The resulting blends were then mixed in a 1% by weight concentration in polyethylene of density 0.9200 g/cc. The blending characteristics of various concentrations of the perfume in percent by weight in the high density polyethylene are shown in Tables 1 through 3 for different polyethylene particle sizes. These blending characteristics are given in terms based on the subjective evaluation of the applicant.

Good in terms of mixing and adsorption was given to mixes having even dispersion in polyethylene which is substantially free of lumps. Good in terms of pourability was given to mixes having a substantially constant viscosity. The column showing the degree of detection of perfume over a given storage period is based on a composition consisting of a mixture of 1% by weight of the corresponding perfume blend in low density polyethylene (density = 0.9200 g/cc).

Table 1 describes the perfume blended with high density polyethylene (density = 0.9600 grams per cubic centimeter) particles that are substantially completely retained by a 20 mesh sieve.

TABLE 1

Perfume Concentration in Percent by Weight of Polyethylene	Mixing	Pourability	Absorption of Perfume	Detection of Perfume in Total Composition
5	Good	Fair	Good	None after 30 days.
10	Good	Fair	Good	Slight after 30 days.
20	Good	Fair	Poor	None after 30 days.
30	Good	Good	Poor	None after 30 days.
40	Good	Good	Very poor	Slight after 30 days.

Table 2 describes the perfume blended with high density polyethylene particles that pass through a 20 mesh sieve but are substantially completely retained in a 50 mesh sieve.

TABLE 2

Perfume Concentration in Percent by Weight of Polyethylene	Mixing	Pourability	Absorption of Perfume	Detection of Perfume in Total Composition
5	Good	Fair	Good	None after 30 days.
10	Good	Fair	Good	Slight after 30 days.
30	Good	Good	Good	Slight after 30 days.
40	Good	Good	Good	Slight after 30 days.

Table 3 describes the perfume blended with high density polyethylene particles that pass through a 250 mesh but are substantially completely retained by a 350 mesh sieve.

TABLE 3

Perfume Concentration in Percent by Weight of Polyethylene	Mixing	Pourability	Absorption of Perfume	Detection of Perfume in Total Composition
5	Good	Fair	Good	Slight after 6 months.
10	Good	Fair	Good	Slight after 6 months.
20	Good	Good	Good	Good after 6 months.
30	Good	Good	Good	Good after 6 months.
40	Good	Good	Good	Strong after 6 months.
60	Good	Good	Good	Strong after 6 months.

From the results of Tables 1 and 2, it will be seen that with the coarser grades of polyethylene powder, it was not possible to retain the perfume odor long even at the higher concentrations. For instance, in the case of the polyethylene powder of Table 1, there was only slight extrudation of perfume after thirty days' storage even when the perfume was incorporated in the blend to an extent as high as 40% by weight based on the total weight of the resulting blend. Similarly, in the case of the medium coarseness grade of high density polyethylene powder of Table 2, there was slight extrudation of perfume after thirty days' storage at the 10% by weight incorporation level.

By way of contrast, in the case of the fine polyethylene powder for which the results are given in Table 3, it will be seen that, even at the relatively low level of 5% by weight perfume, there were detectable traces of the perfume after 6 months' storage.

Retarded Vaporization Compositions

H.A. Segal; U.S. Patent 3,767,787; October 23, 1973 describes a retarded vaporization composition in which odoriferous material is retained in a nonaqueous colloid, in which state there is relatively little volatilization of the odoriferous material, but which on contact with moisture changes to an aqueous system in which the nonpolar volatile materials are released to the atmosphere (relatively rapid volatilization).

The compositions include finely divided fumed amorphous silica; in particular, powdered Cab-O-Sil, which is more than 99 weight percent of fumed amorphous silica, having an average particle size of about 0.011 micron and an approximate surface area of about 160 square meters per gram. The fumed amorphous silica constitutes the gelling agent for the nonaqueous colloid. The retarded vaporization composition also includes a gelatinizing agent which is capable of being suspended in a nonaqueous colloid, and which is also capable of forming an aqueous colloidal gel on contact with water.

The retarded vaporization compositions are prepared by blending the components using mild agitation. In particular, the fluffy nature of the fumed amorphous silica requires mild agitation. The blending can be performed at room temperature. For ease of handling, it is convenient to first mix all of the liquid components, and then with slow agitation, add the fumed amorphous silica and gelatinizing agent, and other solids.

After the composition has been blended as aforesaid, it is necessary that it be cured at a temperature of from 110° to 160°F or more. The time duration of curing is inversely related to the temperature of curing. At 160°F, an appropriate time duration of one-quarter hour can be used for curing. At a temperature of 110°F, 8 hours is a suitable time duration for curing.

A curing temperature of 160°F is not to be considered as an absolute maximum, since higher temperatures could be employed. However, temperatures above 160°F are not necessary and may not be suitable where low boiling point components are present or where low melting point containers are used. The curing can be accomplished in the final vessel. Thus, the components of the composition can be blended, and the blended mixture poured into the storage vessel. The composition can then be cured in the storage vessel.

The following examples are illustrative of compositions of the process. In each case, the procedure set forth above is followed, namely the liquids are first blended and then the solids added slowly with very mild agitation to form the nonaqueous colloid.

Example 1: A deodorant for usage in bedpans and urinals, which releases its odoriferous material and nasal suppressant upon contact with fecal matter or urine may be prepared by blending:

	Pounds
Amyl acetate	0.6
Oil of wintergreen	3.4
Isopropanol	8.0
Glycerin	68.0

To this liquid mixture may be added:

Cab-O-Sil M5	5.0
K & K 275 Bloom edible porkskin gelatin	15.0
Chlorophyllin	0.025
Hexachlorophene	0.25

The mixture should be mixed very slowly until homogeneously blended. The final product can be extruded or spooned into suitable containers. When sealed, it is cured at a temperature of 160°F for 15 minutes. It can be stored under ambient conditions for extended periods of time without releasing either the odoriferous material (oil of wintergreen) or the nasal suppressant (amyl acetate). However, on contact with moisture, both the oil of wintergreen and the amyl acetate are slowly released.

Example 2: A suitable colloidal composition for use in a steam vaporizer consists of:

	Percent
Cab-O-Sil	4.5
Gelatin	13.5
Vicks Vaposteam commercial vaporizer base	23
Glycerin	49
Tween 20	10

The resultant mixture should be mixed very slowly until homogeneously blended. It can be extruded or spooned into suitable containers. When sealed, it can be cured at a temperature of 150°F for 4 hours.

OTHER PRODUCT APPLICATIONS

Bath Oil

M.F. Emory; U.S. Patent 3,150,049; September 22, 1964 describes a bath oil composition for use in bathing water, which contains pine oil or any other perfume oil of any desired fragrance in homogeneous colloidal distribution. The bath oil is clear and stable on storage and, when added to water is evenly and substantially dispersed to very fine particles capable of being taken up by wet human skin. Moreover, the product leaves a very thin, substantially uniform layer of oil on the surface of the human skin, when added to, and used in the bath. The following examples illustrate the process.

Example 1: 12.5 parts by weight of pine oil and 1.5 parts by weight of lecithin are mixed under stirring at a temperature of 60° to 80°C with 50 parts by weight of isopropyl palmitate and 36 parts by weight of isopropyl myristate, to form a uniform mixture. To the latter 100 parts by weight of liquid petrolatum having at 60°F a specific density of 0.830 to 0.880 are added under stirring and the mixture is filtered, if necessary, in order to obtain a clear liquid.

Example 2: A bath oil composition is prepared by mixing under stirring at a temperature of 75°C the following ingredients:

	Parts by Weight
Pine oil	12.5
Lecithin	1.5
Isopropyl palmitate	40.0
Isopropyl myristate	46.0
Liquid petrolatum (as used in Example 1)	50

Example 3: A bath oil composition is prepared in the manner described in the above Example 1, from the following ingredients:

	Parts by Weight
Pine oil	10.0
Lecithin	1.5
Isopropyl palmitate	48.5
Isopropyl myristate	40.0
Liquid petrolatum (as used in Example 1)	100

Bath Capsule

S. Benford; U.S. Patent 3,520,971; July 21, 1970; assigned to R.P. Scherer Corporation describes a bath capsule containing a bath oil, such as mink oil, and having an outer shell made of a gelatin capsule formulation which includes a finely divided titanium oxide coated mica as a pigment. The following examples illustrate specific capsules made by the process.

Example 1: A capsule formulating composition was made with the following ingredients:

Material	Percent
Gelatin	41.7
Glycerin	11.0
Sorbitol special (plasticizer)	13.6
Added water	32.0
Methyl-propyl-paraben blend (methyl-p-hydroxy benzoate, a gelatin preservative)	0.2
Titanium oxide coated mica (pigment)	1.5

Following the usual capsule making techniques, sheets were made from the formulation. The sheets were then processed in capsule making machines in the usual manner and mink oil was added to the capsules. The final product was dried until 12 to 15% moisture remained in the outer shell of the capsule. The capsules had the external appearance of natural pearls.

Example 2: A capsule formulation was made in accordance with the following formula shown on the next page.

Material	Percent
Gelatin	40.1
Glycerin	10.1
Sorbitol special (plasticizer)	12.5
Added water	35.7
Methyl-propyl-paraben blend (methyl-p-hy-droxy benzoate, a gelatin preservative)	0.2
Titanium oxide coated mica (pigment)	1.5

Sheets of gelatin having the above formulation were made according to usual procedures. The sheets were then passed through a capsule making machine and mink oil was added to the capsules. The capsules were dried and capsules having an outer shell with a moisture content of 12 to 15% resulted. The capsules had the size, shape, and appearance of natural pearls.

Fragrance-Releasing Flowerpot

F.E. Gould; U.S. Patent 3,596,833; August 3, 1971; assigned to National Patent Development Corporation describes a decorative article fabricated to resemble a flowerpot and incorporating a synthetic hydrophilic hydrogel capable of releasing fragrance in the presence of a solvent.

The process takes advantage of the capability of certain synthetic chemical compositions to absorb liquid solutions of fragrances and aromas and to store the solid elements of these fragrances for an indefinite period of time so that upon the later addition of solvent, the fragrance may be released to the surrounding atmosphere.

Decorative articles of this type may also be made from certain of these synthetic chemical compositions which, in turn, may include fragrances in their solid form incorporated therein prior to the molding, or shaping, of the finished article; the fragrance itself being released when contacted by the appropriate solvent.

Compositions having these characteristics are described in U.S. Patents 2,976,576 and 3,220,960. Such compositions may be generally defined as consisting of a nonswollen, mechanically workable, infrequently cross-linked hydrophilic polymer.

An article which resembles a conventional flowerpot such as is commonly used to display living plants, shrubs or flowers is described. It consists essentially of an open vessel having a generally cylindrical sidewall and a flat bottom. A portion of the interior wall of the vessel may be formed of a hydrogel material made in accordance with the teachings of the above noted patents, while the remainder of the vessel, or pot, may be formed of any other material such as: plastic, metal, wood or the usual clay from which flowerpots are ordinarily made.

It will be understood that the hydrogel liner will be fabricated so as to be capable of including the solid constituents of the particular fragrance desired. Thereafter, in use, when it is desired to liberate the fragrance, the pot will simply be filled with the appropriate solvent. For example, if it is desired to simulate the fragrance of violets, the liner material would have incorporated therein the solid material of violet essence, which would remain therein indefinitely so long as no solvent were applied to it. However, if the liquid in the vessel were the appropriate solvent, such as water or alcohol, it would penetrate into the hydrogel material and the violet fragrance would be gradually liberated so long as any such solid constituents remained therein.

Pine Needle Fragrance

E.-R. Detert; U.S. Patent 3,565,831; February 23, 1971; assigned to Eduard Gerlach GmbH, Chemische Fabrik, Germany describes a strongly adherent fragrance composition suitable for application by spraying to artificial Christmas trees to provide them with a natural pine needle odor which is provided by a mixture of pine needle oil, oil of lavender, cedar oil, in a volatile organic solvent, together with a cellulose ether fixative.

Example: A formulation suitable for a strongly adherent pine fragrance composition was prepared by dissolving in a vessel equipped with stirrer, 35% of methanol, 5% lavender oil, 15% dwarf pine oil, 5% pine needle oil, and 10% cedarwood oil, all percentages being by weight. After thorough mixing, there was added 20% by weight of ethylcellulose and 10% by weight of powdered rosin, and mixing was continued until a homogeneous, viscous, yellowish solution was obtained. This concentrate solution is adapted, upon dilution, for spraying on artificial trees or foilage. It can be diluted to any desired concentration by further addition of a volatile organic solvent, such as methanol or isopropanol, in a ratio of about 1 part concentrate to about 4 parts solvent, by weight. It can also be put up in aerosol spray cans upon mixing with a suitable propellant.

Silicate Esters of Essential Oils for Treating Textiles

T.C. Allen and H.J. Watson; U.S. Patent 3,215,719; November 2, 1965; assigned to Dan River Mills, Incorporated describe the preparation of silicate esters of the essential alcohols, including the essential isoprenoid alcohols, the essential aryl-substituted aliphatic alcohols and the essential aliphatic-substituted phenols. A silicate ester as described above is best fitted for treating textiles to impart a long-lasting fragrance which is strongly renewable upon moistening or wetting when the molar ratio of essential alcohol to silicon in the silicate ester is about 1.0 to 2.5 and the molar ratio of silicon-bonded lower alkoxy groups to silicon is 1.0 to 3.0.

Silicate esters containing less than 1.0 mol of essential alcohol per mol of silicon or less than 1.0 lower alkoxy group per silicon atom are useful for other purposes, e.g., in sachets and the like although such silicate esters can be used in treating textiles, if a lower degree of original and/or renewable fragrance imparted to the textile is desired.

The silicate esters are formed in effect by the replacement of one or more alkoxy group or alcoholyzable group, e.g., silicon-bonded halogen, hydrogen (with chloroplatinic acid, sodium, alkoxide, lithium alkoxide, hydrogen chloride or zinc chloride catalysts), or amino groups, of a silane with the desired number per silicon atom of organic oxy groups of an essential alcohol and, if desired, any remaining silicon-bonded alcoholyzable groups can be replaced with the desired number of lower alkoxy groups of lower alkanols.

Silicate esters of this process in the form of silanes include those represented by the formula: $(RO)_a Si(OR')_b (R'')_{(4-a-b)}$ where RO is the organic oxy group of an essential organic hydroxy compound having the formula ROH where R is an organic group; R' is an alkyl group, preferably lower alkyl having 1 to 6 carbon atoms, or can be phenyl; and R'' is a monovalent organic group which is a part of the starting silane, e.g., such as any of the well-known hydrocarbon-substituted or other organic-substituted silanes; a is an integer from 1 to 4; b is an integer from 0 to 3; and a + b is not more than 4.

For purposes of treating textiles, it is preferred to employ a silicate ester of the above formula where R' is an alkyl group having 1 to 6 carbon atoms and b is an integer of at least one. Silicate esters of this process in the form of siloxanes include those containing groups represented by the formula:

$$(RO)_m Si \underset{\overline{2}}{O_{4-m-n}} \overset{R''_n}{\underset{|}{}}$$

where R and R'' are as defined above, m is an integer of 1 to 3, n is an integer of 0 to 2, and m + n is an integer of 1 to 3, as the only groups of the siloxane or in combination with other siloxane units, e.g., dimethylsiloxy, methylsiloxy, trimethylsiloxy, phenylsiloxy and phenylmethylsiloxy, groups. The following examples illustrate the process.

Example 1: Two mols of beta-phenylethyl alcohol and 1 mol of tetraethyl silicate, with 0.5 gram of silicon tetrachloride as catalyst, were placed in a distilling flask equipped with a fractionating column and a condenser. This mixture was then refluxed until 2 mols of ethyl alcohol were collected. The reaction temperature during this time did not exceed 150°C and the time of refluxing was approximately 2 hours. The product in the flask was a light yellow liquid having 6.66% silicon and comprised predominantly bis(beta-phenyl-ethoxy)diethoxy silane.

The product was easily emulsified in water with Triton X-100 (an alkaryl monoether of polyoxyethylene glycol) to form an emulsion containing 1.6 weight percent of the product. The emulsion was then applied to cotton cloth by padding to a 60% wet pickup. The cloth was then air dried, and had a fragrance of roses. Immediately after washing and drying the treated cloth, the fragrance of roses became stronger. This fragrance gradually decreased with time, becoming very faint when the fabric was extremely dry and increasing in the presence of a small amount of moisture. The rose fragrance was still present and strongly renewable by contact with water, even after 20 home launderings.

Example 2: Two mols of terpineol and 1 mol of tetraethyl silicate, with 0.5 gram of silicon tetrachloride as catalyst, were mixed and refluxed as described in Example 1. The reaction was slow in starting so an extra 0.5 gram of silicon tetrachloride was added. Two mols of ethyl alcohol were collected at 77° to 79°C in about 7 hours. The product in the flask was a golden brown liquid having 8.71% silicon and comprised predominantly bis(terpineoxyl)diethoxy silane, $(C_{10}H_{17}O)_2(C_2H_5O)_2Si$.

The product was easily emulsified in water with Triton X-100 to form an emulsion containing 10 weight percent of the product. The emulsion was applied to cotton cloth in the same manner and to 60% wet pickup. After air drying the treated cloth had the fragrance of pine oil which was stronger when the fabric was in the presence of moisture and fainter as the fabric became drier. The pine oil fragrance persisted and was strongly renewable by washing even after 5 home launderings.

Example 3: Two mols of d,1-menthol and 1 mol of tetraethyl silicate, with 0.33 gram of silicon tetrachloride as catalyst, were mixed and refluxed according to the procedure in Example 1. One mol of ethyl alcohol distilled off very fast with the reaction temperature not exceeding 95°C. The second mol of ethanol did not begin distilling until the reaction temperature reached 190°C. The temperature then rapidly rose to 250°C whereupon the evolution of the second mol of ethanol was completed. The resulting product was a golden brown liquid having 5.11% silicon and comprised predominantly bis(menthoxy)diethoxy silane $(C_{10}H_{19}O)_2(C_2H_5O)_2Si$.

Nail Enamel

R. Charle, C. Zviak and G. Kalopissis; U.S. Patent 3,729,569; April 24, 1973; assigned to SA dite L'Oreal, France describe a cosmetic composition for removing nail enamel which comprises microencapsulated solvent nail polish remover with a perfume to mask the solvent odor, either as aqueous drops adapted to be applied with cotton wad or cloth, or as an aqueous paste adapted to be stored in a jar or in a flexible tube, and to be applied with a spatula. In the examples values given represent parts.

Example 1: Liquid Solvent — A cosmetic composition is prepared which is constituted by a dispersion of microcapsules in an aqueous phase, optionally in the presence of thickeners, to obtain dropwise application. The composition comprises an aqueous phase: carboxymethylcellulose, 2.5 and water 97.5.

The capsules contain the solvent agent and a perfume, in the form of the following mixture: acetone, 84.8; ethylene glycol monoethylether, 10; butyl stearate, 5; and perfume, 0.2. The capsule envelope is constituted by a natural wax, an acrylic resin or casein. The capsule dimension is from 50 to 250 microns. The composition is prepared by dispersing the capsules in the aqueous phase. To use the composition, a drop is allowed to fall on the nail from which the polish is to be removed and rubbed with a small wad of hydrophilic cotton or a cloth to crush the capsules, releasing their solvent mixture.

Example 2: Solvent Paste — A solvent cosmetic composition constituted as a paste and containing two kinds of solvent capsules C_1 and C_2 is prepared. The aqueous phase is constituted by: ethyl cellulose, 3; stearic acid, 10; 20% ammonia solution, 4; and water in sufficient quantity to obtain a paste of the desired consistency.

Capsules C_1 contain the following solvent mixture: γ-valeroacetone, 50; ethylene glycol monoethylether, 15; and ethanol, 35. The envelope of the capsules C_1 is constituted by natural wax, their dimension being from 150 to 250 microns.

Capsules C_2 contain the following solvent mixture: ethyl acetate, 50; acetone, 49.8; and perfume, 0.2. The envelope of the capsules C_2 is constituted by a styrene polymer/maleic acid, completely hydrolyzed, the dimension being from 50 to 100 microns. Capsules C_1 and C_2 are incorporated in equal quantities in the previously prepared paste and the whole is then stored in a jar or in a flexible tube with a spatula applicator. Release of the solvents is effected as indicated in the preceding description.

Stabilized Compositions

A.A. Levinson, L.C. Radtke and K.B. Basa; U.S. Patent 3,385,713; May 28, 1968; assigned to H.B. Taylor Co. describe a stabilized liquid, flavoring, odorant and perfume composition comprising from $\frac{1}{8}$ to 90% by weight in relation to solvent of a carbonyl containing compound, an aliphatic polyhydroxy, alcohol carrier and solvent containing at least two hydroxy groups which are substituted in the 1,2-; 1,3-; and 1,4-positions and an alkaline material present in an amount sufficient to substantially inhibit dioxolane formation and less than the amount required to promote alkali catalyzed side reactions.

Example 1: Compositions of 5% cinnamaldehyde in 1,3-butanediol with and without stabilizer were prepared and analyzed by gas chromatography, both initially and at various intervals during the test period. The stabilized composition contained 1% v/v of 0.5 M $NaHCO_3$ (0.033% by weight $NaHCO_3$ in polyol). The results are reported in the following table as a percent ratio of concentration of aldehyde in unstabilized solution to concentration of aldehyde in stabilized solution, after storage aging at about 25°C. The lower numbers show that the rate of conversion of the aldehydes to the dioxolane form proceeds at an accelerated rate in the unstabilized composition as compared to the stabilized. The percent values given are calculated using the following: (unstabilized/stabilized) x 100.

Storage Time (days)	Percent
0	88
1	72
7	15
14	2
241	2

Example 2: Compositions similar to Example 1 were prepared using, however, 1% of a 0.1 N solution of glycine as stabilizer. The percent values given are calculated using the following: (unstabilized/stabilized) x 100.

Storage Time (days)	Percent
0	95
1	79
7	21
14	14

Example 3: Compositions were prepared and tested as in Example 1 using 5% vanillin in place of cinnamaldehyde and a 50/50 mixture of 1,3-butanediol and 1,2-propanediol. The stabilizer was 1% of 0.01 M $NaHCO_3$ showing inhibition at very low concentrations. The

percent values given below are calculated using the following: (unstabilized/stabilized) x 100.

Storage Time (days)	Percent
0	90
7	81
14	69

Complete inhibition was obtained using concentrations of alkaline material of 0.1 M or 0.5 M NaHCO$_3$.

COMPANY INDEX

The company names listed below are given exactly as they appear in the patents, despite name changes, mergers and acquisitions which have, at times, resulted in the revision of a company name.

Allied Chemical Corp. - 236
Badische Anilin- & Soda-Fabrik AG - 39, 40, 219
Bush Boake Allen Ltd. - 30, 31, 210
NV Chemische Fabriek Naarden - 34, 153
Chevron Research Co. - 258
Chugai Seiyaku KK - 101
Collins Chemical Co., Inc. - 211
Dan River Mills, Inc. - 287
Diamond Alkali Co. - 93
Dow Chemical Co. - 203
Drackett Co. - 277
E.I. du Pont de Nemours and Co. - 255
Eastman Kodak Co. - 121, 226, 236
Eduard Gerlach GmbH - 286
Esso Research and Engineering Co. - 143
Etablissements Roure-Bertrand Fils & Justin Dupont - 45, 134
Ethyl Corp. - 222, 250, 251
Firmenich et Cie - 38, 45, 111, 125, 126, 157, 168, 223
Fritzsche Brothers, Inc. - 133, 247
Fritzsche Dodge & Olcott Inc. - 160
General Electric Co. - 234
General Mills, Inc. - 217
Givaudan Corp. - 21, 57, 62, 63, 74, 76, 87, 90, 108, 109, 118, 119, 123, 125, 130, 146, 155, 162, 173, 176, 185, 187, 206, 223, 241, 254
Glidden Co. - 22
Gulf Oil Corp. - 261
Haarmann & Reimer GmbH - 26, 183
Hoffmann-LaRoche Inc. - 103, 120, 176, 178, 193, 203, 205, 246, 252
International Flavors & Fragrances Inc. - 24, 25, 27, 41, 43, 47, 49, 50, 51, 52, 55, 64,

68, 73, 79, 80, 91, 96, 99, 100, 106, 113, 114, 148, 152, 163, 165, 186, 189, 196, 199, 201, 207, 209, 227, 229, 231
Johnson & Johnson - 275
Lever Brothers Co. - 128, 265, 267, 268
SA L'Oreal - 288
MacMillan Bloedel Ltd. - 170
May & Baker Ltd. - 65, 115
Monsanto Co. - 58, 59, 61, 215
National Patent Development Corp. - 279, 286
National Starch and Chemical Corp. - 278
Norda Essential Oil and Chemical Co., Inc. - 36, 174
Olin Mathieson Chemical Corp. - 239, 240
Chas. Pfizer & Co., Inc. - 93, 167
Pfizer Inc. - 37, 110, 179
Philip Morris Inc. - 249
Pillsbury Co. - 271
Procter & Gamble Co. - 3, 6, 9, 10, 11, 13, 16, 20, 31, 138, 140, 190, 191, 192, 240, 242, 243
Reichhold Chemicals, Inc. - 188
R.J. Reynolds Tobacco Co. - 199, 238
Rhodia, Inc. - 35, 145, 157
Rhone-Poulenc SA - 59, 116, 135, 171, 194, 220
Rohm & Haas Co. - 232
SCM Corp. - 122, 231, 232
Sandoz Ltd. - 255
R.P. Scherer Corp. - 285
Shell Oil Co. - 154
Smith Kline & French Laboratories - 237
Stepan Chemical Co. - 124
Studiengesell ~haft Kohle mbH - 127, 129, 142

291

INVENTOR INDEX

U.S. PATENT NUMBER INDEX

NOTICE

Nothing contained in this Review shall be construed to constitute a permission or recommendation to practice any invention covered by any patent without a license from the patent owners. Further, neither the author nor the publisher assumes any liability with respect to the use of, or for damages resulting from the use of, any information, apparatus, method or process described in this Review.

HAIR DYES 1973

by J. C. Johnson

Chemical Technology Review No. 4

It has been estimated that the U.S. consumer spends over $100 million annually on hair color preparations. This does not include the very sizable sales made to professional beauty parlors and similar establishments.

Today the number of hair dyes and adjuvants available to the manufacturer of hair preparations cannot be counted. This book describes what has been patented in recent years.

152 methods are presented. A partial and condensed table of contents follows. Numbers in parentheses indicate the number of patents per topic. Chapter headings are given, followed by examples of important subtitles.

ISBN 0-8155-0477-2

368 pages

FURANS 1973
Synthesis and Applications

by Alec Williams

Chemical Technology Review No. 18

In large scale production processes, most furans are obtained from the key chemical furfural (2-furaldehyde) which is prepared commercially from cereal straws and brans, especially corncobs, oat hulls, cottonseed hulls, and rice hulls. Treatment with sulfuric acid hydrolyzes the pentosan components of these agricultural residues and dehydrates the freed pentose sugars to furfural.

In this sense, furans are products of agriculture, yielding an abundant harvest crop each year.

Tetrahydrofuran is an important solvent and intermediate in the manufacture of printing inks, lacquers, adhesives and other coating compositions. It is also used in polyurethane technology.

Benzofuran (coumarone) and reduced benzofurans are of considerable importance in pharmaceutical, insecticidal and photochromic applications.

Furan polymers and resins are inexpensive and have great potential use where products with their characteristics are required.

This book describes synthetic routes, products and end use applications of the furans. Over 100 different patent-based syntheses are provided covering the many derivatives of this family of commercially valuable materials.

A partial and condensed table of contents follows. Numbers in ( ) indicate the number of processes per topic. Chapter headings are given, followed by examples of important subtitles.

ISBN 0-8155-0506-X

303 pages

ORGANIC PEROXIDE TECHNOLOGY
1973

by Louis F. Martin

Chemical Technology Review No. 15

Some 40 to 50 different peroxide compounds are commercially available at present, and many are used as initiators in the polymerization of polyethylene, polyvinyl chloride, polyester thermosets, styrene-butadiene rubber, and for in-process cross-linking of ethylene-propylene copolymers and silicone rubbers.

Benzoyl peroxide, used in polystyrene and polyester markets such as toys, furniture, automobiles, trucks, airplanes and ships, is by far the largest volume product. Methyl ethyl ketone peroxide is also used in large volumes for glass fiber reinforced plastics applications such as pleasure craft, shower stalls, tub components and sports equipment. The so-called per esters are growing more slowly, because of some substitution with the cheaper peroxydicarbonates and azo compounds.

Research efforts are toward high performance specialty compounds, offering added value at reasonable prices. The development of safer, easily handled, and more efficient initiators is a major goal.

This book describes some 140 different, patented processes relating to all aspects of peroxide manufacture, and over 600 specific, detailed examples are provided. The very significant interest the world over is reflected in the 40 processes developed in Europe and Japan. A partial and condensed table of contents follows. Numbers in ( ) indicate the number of processes per topic. Chapter headings are given, followed by examples of important subtitles.

ISBN 0-8155-0499-3

TABLET MANUFACTURE 1974

by J.C. Johnson

Chemical Technology Review No. 30

Tablets are considered to be formed by compaction of powders, crystals or granulations into small cakes. They consist of excipients or carriers and active ingredients. In this review the definition has been extended to include other solid forms such as pills, pellets, dragees, lozenges, and the like.

Although tabletting is usually a pharmaceutical process for subdividing medicaments into dosage forms, the technique is also used by other industries for catalysts, metallurgical pellets, enrichment wafers, etc.

Most of today's tablets have a complex structure. Laminated, core-in-core, multiple layered and bonded pilules or pellets are examples. Many formulations are directed toward the controlled release of the active material. For detailed designs the interested reader is referred to the companion volume entitled CONTROLLED ACTION DRUG FORMS by J.C. Colbert. A separate volume on CAPSULE TECHNOLOGY AND MICROENCAPSULATION is also available.

This review covers 211 patents issued since January 1976 on the advances in tabletting techniques and materials. 99 methods involve matrix materials or binders, also coating materials and lubricants. Others cover tablet structure and manufacturing processes. 67 techniques treat the tabletting of specific drugs. An additional 19 reviews discuss the preparation of nonmedicinal tablets.

A partial and condensed table of contents follows here. Numbers in parentheses indicate the number of patents per topic. Chapter headings are given, followed by examples of important subtitles.

ISBN 0-8155-0530-2

270 pages

CONTROLLED ACTION
DRUG FORMS 1974

by J. C. Colbert

Chemical Technology Review No. 24

Speedy antacids and quick-acting analgesics have long been extolled for their fast remedial performance in all forms of advertising. Enteric coatings for specific release along the intestinal tract have been known to pharmacists since the early 1900's. Even the 12-hour cold capsule is now commonplace.

All this is a far cry from today's sophisticated drug design. Hydrophilic polymers and biological binding substances, such as select proteins and polysaccharides, enable the medicinal chemist and pharmacologist to design drug systems by which simple implants will release measured low doses of a hormone or contraceptive continuously for as long as one year. By means of skillful lamination techniques it is possible to withhold release or absorption until a certain poison enters or is generated within the body.

This review covers 211 patents issued since 1956 covering numerous methods of preparing practical dosage forms of human or veterinary drugs having some means of controlling the action or release of the active ingredients. Numbers in parentheses indicate a plurality of processes per topic. Chapter headings and some of the more important subtitles are given in the partial and condensed table of contents that follows here.

ISBN 0-8155-0520-5

340 pages

PROSTAGLANDINS 1973

Isolation and Synthesis

by J. C. Colbert

Chemical Technology Review No. 17

Prostaglandins are a family of chemical compounds with a wide spectrum of physiological responses, and medical research here is still in its early, and perhaps fastest growing, stages.

Since analogs and homologs are also physiologically active, many potentially useful medicinal agents can be prepared in order to study, prevent, control, or alleviate a wide variety of diseases and undesirable bodily conditions.

How to prepare these compounds by isolation from natural products such as coral, by enzymatic conversion of unsaturated fatty acids, or by total synthesis, are the subjects of this book.

Altogether 60 processes are described. The book also contains a valuable introduction to the stereochemistry and nomenclature of these amazing substances.

A partial and condensed table of contents follows. Numbers in parentheses indicate the number of patents per topic. Chapter headings are given, followed by examples of important subtitles.

ISBN 0-8155-0501-9

279 pages

CHEMICAL GUIDE TO EUROPE 1973

Sixth Edition

This sixth, expanded edition describes approximately 1,160 companies in the 19 countries of Western Europe which together constitute a market almost as large as that of the United States. Includes all the major European chemical companies. Gives all this information (where pertinent and available):

Name and Address
Telephone and Telex Numbers
Ownership
Plant Locations and Products
Internal Structure
Local Subsidiaries and Affiliates
Foreign Subsidiaries and Affiliates
Principal Executives
Annual Sales
Number of Employees

A valuable marketing guide.

Even companies which are predominantly non-chemical, but which nevertheless have important chemical interests, are included. Also included are groups which hold substantial chemical interests through a number of subsidiaries. This allows you to concentrate your efforts in the most profitable direction.

Describes the 1,160 major chemical firms in these 19 countries.

Austria	30	Luxembourg	4
Belgium	88	Netherlands	89
Denmark	23	Norway	21
Finland	18	Portugal	8
France	130	Spain	136
Germany	179	Sweden	31
Greece	17	Switzerland	37
Iceland	1	Turkey	6
Ireland	12	U.K.	186
Italy	144		

These are the firms that have the most to offer in the way of sales contracts, licensing arrangements, joint ventures, and the obtaining of research and development know-how. In order to give you an indication of the size of each firm we have included, where available, the annual sales figures and/or the number of employees.

The basis of selection was size, although this criterion was not applied indiscriminately since this would have meant the exclusion of some of the companies in smaller countries which, although not large on a European scale, are nevertheless very important in their own countries. Consequently companies which have been included in the entry for Finland, for example, would not have qualified had they been in, say, Germany or the United Kingdom.

ISBN 0-8155-0497-7
326 pages.

CHEMICAL GUIDE TO THE U.S. 1973

Seventh Edition

This seventh edition describes over 400 of the largest United States chemical firms:

Name and Address
Ownership
Annual Sales
Number of Employees
Plant Locations
Products
Domestic Subsidiaries and Affiliates
Foreign Subsidiaries and Affiliates

This guide is a valuable research and marketing tool. The companies described in this book are those who actually undertake chemical reactions in their plants. Not included are companies producing paint, printing ink, etc. which primarily process chemicals physically rather than chemically. Pharmaceutical firms are included only if they are also producers of commercial chemicals and intermediates.

This book also gives information on closely held firms, joint ventures, and others that do not publish annual reports.

. . . a valuable market research tool
. . . find information quickly
. . . increase your sales to the
        chemical industry
. . . search for potential acquisitions
        and divestitures
. . . know whom to contact
. . . a valuable employment guide
. . . pinpoint your sales effort to the
        BIG BUYERS
. . . describes joint venture companies
. . . contains hard-to-get information
        on medium sized and smaller firms
. . . gives a broad picture of the
        United States chemical industry
. . . includes all the latest mergers
        and joint ventures
. . . find out who owns whom.

An index is included to enable you to quickly locate the firm, subsidiary or division in which you are interested.

ISBN 0-8155-0498-5
210 pages.

POLLUTION CONTROL
IN THE ORGANIC CHEMICAL INDUSTRY
1974

by Marshall Sittig

Pollution Technology Review No. 9

Wastes from plants manufacturing identical compounds may be quite dissimilar, because of the difference in processes and raw materials. Since the organic chemical industry is now largely petrochemical, preference has been given to waste treatment from such operations.

Detailed treatability evaluation of each waste stream has become a prerequisite for any profitable product.

Physical methods for waste and by-product removal include gravity separation, air flotation, filtration, evaporation and adsorption techniques.

Chemical methods include precipitation, polyelectrolyte treatment, oxidation and other chemical conditioning such as neutralization.

Biological treatment methods comprise activated sludge and its modifications, trickling filters, aerated lagoons, and waste stabilization ponds.

This book intends to assist the chemical engineer in treating chemical waste products and effluents in conjunction with prudent raw material choices and thus bring about process economics. It presents condensed vital data from government and other sources of information that are scattered and difficult to pull together.

A partial and condensed table of contents follows here.

Dinitrotoluene from Nitrotoluene

Disulfoton from Ethanol

Dyes and Pigments from Aromatics

Epichlorohydrin from Allyl Chloride

Ethylbenzene from Benzene

Ethyl Chloride by
Hydrochlorination of Ethylene
Chlorination of Ethane
Hydrochlorination of Ethanol

Ethylene or Propylene from Paraffins

Ethylene Dichloride from Ethylene

Ethylene Glycol from Ethylene Oxide

Ethylene Oxide from Ethylene

Formaldehyde from Methanol

Long Chain Alcohols from
Ethylene Oligomers

Malathion® from Methanol

Methanol from Natural Gas

Methylamines from Methanol + Ammonia

Methyl Bromide from Methanol

Methyl Methacrylate from
Acetone Cyanohydrin

Nitrobenzene from Benzene

Nitrochlorobenzene from Chlorobenzene

Nitroparaffins from Paraffins

Oxo Products from Olefins

Parathion from p-Nitrophenol

Perchloroethylene from Propane

Phenol from Chlorobenzene

Phenol from Cumene

Phorate from Ethanol

Phosgene from $CO + Cl_2$

Phthalic Anhydride from
Naphthalene or Xylene

Propylene Glycol from Propylene Oxide

Propylene Oxide from Propylene

Styrene from Ethylbenzene

SNG from Crude Oil

2,4,5-T from Trichlorophenol

Terephthalic Acid from Xylene

Tetraethyl Lead from Ethyl Chloride

Trichloroethane from Vinyl Chloride

Trichloroethylene by
Chlorination, then by
Dehydrochlorination of Acetylene
or by Oxyhydrochlorination
of Dichloroethane

Trifluralin from Perfluoromethylchloro-
benzene

Vinyl Acetate from
Ethylene and Acetic Acid

Vinyl Chloride from Acetylene

Vinyl Chloride from Ethylene Dichloride

AIR POLLUTION CONTROL
Halogen Acids
Halogenated Hydrocarbons
Halogens
Hydrocarbons
Particulates
Sulfur Compounds
Coking of Coal

WATER POLLUTION CONTROL
Primary
Oil Separation
Equalization
Neutralization
Sedimentation
Flotation
Flocculation
Nutrient Addition
Secondary
Activated Sludge
Extended Aeration
Trickling Filters
Aerated Lagoons
Waste Stabilization Ponds
Chemical Oxidation
Nitrification—Denitrification

Tertiary
Chemical Precipitation
Gas Stripping
Microstraining
Carbon Adsorption
Electrodialysis
Ion Exchange
Evaporation
Reverse Osmosis
Chlorination
Rapid Sand Filtration
Sludge Handling
Aerobic Digestion
Anaerobic Digestion
Wet Oxidation
Thickening
Lagooning
Sand Drying Beds
Vacuum Filtration
Filtration
Land Disposal
Incineration
Sea Disposal
Ultimate Disposal
Thermal Oxidation
Deep Well Disposal

OVERALL WATER POLLUTION
CONTROL MODELS
BPCTCA: Best Practicable Control
Technology Currently Available
BATEA: Best Available Technology
Economically Available
BADCT: Best Available Demonstrated
Control Technology

THE ECONOMICS OF POLLUTION
CONTROL

FUTURE TRENDS

ISBN 0-8155-0536-1   305 pages